Instructor's Manual and Test Bank to Accompany

CLINICAL TEXTBOOK *for* VETERINARY TECHNICIANS

Instructor's Manual and Test Bank to Accompany

CLINICAL TEXTBOOK *for* VETERINARY TECHNICIANS

SIXTH EDITION

DENNIS M. McCURNIN, DVM

Professor, Department of Veterinary Clinical Sciences
Hospital Director, Veterinary Teaching Hospital and Clinics
School of Veterinary Medicine
Louisiana State University, Baton Rouge, Louisiana

JOANNA M. BASSERT, VMD

Professor and Director
Program of Veterinary Technology
Manor College, Jenkintown, Pennsylvania

Prepared by

REBECCA SWEENEY, DVM

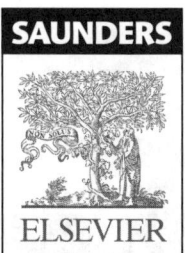

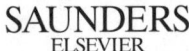

11830 Westline Industrial Drive
St. Louis, Missouri 63146

Instructor's Manual to Accompany Clinical Textbook for Veterinary Technicians
Copyright © 2006, Elsevier Inc.

All rights reserved. No part of this publication may be reproduced or transmitted in any form or by any means, electronic or mechanical, including photocopying, recording, or any information storage and retrieval system, without permission in writing from the publisher. Permissions may be sought directly from Elsevier's Health Sciences Rights Department in Philadelphia, PA, USA: phone: (+1) 215 239 3804, fax: (+1) 215 239 3805, e-mail: healthpermissions@elsevier.com. You may also complete your request on-line via the Elsevier homepage (http://www.elsevier.com), by selecting 'Customer Support' and then 'Obtaining Permissions'.

Notice

Knowledge and best practice in this field are constantly changing. As new research and experience broaden our knowledge, changes in practice, treatment, and drug therapy may become necessary or appropriate. Readers are advised to check the most current information provided (i) on procedures featured or (ii) by the manufacturer of each product to be administered, to verify the recommended dose or formula, the method and duration of administration, and contraindications. It is the responsibility of the practitioner, relying on their own experience and knowledge of the patient, to make diagnoses, to determine dosages and the best treatment for each individual patient, and to take all appropriate safety precautions. To the fullest extent of the law, neither the Publisher nor the Authors assume any liability for any injury and/or damage to persons or property arising out or related to any use of the material contained in this book.

The Publisher

ISBN-13: 978-1-4160-2453-8
ISBN-10: 1-4160-2453-0

Publishing Director: Linda L. Duncan
Managing Editor: Teri Merchant
Publishing Services Manager: John Rogers
Senior Project Manager: Beth Hayes
Senior Designer: Julia Dummitt

Printed in the United States of America
Last digit is the print number: 9 8 7 6 5 4 3 2

Preface

Designed as a companion for *Clinical Textbook for Veterinary Technicians*, sixth edition, the Instructor's Manual was developed to provide an organizing framework for developing teaching strategies for instructors of veterinary technology.

Each chapter in the Instructor's Manual contains teaching/learning objectives, vocabulary, chapter outlines with teaching strategies keyed to the headings, suggested activities and critical thinking challenges, and a chapter quiz.

This manual contains a comprehensive test bank intended to accurately evaluate students of all levels. Its multiple-choice, true/false, and short-answer questions cover both factual topics and practical skills. Real-world scenarios are included to test the students' ability to solve problems as they might occur in the animal hospital. The use of all questions for a given chapter will provide a comprehensive evaluation of all subjects in that chapter. However, the questions are designed to stand alone, which allows you to custom-design tests covering specific topics or containing a preferred question format. Both written and interactive class exercises are provided for chapters not lending themselves as well to test questions.

Extra-credit questions are also included. We attempted to add a bit of humor to each of these questions; this was done not only to relieve the tension present at the end of a test but to remind everyone to keep his or her sense of humor in the face of the stress that accompanies an intensive education program in a health profession. We have found it immeasurably helpful to remember the lighter side of our work with animals, and we hope our humor helps you and your students to do so, as well.

Elsevier has created an Evolve website dedicated solely to supporting this teaching package. In addition to an electronic version of the Instructor's Manual and Test Bank, a comprehensive electronic image collection is provided that will allow the instructor to download any image, table, or box from the book into a PowerPoint presentation.

This Evolve website also includes features that students can access, including student activities, games, and crossword puzzles using some of the chapter vocabulary.

Along with the instructor's package, the Evolve course management tools include:

- **Discussion Board** Allows users to post new messages and respond to posted messages
- **Send E-mail** Allows users to send e-mail to others in the course
- **Virtual Classroom** A chat/whiteboard tool that allows real-time discussions and content sharing
- **Calendar** Allows for the posting and viewing of events by date and time
- **Address Book** Allows for the storing and retrieval of contact information
- **Task Manager** Allows for the organization of assignments and their completion status
- **Group Pages** Allows instructor-assigned groups to have private access to tools for group assignments
- **Digital Drop Box** Allows students to submit electronic files to the instructor and vice versa
- **Edit Homepage** Allows students to create a webpage about themselves for classmates to view
- **Check Grade** allows students to view their grades in the course's Online Gradebook
- **Electronic Blackboard** Allows users to make notes and store them online
- **Assessment Manager** Allows for the custom creation of online tests with seven different question types: multiple choice, true/false, fill-in-the-blank, multiple answer, matching, ordering, and short answer/essay
- **Pool Manager** Allows for the creation of question groups for easy retrieval and online test building
- **Online Gradebook** Allows for automatic online test scoring, easy grade retrieval, export to Excel, and much more
- **Online Statistics** Allows for detailed tracking of student usage (and nonusage) of course content

This Instructor's Manual was developed to complement the growth and success of its accompanying textbook, and we hope it enhances and simplifies your teaching experience. We welcome your suggestions for future editions.

Acknowledgment

The authors and publisher recognize and appreciate the original contribution of Heather McLaughlin McKelvey, DVM, who created the original Test Bank for the fifth edition of *Clinical Textbook for Veterinary Technicians*.

Contents

**SECTION ONE
INSTRUCTOR'S MANUAL, 1**

An Introduction to the Profession of Veterinary Technology, 1

Part One
Clinical Procedures

1. Restraint and Handling of Animals, 5
2. History and Physical Examination, 10
3. Diagnostic Sampling and Therapeutic Techniques, 13
4. Wound Healing, Wound Management, and Bandaging, 19
5. Basic Necropsy Procedures, 23

Part Two
Clinical Sciences

6. Clinical Pathology, 26
7. Parasitology, 31
8. Clinical Microbiology, 36
9. Diagnostic Imaging, 41
10. Veterinary Oncology, 47

Part Three
Patient Management and Nutrition

11. Preventive Health Programs, 50
12. Neonatal Care of Puppy, Kitten, and Foal, 54
13. Geriatric Medicine in Companion Animals, 58
14. Animal Behavior, 60
15. Companion Animal Clinical Nutrition, 65
16. Concepts in Livestock Nutrition, 71
17. Animal Reproduction, 74
18. Care of Birds, Reptiles, and Small Mammals, 80

Part Four
Anesthesia and Pharmacology

19. Veterinary Anesthesia, 84
20. Pain Management, 89
21. Pharmacology and Pharmacy, 94

Part Five
Surgical and Medical Nursing

22. Surgical Instruments and Aseptic Technique, 101
23. Surgical Assistance and Suture Material, 106
24. Small Animal Surgical Nursing, 110
25. Small Animal Medical Nursing, 115
26. Emergency and Critical Care Medicine, 122
27. Toxicology, 128
28. Veterinary Dentistry, 133
29. Equine Medical and Surgical Nursing, 137
30. Food Animal Medical and Surgery, 144
31. Nursing Concepts in Alternative Medicine, 152

Part Six
Topics in Practice Management

32. Veterinary Practice Management, 156
33. Medical Records, 160
34. Computer Applications in Veterinary Practice, 163
35. Zoonoses and Public Health, 165
36. Occupational Health and Safety, 169

37 Euthanasia, 173
38 Client Bereavement and the Human-Animal Bond, 175
39 Stress and Substance Abuse in Practice, 177

**SECTION TWO
TEST BANK, 181**

**SECTION THREE
ANSWER KEY, 301**

INTRODUCTION

An Introduction to the Profession of Veterinary Technology

TEACHING/LEARNING OBJECTIVES

1. What are the continuing education requirements for veterinary technicians in Missouri?
2. What is the fee for veterinary technicians to renew their license in Missouri?
3. What is distance education?
4. List the areas in the veterinary clinic/hospital in which the veterinary technician can expect to work upon graduation.
5. What are the duties required of the veterinary technician in each of the areas listed in objective 1?
6. What does the acronym NAVTA stand for and what are the responsibilities of this organization?
7. What does the acronym CVTS stand for and what are the responsibilities of this organization?
8. Describe typical job responsibilities of veterinary technicians who are AALAS certified.
9. What does the acronym VTNE represent?
10. What does the acronym AAVSB represent and what are the responsibilities of this organization?
11. Explain the concept of reciprocity as it relates to the field of veterinary medicine.
12. What four responsibilities are strictly forbidden by law for any member of the veterinary team to perform except the veterinarian?
13. According to the Model Rules and Regulations for Veterinary Technicians, what activities fall within the realm of immediate, direct, and indirect supervision?
14. What is the relationship between a Practice Act and Rules and Regulations?
15. Compare legislative and common law and give an example of each.
16. What is respondeat superior? Give an example.

KEY TERMS

American Association of Veterinary State Boards (AAVSB)
American Veterinary Medical Association (AVMA)
Certified
Committee on Veterinary Technician Specialties (CVTS)
Common law
Continuing education
Direct supervision
Distance education
Immediate supervision
Indirect supervision
Laboratory animal technician
Legislative law
Licensed
Malpractice
National Association of Veterinary Technicians in America (NAVTA)
Personal ethics
Practice act
Professional ethics
Reciprocity
Referral practice
Registered
Respondeat superior
Societal ethics
Specialty practice
Veterinary assistant
Veterinary nurse
Veterinary technician
Veterinary Technician National Examination (VTNE)
Veterinary Technician Oath
Veterinary technologist

INTRODUCTION

Chapter Outline	Teaching Strategies
History of veterinary technology	At the beginning of the semester, ask the students to discuss their views of the role of the veterinary technician, as it relates to the Veterinary Technician Oath. At the end of the semester, ask the students to read the oath again, and present any new or modified thoughts on this topic.
The veterinary technician today	Discuss the relationship between technological advances in the field of veterinary medicine and the role of the veterinary technician.
Jobs, prospects, salaries, and attrition	Review average salaries earned by veterinary technicians, technologists, and assistants, and compare them to other professions that require the same amount of education. Discuss reasons for the high rate of attrition in the field.
Education	Differentiate between 2-, 3-, and 4-year programs. Include differences in job responsibilities and salaries.
Distance education	Explain the concept of distance education.
Continuing education	Discuss continuing education requirements in Missouri and the ways in which one may meet these requirements. Talk about the consequences of not meeting these requirements.
Responsibilities of the veterinary technician	Prepare comprehensive lists of the responsibilities for each of the areas described. Ask a veterinary technician who works at a local clinic to talk to your class and describe his/her average workday. Include the duties of the veterinary technician employed at large animal and mixed animal practices.
Reception area	
Examination rooms and out-patients	
Laboratory and pharmacy	
Radiology	
Treatment room	
Operating room	
Wards	
Hospital management	
Terminology and the veterinary health care team	
Veterinarian	
Veterinary technician specialist	Discuss the three disciplines in which veterinary technicians may become specialized. Include educational requirements, job opportunities, and salaries.
Veterinary technologist	Discuss differences in educational requirements, job responsibilities, and salaries between veterinary technologists, technicians, technologists, assistants, nurses, and laboratory animal technicians.
Veterinary technician	
Veterinary assistant	
Veterinary nurse	
Laboratory animal technicians	
The veterinary technician national examinations	Describe these examinations and include the number of questions, types of questions, how long the tests take, and when/where these are offered.
Laws governing veterinary technology	
Certification, registration, and licensure	Explain that these three words have essentially the same meaning. Review various requirements of different states to become "credentialed."
Scope of practice	Discuss the constantly increasing responsibilities of the veterinary technician in today's practice. Explain that only the veterinarian can legally prescribe, diagnose, prognose, and perform surgery.
Where the confusion lies	
Practice acts	Ask the students to read the NAVTA Model Practice Act for Veterinary Technicians. Discuss the process for amending the Act.
Rules and regulations	Ask the students to read the Model Rules and Regulations for Veterinary Technicians. Discuss how these rules are made and who is responsible for making these rules. Review the function of a state board.
Malpractice and common law	Compare legislative and common law as they relate to the duties of the veterinary technician. List several important common laws.

Copyright © 2006 by Elsevier, Inc. All rights reserved.

Introduction

Chapter Outline	Teaching Strategies
Ethics	Compare the three types of ethics presented. Ask the students to give examples of each. Present real-life situations and encourage the students to debate the various viewpoints. Ask them to empathize with other people involved in the scenarios.
Societal ethics	
Personal ethics	
Professional ethics	
Professional ideals	Ask the students to prepare a list of activities that every technician should perform to promote their profession.
Professional organizations	Stress the importance of actively participating in local, regional, and national organizations that promote the profession of veterinary technology. Provide a list of e-mail addresses, phone numbers, and addresses of important organizations.

CRITICAL THINKING CHALLENGES

1. Present a real-life financial situation of a veterinary technician. Include salary or hourly wage, rent or mortgage, food, utilities, and other expenses that are typically needed to survive for one month. Ask the students to discuss their thoughts on the lifestyle that is attainable for a single person working as a veterinary technician.
2. Ask several students to contact organizations that offer distance education for veterinary technicians and to request literature on these programs. Compare the programs, including cost and time requirements, with your own. What conclusions do they draw after this comparison?
3. Contact the AVMA Professional Liability Insurance Trust (PLIT) and request literature on legal cases that deal with malpractice or professional negligence and respondeat superior. Ask the students to discuss these cases, particularly methods of prevention.
4. Ask the students to read NAVTA's Code of Ethics for the Profession of Veterinary Technology and to write additional codes that they believe are important but missing.

QUIZ

Match each statement with the term that it describes. There is only one correct answer for each statement.

1. _____ This organization has written the Veterinary Technician Oath and the Code of Ethics for the Profession of Veterinary Technology.
2. _____ This person holds a bachelor of science degree (B.S.) in veterinary technology from a 4-year, AVMA-accredited program.
3. _____ Who performs audits to ensure that continuing education requirements are met by veterinary technicians/technologists?
4. _____ Veterinary technicians are not legally able to do this.
5. _____ This is the "umbrella" law that governs the practice of veterinary medicine.
6. _____ Euthanasia can be performed by veterinary technicians under this type of supervision.
7. _____ This type of law has evolved over time based on established professional conduct, customs, and practices.
8. _____ Under this type of supervision, the veterinary technician may administer treatment in the form of intravenous, intramuscular, intraperitoneal, and subcutaneous injection.
9. _____ This organization provides accreditation to programs of veterinary technology in the United States.
10. _____ In veterinary medicine, only this person can legally prescribe medication and perform surgery.

A Practice Act
B State's Board of Veterinary Medical Examiners
C Direct
D National Association of Veterinary Technicians in America (NAVTA)
E Common
F Committee on Veterinary Technician Education and Activities (CVTEA)
G Indirect
H Veterinary Technologist
I Veterinarian
J Diagnose

Answers: (1) D, (2) H, (3) B, (4) J, (5) A, (6) C, (7) E, (8) G, (9) F, (10) I

QUIZ

1. List the potential places of employment for a veterinary technician.
2. What is the role of the Committee on Veterinary Technician Education and Activities in veterinary technical programs today?

Copyright © 2006 by Elsevier, Inc. All rights reserved.

INTRODUCTION

3. In addition to animal care, what other roles might veterinary technicians assume in a practice?
4. How does the veterinary technician help with animals scheduled for surgery?
5. What are the requirements for becoming a veterinary technician specialist?
6. What is the difference between a veterinary technician and veterinary technologist?
7. Compare and contrast *licensing, registered,* and *certified.*
8. Name four activities in practice that can only be performed by the veterinarian.
9. What is the purpose of the Model Practice Act for Veterinary Technicians?
10. Who is responsible for writing the rules and regulations?
11. Explain when a veterinary technician is covered by malpractice insurance.
12. Name three items on NAVTA's list of ideals and recommended behaviors for veterinary technicians.
13. What are the requirements to be a member of NAVTA?
14. When and where was the first animal technician program established in the United States?
15. When was NAVTA formed?
16. How many accredited programs (by the AVMA) were there in 2003?
17. What is the difference between a veterinary technician and veterinary technologist?
18. What does it mean to be "credentialed"?
19. Define *extralabel* use of a drug.
20. What is an "impaired veterinarian"?
21. What is the purpose of a Board of Veterinary Medicine?
22. What are the requirements to be a board member?
23. Name five reasons why the board would revoke a license.
24. When is an animal considered to be "abandoned" according to law?
25. What is the veterinarian allowed to do with animals that are abandoned at the clinic?

1

Restraint and Handling of Animals

TEACHING/LEARNING OBJECTIVES

1. List common situations that require animal restraint in the clinic.
2. Explain the importance of appropriate restraint techniques in terms of safety and legal implications.
3. Explain how horses and bulls might react to unfamiliar smells.
4. Describe ear positions of the horse, llama, dog, and cat that indicate the need to approach with caution.
5. Explain adaptations of hearing, vision, smell, and touch in animals that are different from humans.
6. Describe physiologic responses and physical actions commonly seen in a fight-or-flight response.
7. List various categories of aggression, and give an example of each. Explain how to avoid injury when handling animals exhibiting these types of aggression.
8. Compare and contrast the fight-or-flight distances of dairy and beef cattle. How would this affect the handling of these animals?
9. Describe body behavior of dogs in dominant and submissive situations.
10. List possible physical responses of a horse to a perceived threat.
11. Give the length in meters of the horse's normal flight distance and kicking zone.
12. Place a halter and tie a horse to an object of the appropriate height using a rope of the appropriate length.
13. Know the appropriate place to stand in order to hold a horse for assessment and treatment.
14. Lift a horse's foreleg for restraint.
15. Lift a horse's hind leg for restraint.
16. Lift a horse's hind leg for examination.
17. Demonstrate the proper use of a scotch hobble.
18. Demonstrate the proper use of mouth gags, wedges, and speculums.
19. Explain why protection of the down side of a horse's head (in lateral recumbency) is crucial.
20. Demonstrate the use of a bovine halter.
21. Explain the differences in the ways that horses and cattle kick and the logical place to stand while handling them.
22. Demonstrate proper restraint of sheep and goats.
23. Explain the differences in restraining adult pigs versus piglets.
24. Demonstrate proper lifting of a small-, medium-, and large-breed dog.
25. Demonstrate appropriate restraint techniques of a dog for venipuncture from the jugular, cephalic, and lateral saphenous veins.
26. Make a gauze or rope muzzle for a dog.
27. Make a slipknot and a quick-release knot, and explain when these might be used.
28. Demonstrate the appropriate way to carry a cat.
29. Demonstrate the proper way to handle/restrain psittacines and passerines.
30. Explain the proper handling techniques for reptiles.
31. Know the following websites and reasons for using them: www.aphis.usda.gov and www.avma.org/grd/lac/Air)_Transport.

VOCABULARY

Active and passive defense reflex
Agnostic behavior
Automization
Binocular field of vision
Blind spot
Brachiocephalic
Chelonian
Cradle
Elapid snake
Elizabethan collar
Ethology
Fight-or-flight distance
Fight-or-flight response
Flanking
Frick speculum
Hazing
Hobbles

Copyright © 2006 by Elsevier, Inc. All rights reserved.

Hock
Jacking
Near side
Pastern
Pinnae
Predatory aggression
Ramphotheca
Rooting

Snare
Tailing
Tapetum
Throatlatch area
Twitch
Withers
Zygomatic arch

Chapter Outline	Teaching Strategies
Indications for restraint	Discuss situations that require restraint in any veterinary clinic.
Animal perception and behavior	Identify specific characteristics of various species' senses that affect their behavior.
Smell	
Hearing	
Vision	
Touch	
Agnostic behaviors	
Fight or flight	Present a situation in which an animal's fight-or-flight distance is encroached, and discuss hormonally induced responses.
Aggressive behavior	Stress that different forms or aggression are classified according to the stimuli or circumstances giving rise to the ferocity. Show a video of animals exhibiting various types of aggression, and ask the students to identify the category of aggression.
Irritable or pain-induced aggression	
Maternal aggression	
Predatory aggression	
Territorial aggression	
Fear-induced aggression	
Intermale aggression	
Dominance aggression	
Typical behavior of domestic animals in aggression and avoidance	Illustrate through videos or verbal description animals displaying aggressive/avoidance behavior. Stress that behaviors are species specific.
Cattle	Stress that dairy breed bulls are the most dangerous animals for veterinary personnel to handle.
Calves	Demonstrate the proper way to approach and handle a calf.
Cats	Emphasize the necessity to close all doors and windows when attempting to handle a cat.
Dogs	Show illustrations of dogs in dominant and submissive postures. Point out key features that represent either dominance or submission.
Horses	Using an illustration, show the horse's binocular field of vision, and explain the need to move the head to see objects outside of this field using the term *blind spot*.
Pigs	Provide (in dollar amounts) examples of a farmer's profits from a pig farm. Then show (in dollar amounts) the results of poor housing.
Sheep	Explain the relationship between avoidance behavior in sheep and herding dogs.
Management ethology	Define management ethology and explain its crucial role in the safety of veterinary personnel.
	Through video or in actual clinical or farm settings, demonstrate proper approach, handling, and restraint techniques for the species listed in this chapter.
Capture and restraint of horses	For all techniques, have students demonstrate the technique after you.
Foals	
Halter and leads	Show the students how to restrain a horse using a halter.
Tying the horse	Emphasize the idea that horses must be tied to objects at least shoulder height or above and that the lead should be only 60 cm long.
The twitch	Bring several types of twitches to class and demonstrate their use. Stress the importance of using a humane twitch.

CHAPTER 1 Restraint and Handling of Animals

Chapter Outline	Teaching Strategies
Lifting the foreleg	Demonstrate the proper way to lift a foreleg for restraint. On a diagram or actual horse identify the location of the suspensory ligament.
Lifting the hind leg	Demonstrate the proper way to lift a hind leg for examination. Review anatomy of the limb.
Stocks	Emphasize that the use of stocks is the safest way to restrain a horse.
Tail tie	Demonstrate a tail tie using a quick-release knot.
Hobbles	Demonstrate the use of a scotch hobble.
Restraint of the down horse	Stress the importance of approaching a down horse from the back and padding the down side of the head.
Other head and mouth restraints	Demonstrate the use of a cradle. Bring various types of head protectors and muzzles to class. Demonstrate proper restraint during examination of the mouth. Review oral anatomy. Bring various mouth gags, wedges, and speculums to class.
Manual and chemical restraints	
Capture and restraint of cattle	Visit a cattle ranch or show a video that demonstrates proper herding and corralling techniques, eventually driving cattle into chutes.
Head catch	Demonstrate the use of a bovine halter, how to flank a calf, and how to restrain a bull.
Restraint of the head	Stress the need to stay at least an arm's length away from the head at all time.
Tail restraint	Demonstrate tail tying using a quick-release knot.
Kicking restraints	Show a video or demonstrate the use of hobbles. Explain how cattle kick and have the students explain where they would stand during handling and restraint.
Casting	Visit a farm or show a video to see the proper way to cast cattle. Stress the importance of placing the animal in right lateral recumbency.
Lifting feet	Visit a farm or show a video that demonstrates the proper way to lift a bovine leg. Demonstrate the use of a tilt table.
Driving sheep and goats	Emphasize the economic impact of grabbing certain breeds by the wool or causing bruising underneath. Bring a shepherd's crook to class, and demonstrate its use. Demonstrate (on video or by visiting a farm) proper handling and restraint of sheep and goats.
Capture and restraint of swine	Explain "rooting." Stress that pigs are intelligent and adept at escaping. Reinforce the importance of wearing earplugs when working with swine. Demonstrate (through video or a visit to a farm) proper restraint of adult pigs and piglets. Bring a support sling to class.
Capture and restraint of dogs	Demonstrate the proper use of a snare. Stress the possibility of damaging the trachea using this technique.
Catching dogs	Have several students bring their dogs. Ask the students to demonstrate various techniques of lifting, table restraint, restraint for access to different venipuncture sites, and the placement of muzzles. Have students make and place a gauze or rope muzzle.
Lifting dogs	
Table restraint	
Restraint for venipuncture	
Muzzles and mouth gags	
Mobility-limiting devices	Bring Elizabethan collars to class, explain their utility, and stress the importance of the pet being able to eat and drink while wearing this device.
Chemical restraint	Explain that chemical restraint is the best way to relieve anxiety.
Capture and restraint of cats	Demonstrate proper restraint and carrying techniques on a student's pet or a video. Bring cat muzzles to class and show proper placement.
Carrying cats	
Restraint for examination	
Restraint for venipuncture	
Bathing	
Chemical restraint	
Restraint of exotic animals	Ask the students to bring their exotic pets to class or visit a local wildlife rehabilitation center to demonstrate proper handling and restraint techniques for these species.
Birds	Stress that a bird's chest movements must never be restricted. Explain that pet birds are often in advanced stages of disease when they arrive at the clinic and any additional stress may be fatal. Examination may have to be done in stages.

PART ONE CLINICAL PROCEDURES

Chapter Outline	Teaching Strategies
Psittacines	
Passerines	
Raptorial species	Visit a local bird sanctuary or wildlife rehabilitation center to view proper restraint and handling techniques. Stress that raptors use their talons as their major protection.
Restraint of reptiles	
Turtles and tortoises	Stress that some turtles have very powerful jaws. Always approach turtles from behind.
Snakes	Show how a snake hook is used. Stress the importance of washing hands before and after handling reptiles.
Lizards and crocodilians	
Restraint of ferrets	Explain the phenomenon of hypnosis in ferrets.
Restraint of rabbits	Point out that rabbits must never be carried by their ears and that their hind legs must always be supported during handling and restraint.
Restraint of rodents and small mammals	Stress that gerbils must never be handled by the tail because if skin is removed, the tail must be amputated.
Transportation and shipping of animals	Give students the following websites: www.aphis.usda.gov (for intra- and interstate transportation guidelines); www.avma.org/grd/lac/Air_Transport (for air transportation requirements and regulations).

CRITICAL THINKING CHALLENGES

1. A client brings in a 5-year-old, male, neutered Akita for vaccinations. When you approach the animal in the waiting area, he pricks his ears forward, pulls his lips back in a "smile," and begins to "wag" his tail. As you get closer, the dog lowers his head to avoid eye contact and his tail goes between his legs. The owner claims that he "just wants to play." What do you tell the owner, and what precautions do you take in order to safely handle this pet.

2. On a farm call, a cattle rancher tells you that he is having trouble with a new horse. The horse just keeps "acting up" every time the rancher walks toward her. You watch as the man walks directly up to the front of the horse and she becomes very agitated, pawing the ground. Imagine that you are the veterinary technician on the call. What suggestions would you have for this client?

3. At a farrowing house, you observe one sow with her piglets. The piglets appear unthrifty. You keep an eye on them for a while and notice that they never suckle. You are concerned. You are the senior veterinary technician on the call along with a trainee, and the veterinarian is in the field talking with the owner of the operation. The new technician walks toward the piglets and bends over to pick one up, and the sow begins to vocalize extremely loudly, obviously very upset. What recommendations do you have for your co-worker?

4. One of your favorite clients manages to bring in a feral cat that she found in her barn. She requests that the veterinarian "check the cat out" because she wants to bring the animal into her house to live with her other cats. The cat presents in a crate. She is a domestic shorthair breed and is hissing and thrashing. Every time that you approach the crate the animal becomes so violent that the whole crate shakes. You and the veterinarian discuss the safest approach. Describe your approach.

5. The veterinarian has asked you to make a video of proper handling and restraint techniques along with other laboratory procedures for new employees. You have three species left to film: ferret, bird, and rabbit. Write the narrative that will accompany each of these three parts of the film.

6. Working in pairs, take turns describing in detail how you would restrain a beagle for venipuncture of the cephalic vein, a domestic shorthair cat for venipuncture of the medial saphenous vein, a horse for examination of the right forelimb, and a snake. Use as many of the following words as possible, as many times as is necessary: skull, suspensory ligament, occlude, muzzle, fetlock, recumbency, and elbow.

7. Have students make a list of actions that they should never take when attempting to handle various species. For example, "never approach a horse from the blind spot." Ask them to give a reason for each statement.

PRACTICAL SITUATIONS

Describe a situation in which a technician is attempting to restrain an animal for a particular technique. Provide a brief history of the animal, including reason for restraint, signalment, etc. Intentionally include mistakes that the technician makes either in his/her thought process or actions. The student must underline each incorrect statement and either rewrite the sentence or explain why it is inaccurate.

Copyright © 2006 by Elsevier, Inc. All rights reserved.

EXAMPLE

Bingo, an 8-year-old, female, spayed Pomeranian has escaped from her cage in the clinic. She was admitted in order to have dental prophylaxis performed. Mary, the technician must capture and restrain the pet in order to draw blood for a preanesthesia workup. Mary finds Bingo in the supply closet backed into a corner with her ears laid back, lips pulled back horizontally, tail between her legs, and her head lowered thereby avoiding direct eye contact. *Mary interprets this posture as playful.* (Underline this sentence because this is a classic fear-induced stance.) *Approaching Bingo slowly, Mary offers the palm of her hand to the dog's muzzle.* (Underline this sentence because it is recommended to offer the back of the hand.) Bingo attempts to bite, but Mary quickly pulls her hand back, avoiding contact. Mary kneels on the floor just outside of the closet and slowly offers the back of her right hand to Bingo. Bingo comes out to sniff her hand, and while Bingo is sniffing, Mary grasps Bingo's scruff with her left hand. *She places Bingo on an exam table while she goes off to gather supplies to draw blood and place a catheter.* (Underline this sentence because a pet should never be left unattended on a table as it may jump off and injure itself.) The veterinarian wants to draw blood from Bingo's jugular vein in order to save the cephalic veins for catheter placement. *Mary positions Bingo in lateral recumbency grasping the scruff with one hand and holding the upper hind leg in a flexed position using her little finger to hold off the vein on the lower leg.* (Underline this sentence because this is the restraint position used to draw blood from a cat's medial saphenous vein.)

QUIZ

Circle T (true) or F (false) for each statement.

1. T F When mating rabbits, the buck must always be taken to the doe's cage because of the doe's strong characteristic of predatory aggression.
2. T F The horse and dog have nearly circumferential fields of vision.
3. T F The horse has an increased ability to accommodate the lens on near objects and this accounts for their fractious and spooked behavior as the handler approaches.
4. T F Cattle are less likely to bloat while in sternal recumbency than in lateral recumbency.
5. T F When attempting to restrain birds for examination, it is best to leave the lights on so that their vision cannot accommodate as rapidly.
6. T F If a bovid must be placed in lateral recumbency, the right side should be down.
7. T F It is safest to stand directly in front of a horse when handling it.
8. T F When carrying a rabbit, always control the hind legs to avoid potential neural injuries to the animal.
9. T F Horses should be tied to objects at least as high as the shoulder.
10. T F Horses, cattle, dogs, and cats must all be vaccinated against rabies in order to legally be transported across state lines.
11. T F Snakes have poor olfactory capability and attack on the basis of vision.
12. T F Sheep have a tendency to flock together to avoid stimuli from outside making herding easier for some dogs.
13. T F The "ears back" position on a llama indicates that the animal is upset or potentially aggressive.
14. T F Blood is often drawn from the lateral saphenous vein of dogs with the animal in sternal recumbency.
15. T F When working with swine, it is strongly recommended to wear ear protection.
16. T F When tail tying a horse, it is recommended to only tie the tail to the horse itself and never to a stationary object.
17. T F Ferrets may be restrained by grasping the scruff and suspending the animal with one hand while stroking the body with the other hand.
18. T F Always handle suckling pigs in full view of the sow so that she is fully aware of you at all times.
19. T F Hydraulic chutes are outdated and have been replaced by halters and prodding.
20. T F Always wear gloves when handling psittacines in the clinical setting so that they cannot smell you.

Answers: (1) F, (2) F, (3) F, (4) T, (5) F, (6) T, (7) F, (8) T, (9) T, (10) F, (11) F, (12) T, (13) T, (14) F, (15) T, (16) T, (17) T, (18) F, (19) F, (20) F. ∎

2

History and Physical Examination

TEACHING/LEARNING OBJECTIVES

1. Demonstrate appropriate history-taking skills by knowing how to ask questions that are not leading and that the client can understand. Be able to paraphrase what the client has said.
2. Explain why paraphrasing is important.
3. Ask at least two questions regarding each body system.
4. Determine if medical records have been completed accurately.
5. Determine the rectal temperature of a cat and dog and know the average ranges for these species.
6. Determine the pulse rate of a cat and dog (via the femoral artery and auscultation) and know the average ranges for these species.
7. Take the respiratory rate of a cat and dog and know the average for these species.
8. Complete an assessment of all 12 body systems of a cat and dog and accurately complete a medical record to reflect findings. Identify normal versus abnormal characteristics.
9. Describe the location, timing, duration, and character of heart murmurs.
10. Categorize heart murmurs according to the grading system described in the chapter.
11. Assess the following spinal reflexes: triceps, quadriceps, patellar, and gastrocnemius. Explain the significance of each.
12. Assess the panniculus reflex on a dog or large animal and explain its importance.
13. Assess superficial and deep pain and the implications of the presence or absence of each.
14. Assess anal tone and the perineal reflex.
15. Identify the location of the prescapular, submandibular, popliteal, axillary, and inguinal lymph nodes on a picture of a dog or cat, and explain which ones are typically not palpable in a healthy animal.
16. Palpate the prescapular, submandibular, and popliteal lymph nodes on a dog and cat.
17. Characterize the ear debris typically seen with bacterial otitis, ear mites, and yeast infections.
18. Draw a simple line drawing of a dog's or cat's outer, middle, and inner ear.
19. Perform an otoscopic exam of a cat or dog.
20. Draw a simple line drawing of a globe and include the eyelids and optic nerve.
21. Perform an ocular exam that includes external structures and the anterior chamber, iris, and lens.

KEY TERMS

Alopecia
Anterior chamber
Aortic valve
Auscultate
Axillary lymph nodes
Capillary refill time (CRT)
Comedones
Cornea
Crackles
Crepitus
Crescendo
Crescendo-decrescendo
Crusts
Decrescendo
Diastole
Dropped pulse
Ectropion
Entropion
Epiglottis
Erythema
Gastrocnemius reflex
Gingival mucosa
Heart murmur
Hematoma
Holosystolic murmur
Inguinal lymph nodes
Injection type murmur
Iris
Irregularly irregular rhythm
Jugular furrow
Labial mucosa

Lens
Machinery murmur
Macules
Mitral valve
Nares
Nictitating membrane
Nonpruritic
Panniculus reflex
Pansystolic murmur
Papules
Paraphrase
Patellar reflex
Perineal area/reflex
Pharyngeal area
Pinnae
Polydipsia
Polyuria
Popliteal lymph nodes
Postural reactions
Prescapular lymph nodes
Pulmonic valve
Purulent
Pustules
Quadriceps reflex
Sclera
Spinal reflexes
Stenotic
Stifle joint
Submandibular lymph nodes
Systole
Triceps reflex
Tricuspid valve
Wheezes

Chapter Outline	Teaching Strategies
Obtaining an accurate history	Provide a list of questions that might be asked when obtaining historical information or show a video of a veterinary technician taking a history from a client and ask the students to determine if questions are appropriately worded. Stress the importance of paraphrasing what the client has said and of not asking leading questions.
Signalment of the animal	Provide examples of various signalments and discuss how rule outs are made based on this information.
Chief complaint	Point out that although the chief complaint is the main reason for the client's visit, questions that may seem unrelated to the chief complaint according to the client may need to be asked.
History of the present illness	Provide examples of history taking situations that illustrate good questions regarding the present illness.
Past medical and surgical history	Provide examples of history taking situations that illustrate good questions regarding the past medical and surgical history.
Environmental history	Explain the importance of taking an environmental history by providing actual case samples whose resolution depended upon asking these questions.
Medication history	Explain the importance of taking a medication history by providing actual case samples whose resolution depended upon asking these questions.
Dietary history	Explain the importance of taking a dietary history by providing actual case samples whose resolution depended upon asking these questions. Stress that a dietary history includes questions regarding potential toxin, garbage, or foreign body ingestion.
Systems review	Emphasize that although a chief complaint may appear to relate to one body system (for example, vomiting and the gastrointestinal system), disorders of other systems may actually be causing the clinical signs. Provide examples.
Recording the information	Compare actual medical records that have the names of the patients obscured. Ask the students to find errors and provide suggestions for improvement. Stress that the medical record is a legal document.
Components of a complete physical exam	Have anatomical charts available for this section.
Temperature, pulse, and respiration	Ask several students to bring in their pets and have the students practice taking their temperature, pulse, and respiratory rates. Restraining techniques can be reinforced.
Systems assessment	Show a video or perform a systems assessment on a normal cat and dog. Then show a video of a systems assessment of abnormal findings. Provide examples of medical records that have already been completed to reflect the systems assessment.

Chapter Outline

- Integument
- Respiratory system
- Cardiovascular system
- Gastrointestinal system
- Urogenital system
- Musculoskeletal system
- Nervous system
- Peripheral lymph nodes
- Ears
- Eyes

Teaching Strategies

Play an audiotape of a normal heartbeat/rhythm and various heart murmurs. Ask the students to describe the murmurs.

Review common reflexes and implications of abnormal responses.
Review the function of lymph nodes and which ones can and cannot normally be palpated.
Show a video or pictures (gross and microscopic) of exudate seen with various etiologies along with otoscopic pictures of foreign bodies, redness, polyps, etc.

CRITICAL THINKING CHALLENGES

1. For each example below, ask two students to role-play with one being the veterinary technician taking a history and the other being the client. The rest of the class must determine if questions are asked appropriately and if all pertinent information has been gathered. If a classmate thinks that a question is inappropriate, he or she must provide an alternative question.
   A. An 8-year-old female, spayed Cocker Spaniel presents with a pendulous abdomen, panting. You observe patches of alopecia bilaterally on the abdomen. The owner's chief complaint (in addition to the abdomen) is that her pet is lethargic with an increased appetite.
   B. A 6-year-old male, intact domestic shorthair cat presents with a painful abdomen. The owner's chief complaint is that he strains in the litter box.
   C. A 10-year-old male, neutered Miniature Schnauzer presents for vomiting. In addition to vomiting, the owner's chief complaint is that her pet has been drinking more water than normal. The pet was diagnosed with diabetes mellitus 1 year ago.
2. Ask the students to work in pairs and role-play with one student being the client and another the veterinary technician. Provide blank medical history forms for them to complete as they take the history. When the history is taken, the other student must "grade" the form.
3. Provide the following information and ask the students to describe the heart murmur, including location, timing, duration, and character: location of maximum intensity, sound on an audiotape.

QUIZ

Fill in the blanks.
1. Collectively, the age, breed, gender, and reproductive status of an animal is called the _____.
2. The _____ is the reason that that the client brought the animal to the clinic.
3. The _____ history must include questions regarding the potential for the ingestion of garbage, foreign bodies, and toxins.
4. The average temperature range for cats is _____ °F to _____ °F.
5. The respiratory rate cannot be assessed while an animal is _____.
6. The pulse rate should be taken from the _____ artery on the _____ aspect of the thigh.
7. Redness of the skin is called _____.
8. Short, popping noises heard on auscultation are called _____ and longer, musical sounds are described as _____.
9. The average capillary refill time in dogs and cats is _____ to _____ seconds.
10. In the dog, the urinary bladder feels pear-shaped and in the cat it feels _____.
11. The _____ kidney is more cranial in the abdomen and can rarely be palpated in the dog.
12. The _____ and inguinal lymph nodes cannot normally be palpated in the dog and cat unless they are enlarged.
13. The ear exudate typically seen with ear mites is dark brown and _____ and with bacterial otitis it is _____.
14. Inward rolling of the eyelids is called _____ and outward rolling of the eyelids is called _____.
15. A yellow sclera is indicative of _____ and a _____ sclera is indicative of inflammation.

Answers: (1) signalment, (2) chief complaint, (3) dietary, (4) 100.5° F to 102.5° F, (5) panting, (6) femoral/medial, (7) erythema, (8) crackles/wheezes, (9) 1, 2, (10) spherical or round, (11) right, (12) axillary, (13) flaky/purulent, (14) entropion/ectropion, (15) jaundice/red. ∎

3

Diagnostic Sampling and Therapeutic Techniques

TEACHING/LEARNING OBJECTIVES

1. List the steps to obtaining a blood sample.
2. Explain the differences between obtaining a sample for a CBC versus obtaining a sample for blood culture.
3. Describe reasons why blood may stop flowing into the syringe during venipuncture and how to remedy the problem.
4. Explain what to do if a hematoma forms during venipuncture.
5. Explain when it might be appropriate to use a Vacutainer collection device and how it differs from venipuncture with a needle and syringe.
6. List reasons to collect a blood sample from the marginal ear vein and name two other sites from which a peripheral capillary sample may be obtained.
7. List sites from which arterial blood samples may be taken and the reasons for their collection.
8. Describe indications for manual expression, cystocentesis, and catheterization for urine sample collections.
9. Describe indications for and methods of collecting a fecal sample.
10. Describe indications for and methods of performing thoracocentesis.
11. Describe indications for and methods of performing abdominocentesis.
12. Describe indications for and methods of performing a transtracheal wash with a percutaneous tube and endotracheal tube technique.
13. Describe indications for and methods of obtaining synovial fluid in various joints.
14. Describe the indications for and methods of performing bone marrow aspirates in various joints.
15. Describe the indications for and method of collecting vaginal cytologic samples.
16. Describe the indications for and method of collecting a fine needle aspirate.
17. Describe the indications for and method of placing a central catheter.
18. List the advantages of placing a through-the-needle catheter.
19. List signs that an injected drug (particularly a chemotherapeutic agent) has extravasated. Explain what action should be taken.
20. Explain the route and method of vaccine administration.
21. Explain indications and contraindications of intraosseous fluid administration.
22. List indications for intraperitoneal administration of fluids and medications.
23. Demonstrate skill at administering medication orally using several techniques.
24. Discuss indications and contraindications for usage of various forms of feeding tubes.
25. List the most common sites used for venipuncture as well as other possible sites in cattle, horses, swine, sheep, and goats.
26. Compare abdominocentesis techniques in ruminants when each of the following is suspected: traumatic reticuloperitonitis, uterine rupture, small bowel rupture, urinary tract obstruction, urinary bladder rupture. List potential complications.
27. On a diagram, describe thoracocentesis of a horse. List and point to the location of structures that must be avoided.
28. List signs of inflammation or infections around a catheter site and explain what is commonly done if any of these signs are present.
29. Compare commonly used sites for medication administration (intramuscularly and subcutaneously) in large animals, sites to avoid, and maximum amounts that may be injected at each site.
30. Discuss steps to follow when performing an intramammary infusion of antibiotics.

KEY TERMS

Abdominocentesis
Arthrocentesis
Balling gun
Bevel
Clean stick
Cricoid cartilage
Cricothyroid membrane
Cystocentesis
Extravasation
Fecal loop
Foley self-retaining catheter
Hemolysis
Marginal ear vein
Milk vein
Olecranon
Over-the-needle catheter
Phlebotomist
Prepuce
Pull slide
Ruminoreticular recess
Streak canal
Synovial fluid
Tail vein
Thoracic inlet
Thoracocentesis
Three-syringe technique
Thromboplastin
Through-the-needle catheter
Tomcat catheter
Tourniquet
Traumatic reticuloperitonitis
Vacutainer collection device
Vesicant
Viscous
Xiphoid process

Chapter Outline	Teaching Strategies
Basic guidelines	Emphasize the importance of having all supplies gathered and labeled before beginning the procedure.
Small animal sampling and therapeutic techniques	Show videos of any of the following procedures. Display anatomical charts to help students visualize pertinent internal anatomy. Stress the indication for each procedure and contraindications, if any. Have collection materials available. Have several students bring their pets to class and practice locating appropriate sampling sites. Review restraint techniques needed for each procedure.
Blood sample collection	
Venous blood sample	
Cephalic venipuncture	
Jugular venipuncture	Demonstrate various tourniquets and their application. Explain the importance of prebending the needle to approximately 150 degrees for venipuncture in small dogs and cats.
Lateral saphenous venipuncture	Discuss the use of this vein in aggressive dogs.
Medial saphenous or femoral venipuncture	Emphasize the importance of applying pressure for at least 30 seconds after venipuncture at this site.
Marginal ear venipuncture	Explain when this vein might be used to collect a sample.
Arterial blood sample	Stress the importance of using a heparinized syringe and review the reasons for collecting arterial samples.
Femoral artery sample	
Dorsal metatarsal artery sample	
Urine sample collection	Students may be able to gently palpate the urinary bladder on their own pets.
Voided collection	
Manual bladder expression	
Cystocentesis	Stress the importance of not redirecting the needle once it is inserted. Review patient positioning for this technique.
Catheterization	On diagrams, point out relevant anatomical structures in the male and female.
Male canine	
Female canine	
Male feline	
Female feline	
Other collection procedures	
Fecal collection	
Thoracocentesis	On students' pets ask them to count to the appropriate rib space and indicate where they would aspirate fluid or air. Bring collection systems to class. Stress the importance of inserting the needle at the cranial aspect of the rib.

Copyright © 2006 by Elsevier, Inc. All rights reserved.

CHAPTER 3 Diagnostic Sampling and Therapeutic Techniques

Chapter Outline	Teaching Strategies
Abdominocentesis	
Gastric peritoneal lavage	
Transtracheal wash	
Endotracheal tube technique	
Arthrocentesis	
Bone marrow aspiration	Explain/demonstrate how a pull slide is prepared. Stress that this is a painful procedure and the animal will require heavy sedation or general anesthesia and possibly local anesthesia.
Iliac bone marrow aspiration	
Humeral bone marrow aspiration	Explain why this site is preferred in heavily muscled or overweight patients.
Femoral bone marrow aspiration	
Fine needle aspiration	
Vaginal cytologic sampling	
Administration of medicine in the small animal	Demonstrate catheter placement and medication administration for each method listed below on a video. Distribute pictures with pertinent anatomy of each method. Stress indications and contraindications (if any) of each method of administration.
Intravenous administration	
Intravenous catheter placement	Stress the importance of placing the catheter in a distal location.
Peripheral vein catheterization	
Jugular vein catheterization	
Arterial catheter placement	Emphasize that medications and fluids should never be administered via an arterial catheter.
Intravenous and intraarterial catheter maintenance	List various problems that may arise after placing these catheters. Ask the students to explain how they would respond to these challenges.
Intravenous chemotherapy administration	Stress the importance of personnel safety when administering chemotherapeutic agents. Show all material/equipment needed when handling these drugs.
Subcutaneous administration	On a diagram, point out locations for administration of vaccinations and subcutaneous fluids. Explain why the intrascapular region should be avoided.
Intramuscular administration	On a diagram, point out the course of the sciatic nerve, explaining how to avoid it and potential complications if it is injured during injection.
Intradermal administration	Remind students not to scrub the skin with anything that might be an irritant before allergy skin testing.
Intranasal administration	
Intratracheal administration	Bring a polypropylene urinary catheter and a rubber feeding tube to class and stress the importance of using this method during CPR.
Intraosseous administration	On a diagram, show the potential placement sites of an intraosseous catheter. Point out pertinent anatomy for each site.
Intraperitoneal administration	List situations in which this route is preferred.
Topical ophthalmic administration	Discuss the administration of ointments and fluids in terms of method and timing. Emphasize the importance of using medication only for the patient to whom it is prescribed.
Aural administration	Ask several students to bring their dog or cat to class. Demonstrate ear cleaning and aural administration of medication.
Transdermal administration	List situations in which this route is preferred.
Intrarectal administration	List situations in which this route is preferred.
Oral administration	Ask several students to bring their dogs and cats to class. Demonstrate methods of administering oral medications using water or a treat.
Orogastric intubation	On diagrams, show the placement of these tubes. Bring various tubes to class. If possible, show videos of their placement.
	Discuss indications and contraindications for each of these methods.
Enteral feeding tubes	On diagrams, point out placement of these tubes; review pharyngeal, laryngeal, and esophageal anatomy.
Nasoesophageal and nasogastric tubes	
Pharyngostomy tube placement	
Esophagostomy tube placement	

PART ONE CLINICAL PROCEDURES

Chapter Outline	Teaching Strategies
Large animal sampling and therapeutic techniques	Provide diagrams of various sites used for venipuncture on cattle, horses, pigs, sheep, and goats. If possible, show videos of these techniques. Stress the importance of proper restraint.
Venous blood sample collection	
Bovine venipuncture	
Jugular venipuncture	
Coccygeal venipuncture	Stress the importance of avoiding coccygeal artery.
Subcutaneous abdominal (milk vein) venipuncture	Stress the need to place the animal in a stanchion when collecting from this vein.
Equine venipuncture	
Porcine venipuncture	
External jugular vein	Show the relationship of the phrenic nerve, cranial vena cava, and exterior jugular vein on the left side and stress the importance of drawing from the right cranial vena cava.
Auricular vein	
Orbital sinus	
Tail vein	
Ovine and caprine venipuncture	
Arterial blood sample collections	Review the reasons for obtaining arterial blood samples.
Urine sample collection	Remind students that the sample should be collected midstream.
Bovine urine collection	
Equine urine collection	
Ovine and caprine urine collection	
Fecal collection	
Rumen fluid collection	Review the anatomy of the bovine stomach and discuss the importance of rumen fluid analysis and transfer.
Abdominocentesis	Compare abdominocentesis sites in large and small animals. Differentiate suspected diseases based on sites used to obtain samples.
Equine abdominocentesis	
Ruminant abdominocentesis	
Thoracocentesis	On a diagram, identify key structures that are important in performing thoracocentesis. Show a video of this procedure.
Transtracheal wash	
Administration of medication in large animals	Review the location of vessels commonly used to administer medication and place catheters in different species. Show videos of catheter placement and various routes of administration, if possible, stressing the importance of proper restraint techniques.
Bovine administration	Remind students that the coccygeal vein is not recommended as the first choice because of possible fecal contamination.
Equine administration	
Ovine and caprine administration	
Porcine administration	
Intramuscular administration	Ask the students to prepare a list of which sites to use and which to avoid in each species. Include maximum volumes recommended to be given. Review indications for intramuscular administration.
Bovine administration	Remind students that the gluteal muscles should be avoided because of the possibility of abscess formation.
Equine administration	Provide pictures of the triangular region used to administer medication in horses and review the anatomy. Stress that the gluteal and pectoral regions should be avoided.
Ovine and caprine administration	List sites commonly used for medication administration and stress that 5 ml is the maximum amount that is recommended for injection.
Porcine administration	
Subcutaneous administration	Ask the students to prepare a list of which sites to use and which to avoid in each species. Include maximum volumes recommended to be given. Review indications for subcutaneous administration.
Bovine and equine administration	
Ovine and caprine administration	
Porcine administration	

CHAPTER 3 Diagnostic Sampling and Therapeutic Techniques

Chapter Outline	Teaching Strategies
Intradermal administration	Review indications for giving intradermal, intraperitoneal, and intranasal injections in large animals.
Intraperitoneal administration	
Intranasal administration	
Oral administration	Review indications for various methods of oral administration. Compare restraint techniques used with each species.
Ovine and caprine administration	
Balling gun	Bring a balling gun to class for demonstration.
Dosing syringe	Bring a dosing syringe to class for demonstration.
Nasogastric intubation	
Nasogastric or orogastric intubation	
Bovine administration	
Balling gun	
Orogastric intubation	
Equine administration	
Syringe administration	
Nasogastric intubation	
Intramammary administration	Discuss mastitis in terms of its economic effects. Ask the students to explain the importance of performing each step listed in the text.

CRITICAL THINKING CHALLENGES

The veterinary technician must be confident in performing various sample collection techniques with minimal supervision. For the following clinical situations, describe in detail how you would accomplish each of these requests from the veterinarian. Include the needle size, restraint technique, collection tube/system, handling of sample, and handling of sampling site after collection.

1. A 10-year-old, female, spayed Beagle is suspected of having immune-mediated hemolytic anemia.
   A. Blood sample for hematocrit and total protein
   B. A urine sample for urinalysis
2. A 5-year-old, male, neutered Abyssinian is suspected of having a urethral obstruction.
   A. Urinalysis
   B. Placement of indwelling urinary catheter in order to measure and assess urine production regularly
   C. Blood sample for complete blood count and chemistry panel
3. A 7-year-old, female, spayed Great Dane presents with gastric dilatation volvulus.
   A. Perform gastrocentesis.
   B. Place two peripheral catheters so that intravenous fluid may be administered.
4. A 2-year-old, male, intact domestic shorthair cat presents after being hit by a car. He has labored breathing. The veterinarian believes that air is accumulating between the cat's lungs and body wall (pneumothorax).
   A. Perform thoracocentesis.
   B. Place a peripheral catheter through which fluid and medications will be administered.
5. A 7-year-old, female, spayed Schnauzer has been diagnosed with cancer. She has had diarrhea and urinary incontinence. She will be hospitalized for several days so that she can be closely monitored.
   A. Place a peripheral intravenous catheter.
   B. The chemotherapy regimen involves administering two medications every 12 hours. Explain how you will do this. Explain how you will maintain the catheter.
   C. During administration, you experience resistance while injecting the chemotherapeutic agent. What is your response?
6. A 2-year-old, male, neutered cat is presented for annual vaccines. Explain where you would administer these vaccines and the route: feline viral rhinotracheitis-calices-panleukopenia, rabies, feline leukemia. The owner also requests that you give a feline infectious peritonitis vaccine. The owner asks why you give the vaccines in these sites. What do you tell the client?
7. On a farm call, the veterinarian suspects peritonitis in a bovid. The owner asks you to explain why the veterinarian is performing abdominocentesis in several sites. When his horse was sick, the doctor only had to stick one site on the belly to obtain a sample. What do you tell the client?
8. You are responsible for making a chart to display in the clinic that addresses venipuncture for blood draws and medication administration for horses, cattle, swine, sheep, and goats. All veterinary technicians and assistants will refer to this chart. For each species, include commonly used vessels or sites (with the most commonly used at the top), maximum volumes that can be administered via each route, and areas to be avoided, explaining why. Include subcutaneous, intramuscular, intradermal, and oral (excluding intubation) routes.

Copyright © 2006 by Elsevier, Inc. All rights reserved.

QUIZ

Match the statement with the appropriate item in the list at the right. Only one answer should be chosen for each statement. Not all choices will be used.

1. _____ For peripheral venipuncture, introduce the needle into the occluded vein as far _____ as possible.
2. _____ This color tube contains an anticoagulant.
3. _____ When performing abdominocentesis, this approach is taken in order to avoid the spleen.
4. _____ To perform venipuncture from the right lateral saphenous vein, the animal is placed in _____ recumbency.
5. _____ This needle size is commonly used to perform venipuncture on the medial saphenous vein.
6. _____ Venipuncture of the marginal ear vein provides a sample from this type of vessel.
7. _____ This method of urine collection is needed in order to collect urine that is free of contamination from the distal urethra and genital tract.
8. _____ A normotensive, normovolemic animal with intact renal function should produce urine at this rate.
9. _____ Thoracocentesis is performed at this intercostal space in dogs.
10. _____ Normal joint fluid appears viscous, clear, and pale _____.
11. _____ This is the route of choice for administering medications if a rapid onset of action is required.
12. _____ Intravenous and intraarterial catheters must not remain in the vessel longer than _____.
13. _____ This area must be avoided when injecting vaccines and insulin.
14. _____ When giving an intramuscular injection into the semitendinosus or semimembranosus muscles, this nerve must be avoided.
15. _____ This amount of blood may be collected from the auricular vein of swine (maximum amount).
16. _____ Blood is commonly collected from this side of the neck in pigs to avoid this nerve.
17. _____ Peritonitis in these animals is often highly compartmentalized.
18. _____ The intercostal vessels and nerves run along this border of ribs.

A. 72 hours
B. Caudal
C. Proximal
D. Intrascapular
E. Seventh or eighth
F. Ruminants
G. Yellow
H. Purple
I. Capillary
J. Phrenic
K. 22- to 25-gauge
L. Cystocentesis
M. 10 ml
N. Umbilical
O. 1 to 2 mg/kg body wt
P. Right paramedian
Q. Intravenous/intraosseous
R. Left lateral
S. Right lateral
T. Sciatic
U. Red
V. Distal
W. 5 ml
X. 12 hours
Y. 18-gauge
Z. Cranial

Answers: (1) V, (2) H, (3) P, (4) R, (5) K, (6) I, (7) L, (8) O, (9) E, (10) G, (11) Q, (12) A, (13) D, (14) T, (15) W, (16) J, (17) F, (18) B. ∎

4

Wound Healing, Wound Management, and Bandaging

TEACHING/LEARNING OBJECTIVES

1. List the phases of wound healing and explain basic events that occur with each phase. Include the approximate time span of each one.
2. List the four types of wound closure and factors that determine which type should be used.
3. Name the layers of a bandage and describe their properties and functions.
4. Describe the advantages of using cast material and their indications.
5. Differentiate between a Robert Jones bandage and a modified Robert Jones bandage in terms of their components and indications.
6. Compare and contrast the indications for the Ehmer sling, 90-90 flexion sling, Velpeau sling, and carpal flexion sling and describe the positions they are intended to prevent or promote.
7. Explain the purpose of the lower limb wound bandage and the lower limb support bandage in the horse.
8. Discuss the placement of casts on horses and cattle. Include proper patient positioning, leg support, managing the frog, and the use of a stockinette.
9. Describe the removal of a cast from a horse or bovid.
10. Describe the indication for placing a claw block and the process.
11. Describe indications for and placement of a modified Thomas splint.

KEY TERMS

90-90 flexion sling
Abrasion
Appositional healing
Avulsion
Carpal flexion sling
Colloid fluid
Contraction and epithelialization
Corticosteroids
Critical number of organisms
Crystalloid fluid
Dead space
Debridement phase
Decubitus ulcer
Degloving injury
Delayed primary closure
Dry-to-dry bandage
Ehmer sling
Elizabethan collar
En bloc wound debridement
Enzymatic wound debridement
Epithelialization
Fiberglass
Fibroblasts
First intention healing
Frog
Golden period
Hobbles
Hydrocolloid bandage
Hydrogel bandages
Hydrophilic dressing
Inflammatory phase
Laceration
Lag phase
Lower limb support bandage
Lower limb wound bandage
Maturation phase
Modified Thomas splint
Myofibroblasts
Peptide growth factors
Polyurethane film
Primary layer of bandage
Primary wound closure
Proud flesh
Puncture wound

PART ONE CLINICAL PROCEDURES

Reepithelialization
Repair phase
Robert Jones bandage
Second intention healing
Secondary closure
Secondary layer of bandage

Semi-occlusive hydrophilic bandage
Splint
Strike-through
Tertiary layer of bandage
Third intention healing
Wet-to-dry bandage

Chapter Outline	**Teaching Strategies**
Wound healing	Outline the phases of wound healing. Provide pictures of wounds at different phases along with pictures of the cells active with each phase.
Factors affecting wound healing	Differentiate between host factors, wound characteristics, and external factors that might delay wound healing. Provide actual case histories and ask the student to discuss reasons for potentially delayed wound healing in each patient.
Host factors	
Wound characteristics	
External factors	
Wound care	Show videos of all types of wound care. Provide photos from actual cases.
Immediate wound care	Stress the importance of using water-soluble antibiotics if antibiotics are to be used.
Wound lavage	Emphasize the importance of culturing a piece of tissue from the wound before lavage if infection is suspected. Also point out that it is the mechanical action of lavage and not of medication added to the fluid that cleans the wound. Demonstrate appropriate pressure using a needle and syringe.
Wound debridement	Compare types of debridement methods including their indications.
Wound closure	Discuss the critical number of organisms per gram of tissue required for a wound to be considered infected. Present actual cases with photos and ask the students to select the appropriate closure. Ask them to justify their answers.
Primary wound closure	Emphasize the time frame of the golden period as it relates to the critical number of organisms.
Delayed primary closure	
Healing by contraction and epithelialization	
Secondary closure	
Wound bandaging	Ask the students to compile a list of reasons to bandage wounds. Emphasize the requirement of keeping the middle two digits exposed during bandage placement on the distal limb. Have actual materials available for the students to feel.
Wound bandaging in small animals	For each bandage, splint, sling, and cast, show a video of them being placed. Practice placing bandages on students' pets (if the pets are calm and will allow it). Practice placing bandages and splints on inanimate objects such as pieces of Styrofoam or wood. Compare and contrast the indications for each.
Casts	Explain why casts must extend one joint above and below the fracture.
Bandages and splints	
Robert Jones bandage	Demonstrate that stabilization comes from the thick cotton secondary layer.
Modified Robert Jones bandage	
Chest or abdominal bandage	Stress that compression bandages must not remain in place longer than 4 hours.
Distal limb splints	Stress the importance of always placing the splint on the caudal aspect of the limb.
Slings	
Ehmer sling	
90-90 flexion sling	
Velpeau sling	
Carpal flexion sling	
Hobbles	

Copyright © 2006 by Elsevier, Inc. All rights reserved.

CHAPTER 4 Wound Healing, Wound Management, and Bandaging

Chapter Outline	Teaching Strategies
Aftercare of casts, bandages, splints, and slings	Ask the students to write instructions for home care that could be sent home with owners explaining what to look for when checking the toes, how to use an Elizabethan collar, and how to walk a pet with a cast, sling, bandage, or splint. The students should be as specific as possible.
Specific wound management	Show videos or photos of all types of wounds listed below. Review means of caring for the wounds.
Abrasions	
Lacerations	
Burns	
Puncture wounds	
Degloving injuries	
Decubitus ulcers	
Wound management of horses	Stress that wound management for horses is similar to wound management for small animals with the addition that the size and nature of the animal and the location of the wound may influence treatment.
Wound care	Review how exuberant granulation tissue forms and stress the need to keep it in check. List treatment methods.
Bandaging and cast Application techniques for horses	Have all bandaging and cast materials in the classroom. Practice bandage, cast, and splint application on pieces of Styrofoam, broom handles, or baseball bats rolled up in towels. Ask the students to grade and critique each other, giving specific details for recommendations.
Bandages	
Lower limb wound bandages	Distinguish between the lower limb wound bandage and lower limb support bandage in terms of purpose and method of placement.
Lower limb support bandages	
Splint application	Discuss the need to cover the leg well above and below the ends of the splint.
Cast application	Show a video of this procedure. Ask the students to list steps in this process.
Cast removal	Emphasize the need to cut the cast on the medial and lateral sides.
Bandaging and cast application techniques for cattle	Explain that this procedure is similar to the procedure for horses with the exception of accommodating the dewclaws.
Application of a claw block	
Modified Thomas splint	Discuss the indications for this splint.

CRITICAL THINKING CHALLENGES

1. Provide cases in which animals presented with wounds. Describe the situation causing the wound, provide a photo (if possible), and include the approximate time of injury. Give the signalment and medical history of each patient. Ask the student to respond to each of the following:
   A. Categorize the wound (laceration, avulsion, abrasion, puncture, burn, degloving injury, decubitus ulcer, or a combination).
   B. What type of closure would allow optimum healing?
   C. Describe each layer of the bandage that should be placed. Justify your choices in terms of wound healing.
   D. Are there any factors that might adversely affect wound healing? Why and how?
2. Present actual cases to your students. Show radiographs if possible. Ask the students to respond to the following:
   A. Would you apply a sling, cast, bandage, or splint? Why or why not?
   B. If yes, which type and why?
   C. If you choose to apply a sling or splint what position are you hoping to achieve or prevent?
   D. Explain to the owners exactly what has been done and why.
   E. Give the owners instructions for home care.

QUIZ

Answer each of the following questions by writing one letter of the answer on each line. The letters in boxes will form the answer to the Super Clue.
1. This is also known as healing by contraction and epithelialization.
2. This apparatus prevents quadriceps contracture after distal femoral fracture repair in young animals.

PART ONE CLINICAL PROCEDURES

3. This phase of wound healing is characterized by the presence of neutrophils and monocytes.
4. This method of wound debridement involves trypsin products that dissolve necrotic tissue.
5. This device is used most frequently to provide maximum support/immobilization externally.
6. This is the most commonly used bandage for temporary immobilization of fractures distal to the elbow or stifle before surgery.
7. This phase of wound healing is characterized by an influx of neutrophils and monocytes.
8. These medications should not be added to wound lavage fluids.
9. This apparatus is placed after ventral coxofemoral luxation to prevent excessive abduction of the legs.
10. This phase of wound healing may last for several years.
11. This is another name for primary wound closure.
12. These bandages are indicated for granulating wounds that are minimally to moderately exudative.
13. These synthetic hormones depress all phases of wound healing.
14. Fibroblasts produce this material that matures into fibrous or scar tissue.
15. This is the most frequently used material for casts today.
16. This type of wound heals by reepithelialization and is a partial-thickness injury of the epidermis that exposes the deep dermis.
17. This is another name for exuberant granulation tissue in horses.

Super Clue: This apparatus helps to prevent animals from chewing their bandages and also prevents them from injuring their eyes, ears, or any other part of the head.

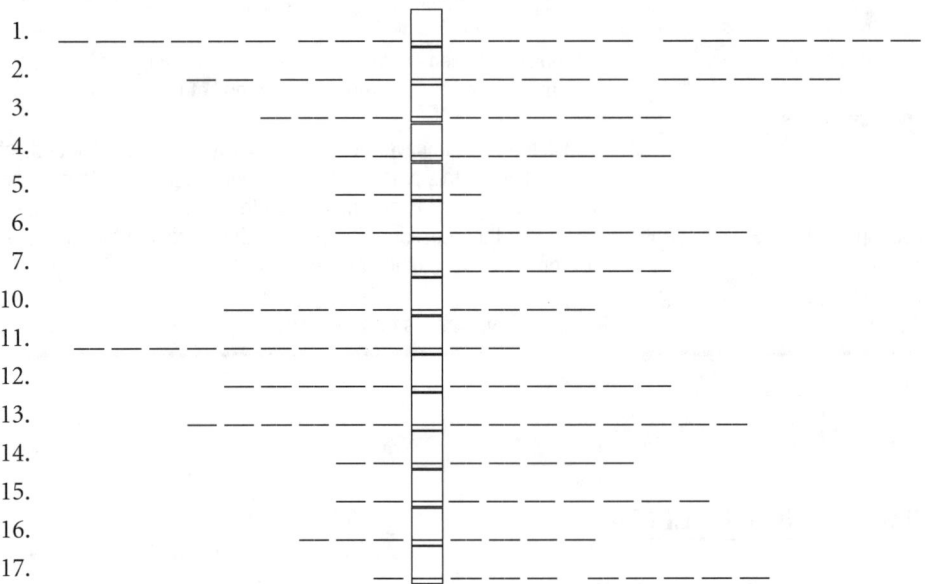

Answers: (1) second intention healing, (2) 90-90 flexion sling, (3) debridement, (4) enzymatic, (5) cast, (6) Robert Jones, (7) tertiary, (8) antibiotics, (9) hobbles, (10) maturation, (11) appositional, (12) hydrocolloid, (13) corticosteroids, (14) collagen, (15) fiberglass, (16) abrasion, (17) proud flesh. ■

Copyright © 2006 by Elsevier, Inc. All rights reserved.

5

Basic Necropsy Procedures

TEACHING/LEARNING OBJECTIVES

1. List four reasons for performing a necropsy.
2. Discuss steps necessary to take before the necropsy begins.
3. Write the recipe for making neutral buffered 10% formalin and explain its advantage over 10% formalin.
4. Write the recipe for making Bouin fixative and explain its advantages.
5. Explain why intestines must always be collected last.
6. Outline the size of the sample required (tissue or fluid), the proper way to fix and store the sample, and the organs to sample for microbiology, virology, and toxicology.
7. List the order in which the body is dissected, beginning with the eye.
8. List the superficial lymph nodes that are collected as skin is dissected.
9. Name the three major body cavities that are examined during a necropsy.
10. Name the major structures of the head that are dissected and examined.
11. Name the major structures of the neck that are dissected and examined.
12. Name the major structures of the heart that are dissected and examined.
13. Describe the order in which the intestines, stomach, liver, spleen, pancreas, and duodenum are examined.
14. Explain the purpose of a dorsal laminectomy and briefly describe the procedure.
15. Describe how to prepare a bird's body for necropsy if psittacosis is suspected.
16. Define morphologic diagnosis.
17. Generally, what ratio of formalin to tissue (by volume) is used to fix tissues?
18. Explain the advantage of completely dissecting each organ immediately upon removing it from the body.

KEY TERMS

Abomasum
Annulus fibrosus
Appendicular skeleton
Atlantooccipital joint
Atlas
Atrioventricular valve
Auricle
Autolysis
Autopsy
Axis
Bouin fixative
Calvaria
Coffin joint
Corticomedullary ratio
Diaphragm
Dorsal laminectomy
Duodenum
Endocardium
Endometrium
Foramen magnum
Forestomachs
Formalin
Frenulum of the tongue
Frontal sinuses
Greater curvature of the stomach
Gross pathology
Guttural pouches
Hematin pigment
Hydronephrosis
Hyoid bones
Ileum
In situ
Intermandibular muscles
Interventricular septum
Laminae
Larynx
Lesions
Maxillary sinuses

Mediastinum
Membrana nictitans
Meninges
Mesenteric root
Mesocolon
Mesometrium
Mesosalpinx
Mesovarium
Morphologic diagnosis
Mucosa
Mummification
Myocardium
Nasal septum
Nasal turbinates
Necropsy
Neutral buffered 10% formalin
Obturator foramina
Omentum
Patella
Pathogenesis

Pathology
Pericardial sac
Pituitary gland
Portal vein
Postcava
Prosector
Psittacosis
Pulmonary artery
Pulmonic vein
Pylorus
Ramus of mandible
Reticulum
Rumen
Sciatic nerve
Serosa
Sternum
Symphysis pubis
Synovium
Tympanic bullae

Chapter Outline

Necropsy reports
Fixatives

Facilities and instruments
Ancillary procedures
Necropsy procedures for a small mammal
Tissue collection

Dissection
Preliminary observations

External examination
Reflection of skin and limbs and examination of superficial organs

Examination of skull and brain
Dissection and examination of the neck and thoracic viscera
Abdominal cavity
Female reproductive tract, urinary tract, and accessory male reproductive organs
Intestinal tract
Abdominal aorta, rectum, and anal glands
Vertebral column and spinal cord
Necropsy variations
Ruminants
Horse
Pig
Fetus
Birds
Laboratory animals
Cosmetic necropsies

Teaching Strategies

Ask the students to read actual necropsy reports to get a feel for the language used.
Compare and contrast various formulations of formalin with Bouin fixative. Review safety procedures.
Show pictures of the required instruments and discuss methods of disinfection.
Emphasize the importance of refrigerating the whole head if rabies is suspected.
Make and present a videotape of necropsies of several species. Discuss variations of technique between species.
Stress the importance of contacting the diagnostic laboratory for specific information. Discuss ways to differentiate sections from paired organs.

List characteristics to be reviewed before necropsy begins and discuss reasons why each is important.

On diagrams, show the structures and organs in the order of dissection recommended by the author. Ask the students to label diagrams. Review the phenomenon of negative pleural pressure as it relates to puncturing the diaphragm during a necropsy.

Discuss the purpose and limitations of this procedure.

CRITICAL THINKING CHALLENGES

1. Create a necropsy report and intentionally omit important information. Ask the students to determine what is missing.
2. As the class watches a videotape of a necropsy, ask them to state the structure being dissected.
3. Discuss reasons why a necropsy is important in some situations. Discuss the legal implications and educational opportunities of this procedure.

ACTIVITY

Describe in story format a necropsy being performed by a technician and intentionally include errors. The student must identify each incorrect statement and either rewrite the sentence or explain why the statement is incorrect.

QUIZ

Fill in each blank.

1. If a necropsy must be delayed, it is best to store the body in a(an) _____ as soon as possible until the procedure can be performed.
2. Slices of tissues to be placed in a fixative should be less than or equal to _____ thick.
3. It takes approximately ___ hours to fix most tissues in formalin.
4. Potential aerosolization of infective agents mandates that the prosector wears a(an) _____.
5. The primary site of the disease and its regional _____ should be collected for microbiology specimens.
6. Always collect the _____ last during a necropsy.
7. When making Bouin fixative, extra caution must be taken when handling _____ because it is explosive.
8. The _____ should always be dissected first because the _____ begins to decompose soon after death.
9. Bone marrow samples are usually taken from the upper midshaft of the _____.
10. Pleural pressure is assessed by puncturing the _____. Normally, pleural pressure is _____.
11. In order to free the tongue, larynx, pharynx, trachea, and esophagus together as a unit, it is necessary to disarticulate the _____ dorsal to the pharynx.
12. The _____ side of the heart is examined first.
13. If ventral or lateral spinal impingements are suspected, a(an) _____ is performed.
14. As a general rule, dogs, cats, ruminants, and horses are placed in _____ recumbency at the beginning of a necropsy and birds are placed in _____ recumbency.
15. Fetal abdominal organs are most easily sampled from the _____ side.

Answers: (1) refrigerator, (2) 1 cm, (3) 24, (4) mask, (5) lymph nodes, (6) intestines, (7) picric acid, (8) eye, retina, (9) femur, (10) diaphragm, negative, (11) hyoid bone, (12) right, (13) dorsal laminectomy, (14) left lateral, dorsal, (15) left. ∎

6

Clinical Pathology

TEACHING/LEARNING OBJECTIVES

1. List the basic equipment necessary for hematologic analyses and the function(s) of each.
2. Interpret a PCV, urine specific gravity on a refractometer, and calculate leucocyte and platelet counts on a hemacytometer.
3. Explain the advantages and disadvantages of automated erythrocyte and leucocyte counts.
4. Identity a heterophil and erythrocyte for a bird and reptile and manually calculate the WBC count for each.
5. Identify platelets and red blood cell clumps from a cat's blood film and manually calculate the RBC count.
6. Prepare a blood film that would be acceptable for determining the platelet count and a differential white blood cell count.
7. Identify *Haemobartonella felis*, *Haemobartonella canis*, *Eperythrozoon* spp, *Babesia*, and *Anaplasma marginale* structures on slides, and determine the species in which they are seen.
8. List the advantages and disadvantages of automated cell counters.
9. Discuss sources of falsely elevated and falsely decreased plasma protein readings.
10. Explain when and why to collect urine for a urinalysis and the reasons for performing the analysis as soon as possible.
11. Perform a urinalysis.
12. List purposes of chemical reagent strips for urinalysis.
13. Perform a urine sedimentation examination.
14. Differentiate epithelial cells, blood cells, casts, and bacteria in urine sediment. Explain the significance (if any) of each.

KEY TERMS

Acanthocytes
Activated partial thromboplastin time (APTT)
Agglutination
Aggregate reticulocytes
Agranulocyte
Alanine aminotransferase (ALT)
Albumin
Alkaline phosphatase (ALP)
Anemia
Anisocytosis
Aspartate aminotransferase (AST)
Bands
Basopenia
Basophil
Basophilia
Basophilic stippling
Beer's law
Bilirubinuria
Blood urea nitrogen (BUN)
Calibration
Central pallor
Cholestatic disease
Citrate anticoagulant
Clot tube
Coagulation factors
Creatinine
Crenation
Cytology
Cytoplasmic vacuolation
Dirofilaria immitis
Disseminated intravascular coagulopathy (DIC)
Döhle bodies
Electrolytes
Eosinopenia
Eosinophil
Eosinophilia
Erythroblast
Erythrocyte
Erythrocytosis
Erythrophagocytosis
Ethylenediamine tetraacetic acid (EDTA)
Feathered edge
Fibrinogen
Fine needle aspirate
Foam test

Granular cast
Granulocyte
Heinz body
Hemacytometer
Hematocrit
Hemoglobin
Hemoglobinuria
Hemostasis
Heterophil
High dry magnification
Howell-Jolly bodies
Hypochromic RBCs
In vitro
Leptocytes
leucocyte
Leucocytosis
Leukopenia
Lipemia
Lithium heparin tube
Lymphoblast
Lymphocyte
Lymphocytosis
Lymphopenia
Macrocytic
Macrophage
Mast cell
Mastocytosis
Mean corpuscular hemoglobin concentration
Mean corpuscular volume
Metarubricyte
Microcytic
Microhematocrit centrifuge
Modified Wright's stain
Monocyte
Mucin clot test
Myeloblast

Neutropenia
Neutrophil
Neutrophilia
Nonregenerative anemia
Nuclear hypersegmentation
Nucleated red blood cell
Oil immersion
Packed cell volume (PCV)
Phagocytosis
Photospectrophotometer
Planachromatic lens
Plasma
Platelet
Poikilocytosis
Polychromatophilic RBC
Postprandial
Prothrombin time (PT)
Punctate reticulocyte
Refractometer
Regenerative anemia
Renal tubular epithelial cells
Reticulocyte
Rouleaux
Serum
Smudge (basket) cells
Spherocyte
Squamous epithelial cells
Squash prep
Standard
Target cell
Thrombocyte
Transitional epithelial cells
Urine protein/creatinine (P/C) ratio
Urobilin

Chapter Outline	Teaching Strategies
Hematology	Discuss maintenance of all types of equipment. Provide examples of repair costs and costs of new equipment.
Equipment	Review the parts of a microscope. Stress the need to use only special lens paper to clean the lens. Demonstrate how the microscope should be left after use. Show slides of microhematocrit tubes of various PCV readings and demonstrate how to interpret results. Emphasize the importance of balancing the samples. Show a slide of a refractometer window with a sample (plasma protein and urine) on it and explain how to interpret results. Demonstrate how to clean the refractometer sample surface to avoid scratches. Show a photo of a hemacytometer grid to be read. Ask the students to determine the WBC and platelet counts.
Sample handling	Show blood work results of samples that were stored or collected inappropriately and compare them to results from the same animal that were stored or collected properly.
Determination of erythrocyte numbers	

Chapter Outline	Teaching Strategies
Determination of leukocyte counts	Show slides of mammalian blood films and ask the students to determine the differential WBC counts. Discuss the effect of platelet clumps on the platelet count.
Avian and reptile leukocyte counts	Ask students to manually determine WBC and platelet counts.
Platelet determination	
Blood film evaluation	Ask a student to bring a pet to class. Draw a blood sample and ask the students to prepare blood films. Demonstrate proper staining techniques.
Erythrocyte evaluation	Show slides of RBCs and platelets from various species for comparison. Discuss poikilocytosis and anisocytosis and categorize cells on slides.
Leucocyte evaluation	Compare slides of leucocytes from various species.
	Categorize WBCs into each of the 5 types.
Neutrophils	Explain the functions of each cell type.
Eosinophils	
Basophils	
Lymphocytes	
Monocytes	
Other cells	
Absolute versus relative numbers	Calculate absolute differential numbers and discuss their significance versus relative percentages.
Automated cell counters	Show a diagram of how electronic cell counters work and illustrate their limitations for veterinary medicine.
Plasma protein determination	Show photos of lipemic, hemolyzed, and turbid plasma protein samples along with results that were obtained from them.
Coagulation testing	Discuss indications for coagulation testing and the collection/storage of the sample.
Clinical chemistry equipment	
Clinical chemistry instrumentation	Illustrate spectrophotometry with diagrams and compare this method of chemical analysis with the principle of reflectance. Discuss the importance of routine maintenance and calibration.
Quality control programs	
Controls	Bring examples of controls for a chemical analyzer to class along with a control log. Ask the students to analyze the log and state concerns.
Sample handling	Bring all collection tubes to class. Help the students to create a user's manual that encompasses tests to be performed using each tube, sample collection technique, handling, and storage.
Urinalysis	Review the anatomy and functions of the kidneys.
	Provide actual urinalysis results from several patients (including urine sediment) and discuss the significance of each parameter. Include case histories and CBC results, if possible.
Equipment	
Urine collection	
Evaluation of physical properties	
Color	
Turbidity	
Specific gravity	
Chemical evaluation	Demonstrate variations in readings using urine samples of different temperatures, colors, and by taking readings at inappropriate times in order to demonstrate the importance of proper technique.
Ph	
Protein	
Glucose	
Ketones	
Bilirubin	
Blood	
Microscopic evaluation	Look at slides of urine sediments and ask students to identify various cells, casts, crystals, and bacteria. Discuss the significance of results.

CHAPTER 6 Clinical Pathology

Chapter Outline

Sample preparation
Epithelial cells
Blood cells
Casts
Crystals
Microorganisms
Miscellaneous findings
Cytology

Equipment
Sample preparation
Fluid analysis
Joint fluid

Teaching Strategies

Show a video to demonstrate a fine needle aspirate of a mass, thoracocentesis, abdominocentesis, arthrocentesis, and the mucin clot test.
Review pertinent anatomy of each site. Discuss the implications of an absent mucin clot formation.

ACTIVITIES

Show hemacytometer fields of an animal's blood and ask students to calculate the corrected WBC count and differential WBC count. Show 10 fields from a monolayer of a blood film and ask the students to calculate the platelets per microliter.

TROUBLESHOOTING EXERCISES

Provide a situation and ask the student to click on possible causes of error.

EXAMPLE

You calculate a cat's platelet count to be 500 platelets/μL. The veterinarian is concerned that this is inaccurately low. What might have caused a falsely low value?

Causes:

Tube was not mixed after blood collection.
There were clots on the sides of the tube.
There were platelet clumps on the feathered edge.
Provide signalment and brief description of an animal's problem(s). Provide results from CBCs with differentials, chemistries, and urinalyses. Ask the student to identify all values that are abnormal and write the word that describes the abnormality. Example: Urine SG = 1.008, PCV = 15%, Platelet count = 88,000/μL, WBC = 44,200/μL in a dog diagnosed with autoimmune hemolytic anemia. The student must write "isosthenuria," "anemia," "leukocytosis," and "thrombocytopenia." Other parameters would probably be abnormal.

CRITICAL THINKING CHALLENGES

1. Abnormalities on blood work results are sometimes the result of technical errors or errors in sample collection, storage, and preparation. Provide blood work results from various species that contain abnormalities caused by such errors and ask the students to troubleshoot the problems by listing potential causes.
2. Present blood films of various species. Ask the students to indicate the species that is most likely represented and why. For example, rouleaux (in a healthy animal) are seen in horses and cats and *Anaplasma marginale* structures are seen in bovine samples.
3. Ask the students to make a chart to display in the laboratory area of their clinic. The chart should list steps for collecting samples for a chemistry profile, coagulation test, and a CBC. The chart must include handling and storage information.

Although veterinary technicians do not make diagnoses, it is helpful for them to understand how or why one arrives at a diagnosis. The more information the technical staff has regarding their patients, the better equipped they will be to treat and care for the pets and to answer some of the clients' questions. Provide case histories and results of physical exams, CBCs with differentials, chemistry panels, and urinalyses. Ask the students to work in pairs to determine the organ system(s) affected and, if possible, the diagnosis. It is unlikely that students will be able to diagnose this early in their coursework; however, attempts may lead to discussions of the importance of differential diagnoses and the processes of elimination.

QUIZ

Answer each of the following questions by writing one letter of the answer on each line. The letters in boxes will form the answer to the Super Clue.

1. _____ is defined as the clumping of red blood cells.
2. A _____ _____ provides a flat field of vision with superior optical properties.
3. One dry chemistry instrument useful for veterinary samples is _____.
4. Commonly seen in conjunction with glucosuria, _____ may indicate a deficiency of carbohydrate metabolism.
5. The _____ determines white blood cell and platelet counts per microliter of blood.
6. Slow drying of a blood film or high temperatures may cause the artifact of _____.
7. An increase in the number of _____ on a film indicates regenerative anemia.
8. The most common type of cast found in animals (probably) are _____.
9. Plasma protein concentration can be determined by measuring the plasma's refractive index using a _____.
10. A urine specific gravity of 1.008 to 1.012 is considered to be _____.
11. Erythrocytes, in dilute urine, may imbibe water and lyse to become _____.
12. Most mammals' red blood cells have less hemoglobin in the center causing _____ _____.
13. As bits of their membrane are removed, erythrocytes lose central pallor and are called _____.
14. _____ have reddish-orange staining granules in the cytoplasm and increase in number during hypersensitivity reaction.
15. The mast cell nucleus is round or oval and the _____ nucleus is segmented thus providing a distinction between the two types of white blood cells.
16. The _____ crudely detects bilirubin in the urine.

Super Clue: The presence of these cells implies severe inflammatory disease, except in cats.

Answers: (1) agglutination, (2) planachromatic lens, (3) IDEXX VetTest, (4) ketonuria, (5) hemacytometer, (6) crenation, (7) reticulocyte, (8) granular, (9) refractometer, (10) isosthenuric, (11) ghost cell, (12) central pallor, (13) spherocyte, (14) eosinophils, (15) basophils, (16) foam test, Super Clue: toxic neutrophils. ∎

Copyright © 2006 by Elsevier, Inc. All rights reserved.

7

Parasitology

TEACHING/LEARNING OBJECTIVES

1. Provide the scientific name for each of the common names of endo- and ectoparasites of cats, dogs, horses, ruminants, and swine discussed in the chapter.
2. Describe how each ecto- and endoparasite is diagnosed, treated, and prevented.
3. Compare and contrast *Dirofilaria immitis* and *Dipetalonema reconditum* in terms of tissues commonly affected, size, shape, intermediate/definitive hosts, the length of time that it takes for each to reach maturity, and characteristics viewed microscopically.
4. Identify microfilaria of *Dirofilaria immitis* microscopically.
5. List ways that cats contract *Toxoplasma gondii* infections.
6. Give the scientific name of the most common flea found on cats and dogs.
7. List advantages, disadvantages, and reasons for performing the following diagnostic methods: fecal flotation, direct fecal smear, Willis-type techniques, and the formalin-ethyl acetate sedimentation technique.
8. Describe the best way to preserve feces that contain parasite eggs and larvae.
9. Describe the best way to preserve ecto- and endoparasites.

KEY TERMS

Anthelmintic
Binary fission
Binary fusion
Brood capsules
Calcareous corpuscles
Cephalopharyngeal skeleton
Cercaria
Coenurus ectoparasite
Coprophagy
Creeping eruption
Cysticercus
Definitive host
Direct life cycle
Endoparasite
Enzootic
First-stage larva
Flagella
Fourth-stage larva
Free-living existence
Gametogony
Glans penis
Grubs
Hydatid cyst
Hydatidosis
Infective larva
Intermediate host
Larva
Lugol solution
Macrogamete
Merozoite
Microfilaria
Microgamete
Miracidium
Nit
Nymph
Occult heartworm infection
Oocyst
Paranasal sinuses
Parthenogenetic
Pathognomonic
Prepatent period
Preputial membrane
Proglottid
Protozoa
Pupa
Quaternary ammonium compounds
Rediae
Schizogony
Schizont
Second-stage larva
Smegma
Sporocyst

Sporogony
Sporozoite
Sporulate
Stigmatal plates
Strobilocercus
Third instar larva

Third-stage larva
Transient host
Trophozoite
Visceral larval migrans
Warbles
Zoonoses

Chapter Outline	Teaching Strategies
Endoparasites	Present diagrams of the life cycle of each endoparasite presented in the chapter. Emphasize clinical signs (if any) that might present if an animal is infected. Review modes of transmission. Stress the importance of thoroughly cleansing kennels, runs, yards, and fomites.
Parasites of dogs and cats	Show photos of the structures that are commonly identified to diagnose the presence of parasites (eggs, oocysts, proglottids, microfilaria, etc.). Provide comparisons of sizes. Show photos with eggs from more than one type of parasite and ask the students to identify each one. If possible, show photos of gross and microscopic pathology associated with each parasite. Bring as many of the preserved specimens as possible to class.
Roundworms (ascarids)	
Hookworm	
Intestinal threadworm	
Whipworm	
Tapeworms	
Heartworm and *Dipetalonema*	
Giardia	
Coccidia	
Parasites of horses	
Roundworm	
Pinworm	
Small and large strongyles	
Intestinal threadworms	
Tapeworms	
Parasites of ruminants	Emphasize the potential economic strain posed by parasitic infections in ruminants and swine and thus the crucial need for prevention.
Strongyles	
Lungworm	
Tapeworms	
Coccidia	
Trichomonas	
Parasites of swine	
Stomach worms	
Ascarids	
Strongyloides	
Oesophagostomum	
Whipworm	
Lungworm	
Kidney worms	
Ectoparasites	Present diagrams of the life cycle of each ectoparasite. Emphasize clinical signs (if any) that might present if an animal is infected. Review modes of transmission. Stress the importance of thoroughly cleansing kennels, runs, yards, and fomites.
Parasites of domesticated animals	
Fleas	Review the relationship between fleas and tapeworms.
Rabbit bots and fox maggots	
Bot flies	

Chapter Outline	Teaching Strategies
Heel flies	
Sheep nasal fly	
Lice	
Mites	
Ticks	
Myiasis-producing flies	
Diagnostic procedures	Demonstrate each technique in the laboratory. Show photos or have microscopic slides available that illustrate advantages and disadvantages of each technique. Discuss advantages, disadvantages, and indications for each method.
Fecal flotation	
Direct fecal smear	
Qualitative fecal examination	Differentiate between qualitative and quantitative tests. Explain the utility of each.
Willis technique	
Disposable fecal flotation kits	
Paper cup technique	
Zinc sulfate centrifugal	
Flotation technique	
Formalin-ethyl acetate	
Sedimentation technique	
Quantitative fecal examination	
Stoll dilution technique	
Stoll centrifugation technique	
Interpretation of quantitative fecal examination	
Specialized diagnostic tests	
Lungworm	
Microfilaria	
Tests for blood microfilaria	Demonstrate all methods of testing blood for microfilaria.
Direct smear	
Saline preparation	
Microhematocrit technique	
Knott technique	
Filter technique	
Pinworms	
Tapeworms	
Adult tapeworms	
Larval tapeworms	
Trematodes	
Protozoa	
Gastrointestinal protozoa	
Trichomonas	
Hexamita meleagridis	
Coccidia	
Giardia spp.	
Entamoeba histolytica	
Endomoeba spp.	
Balantidium spp.	
Histomonas meleagridis	
Trichomonas foetus	
Arthropods	
Mites and chiggers	
Ticks, fleas, and lice	
Diptera	
Preserving parasitic samples	Demonstrate methods of preserving parasites using 10% formalin and 70% alcohol. Show that some eggs and oocysts continue to develop even in 10% formalin.
Parasitology and public health	Ask students to work in pairs to research a zoonotic disease and to present their findings to the class.

GAME: NAME THAT PARASITE

This game can be played by one or two people.
Show four or five pictures of parasites, labeled, at any stage of development that can be taken from the chapter or other books.
Provide a series of clues, one at a time, that would lead to the identification of the parasite.
After hearing or reading the first clue, the student clicks on the picture.
If the student is wrong, he prompts for the next clue.
If the student clicks on the correct picture, he can still go on to read the remaining clues.

EXAMPLE

Provide pictures of *Dirofilaria immitis*, *Giardia* spp., *Isospora* spp., *Fasciola hepatica*, and *Ctenocephalides felis*.

Clue #1: The intermediate host of this parasite is a snail.
Clue #2: This parasite eventually penetrates the liver after leaving the intestines of the host.
Clue #3: This parasite is diagnosed in cattle and sheep.
Clue #4: The egg of this parasite doesn't float upon sedimentation.
Clue #5: Albendazole and Clorsulon are the treatment of choice against this parasite.

CRITICAL THINKING CHALLENGES

1. A 2-year-old, female intact Bichon Frise presents with a flea infestation. The veterinarian makes the diagnosis, and you bathe the pet and topically apply the first dosage of medication in front of the owner. Two days later, the owner calls to thank you for "curing" her dog. The dog is no longer itching at home and literally not one flea can be found on her pet. About three weeks later, the owner calls again and accused the clinic staff of incompetence stating that her dog is once again infested with fleas. The owner herself is now being bitten by fleas at home. How do you explain these events to her? What questions do you ask her?
2. As an exemplary veterinary technician, you are always interested in ways to improve communication with clients and client education. You are keenly aware of the risks posed by exposure to zoonotic agents. Your clientele includes elderly people, women who are pregnant, families with very young children, and even some immunocompromised individuals. You have decided that before each monthly staff meeting you will research zoonotic diseases and present one each month. Research visceral larval migrans, toxoplasmosis, and cryptosporidiosis. Present your findings on their lifecycles, modes of transmission, populations at risk, clinical signs, treatment options for pets and people, and prevention.

QUIZ

Circle T (true) or F (false) for each statement below.

1. T F Hookworm eggs have a thick brown-yellow shell with a clear polar plug at each end.
2. T F The direct fecal smear is commonly used to identify eggs of tapeworms, nematodes, and coccidia.
3. T F *Parascaris equorum* is highly resistant to environmental conditions making control difficult in horses.
4. T F Zoonotic diseases should be a concern to veterinary personnel and requires strict attention to personal hygiene and avoidance of contaminated materials.
5. T F Cattle and sheep lungworms are best diagnosed by using the Baermann funnel technique, which detects eggs from feces, soil, or minced tissues of animals.
6. T F The zinc sulfate centrifugal flotation technique uses Lugol solution to stain certain eggs, larvae, and cysts.
7. T F Organophosphates should never be used on puppies younger than 16 weeks of age or on kittens younger than 6 months of age.
8. T F The Stoll Centrifugation Technique provides a direct correlation between the severity of parasitism and the number of eggs.
9. T F The roundworm's normal mode of infection is skin penetration.
10. T F The complete life cycle of the flea occurs on the dog or cat's body.
11. T F The best control for *Giardia* spp. is to prevent consumption of raw flesh and contact with feces of infected cats.
12. T F The Willis technique is a reliable test for the identification of *Giardia* spp. and lungworms.
13. T F *Oxyuris equi* is effectively performed only by the adhesive tape method.
14. T F All tapeworms use an intermediate host in which a larval stage develops.
15. T F Mites are usually diagnosed by the Baermann funnel technique.
16. T F *Dirofilaria immitis* occurs in the left ventricle and pulmonary arteries of the host.
17. T F The filter and Knott techniques are simple tests commonly used to detect microfiliariasis.
19. T F The most common endoparasite in pigs is *Ascaris suum*.

Copyright © 2006 by Elsevier, Inc. All rights reserved.

20. T F The Willis technique is a qualitative diagnostic technique that takes approximately 10 minutes.

Answers: (1) F, (2) F, (3) T, (4) T, (5) F, (6) T, (7) T, (8) F, (9) F, (10) F, (11) F, (12) F, (13) F, (14) T, (15) F, (16) F, (17) T, (18) T, (19) T, (20) T. ■

8

Clinical Microbiology

TEACHING/LEARNING OBJECTIVES

1. Compare and contrast nucleic acid amplification procedures and culture.
2. List the most common bacterial species associated with infection in animals.
3. Describe and perform each step of the Gram's stain procedure.
4. Discuss requirements of incubation conditions, time, and temperature for cultures.
5. List indications for performing blood cultures.
6. Provide a detailed description of the collection, incubation, and interpretation of results of a blood and urine culture.
7. Identify gram-positive bacteria, gram-negative bacteria, and spores on gram-stained slides.
8. List the gram-negative bacteria along with their sources and the diseases with which they are associated.
9. Explain the role of plasmids in antimicrobial resistance.
10. List the characteristics of bacteria for which susceptibility testing is indicated.
11. Define minimal inhibitory concentration in terms of the broth dilution susceptibility test and the agar diffusion test.
12. Describe the method of collecting a dermatophyte sample for culturing from a cat's skin or hair and a dog's nails.
13. Provide two types of agar on which yeast should be cultured.
14. Explain four sources of antibodies in the serum of an animal.
15. Discuss the ideal protocol for collecting serum samples to test for seroconversion using days as the unit of time.
16. Define failure of passive transfer and explain how it is detected.
17. Give the two main causes of nosocomial infections and the two most common bacterial genera.

KEY TERMS

100× oil immersion
Acid-fast bacteria
Acquired resistance
Aerobic bacteria
Agar diffusion test
Alpha-hemolysis
Anaerobic bacteria
Antibiogram
Antibody
Antigen
Antisera
Bacterial endospores
Bacteriophage
Bacteruria
Bacteriologic loop
Beta-hemolysis
Binocular light microscope
Broth dilution susceptibility test
Complete hemolysis
Convalescent phase (of serum antibody production)
Dermatophytosis
Differential medium
Ectothrix
Enzyme-linked immunosorbent assay (ELISA)
Epidemiology
Erythrocytes
Exudate
Facultative anaerobes
Failure of passive transfer
Gamma hemolysis
Gammopathy
Gram stain
Hyphae
Impression smear
Incomplete hemolysis
Indigenous flora
Inoculating wire
Isolated colonies

CHAPTER 8 Clinical Microbiology

Lactophenol cotton blue stain
Macroconidia
Microconidia
Minimal inhibitory concentration (MIC)
Morphology
Nosocomial infection
Obligate anaerobic bacteria
Opportunistic bacteria
Oxidase test
Phagocyte
Plasmid
Pleomorphism

Polymerase chain reaction (PCR)
Radial immunodiffusion test (RID)
Ringworm
Saprophyte
Scours
Selective medium
Seroconversion
Superinfecting agent
Titer
Transport media
Vector
Vegetative bacteria

Chapter Outline	**Teaching Strategies**
Diagnostic methods	
Collection of specimens	Discuss optimum times, sites, adequate quantity, appropriate collection devices, and proper labeling of samples.
Proper specimen collection	
Special collection and handling procedures	Differentiate between aerobic and anaerobic bacteria and include their individual collection requirements. Explain special requirements of fastidious groups of microorganisms, fungi, and mycobacteria.
Processing specimens	
Conditions of the specimen	
Direct microscopic examination	Show various slides of gram-stained specimens and ask the students to identify gram-positive versus gram-negative species.
Bacterial isolation and identification procedures	
Equipment	Have commonly used equipment available.
Culture media	Review Table 8-2 in class and have plates available for students to see. Demonstrate inoculation techniques.
Purpose of specific media	
Inoculation of media	
Inoculation conditions	
Temperature	
Atmosphere	
Time	
Routine culture system	Show cultured media with a variety of colony isolates to demonstrate the variety of potential results. Explain the source of the specimens and ask the students to determine if the growth is significant.
Primary isolation media	
Preliminary evaluation of cultures	
Recording, interpreting, and reporting results	
Indigenous flora	
Identification procedures	Perform gram-stain, catalase, and oxidase tests in class and ask students to interpret the results.
Gram's reaction	
Catalase test	
Oxidase test	
Presumptive identification	Discuss the differences between a presumptive and a definitive identification and the implications of each in treatment.
Definitive identification	
Commercial identification kits	
Special culture procedures	Outline the steps that must be taken to obtain accurate results for blood and urine cultures.
Blood cultures	
Urine cultures	

Copyright © 2006 by Elsevier, Inc. All rights reserved.

Chapter Outline	Teaching Strategies
Common bacterial species	
Gram-positive cocci	Show slides of gram-positive species. Include slides that demonstrate double-zones of hemolysis, alpha-, beta-, and gamma-hemolysis.
Staphylococcus	
Streptococcus	
Anaerobic cocci	
Gram-positive rods	Show slides of gram-positive species. Include slides with spores and a variety of rods. Stress the importance of reporting *Bacillus anthracis* if it is suspected.
Spore formers	
Small rods	
Filamentous rods	
Anaerobes	
Acid-fast bacteria	
Gram-negative bacteria	Discuss the economic impact of *E. coli* and *Salmonella* spp. outbreaks in food animals. Present actual cases of outbreaks and discuss how these could have been prevented, how they were treated, and the effect they had on the owners' profits.
Coliforms	
Salmonella	
Proteus	
Other enteric organisms	
Aeromonas	
Actinobacillus	
Pasteurella	
Haemophilus	
Pseudomonas	
Bordetella	
Brucella	
Other gram-negative rods	
Anaerobes	
Spirochetes and curved bacteria	Show slides of various spirochetes and curved bacteria. Discuss the clinical signs associated with each and diagnostic tests of choice.
Mycoplasma	Show a stained blood smear of this organism and stress the difficulty of staining this organism due to the lack of a cell wall.
Other fastidious bacteria	
Antimicrobial susceptibility testing	
Indications for susceptibility testing	Reinforce indications by giving examples from actual cases that required susceptibility testing.
Susceptibility test methods	Explain that the simplest tests look for enzymes in the microbes that can inactivate the antibacterial agent. Give the example of *Staphylococcus*' resistance to penicillin.
Diffusion test procedure	Show examples of the set-up and results for both the broth dilution susceptibility test and the agar diffusion test.
Inoculum	
Test procedure	
Measuring zones of inhibition	
Results	
Interpretation and limitations	Stress that these tests have limitations and, in many cases, the interpretive criteria are assumed from results in humans. Have the students discuss the implications for the veterinary team.
Mycology	
Dermatophytes	Show slides of dermatophytes stained with lactophenol cotton blue stain. Point out macroconidia, microconidia, and hyphae structures, if possible.
Specimen collection	
Direct examination	
Culture procedure	
Systemic mycoses	Show slides of systemic mycosis specimens. Emphasize that coccidiomycosis, histoplasmosis, and blastomycosis are caused by zoonotic agents and culture must be carried out in an approved biohazard safety hood.

Copyright © 2006 by Elsevier, Inc. All rights reserved.

CHAPTER 8 Clinical Microbiology

Chapter Outline	Teaching Strategies

Yeasts
  Malassezia pachydermatis
  Cryptococcus neoformans
  Candida albicans
	Show slides of various yeast specimens.

Virology Virus isolation	Review the life cycle of a virus. Emphasize that viruses are obligate intracellular organisms and diagnosis is best made from live tissues.
Microscopic evaluation	Show electron microscopic photos of viruses and virus particles.
Antigen detection	Discuss the advantages of these methods and stress that viral antigens usually remain after the virus dies.
Immunohistochemical staining Solid-phase immunoassays	
Serology	Review Figure 8-12 with the students.
Antibody response to Infection	Differentiate the various reasons for the presence of serum antibodies.
Interpretation of serologic Results	Provide case examples and discuss why serologic testing would or would not be justified in each case. Talk about results that you might expect to obtain.
Collection of serum	
Serologic test procedures	Show photos of test results from various serology kits. Stress the importance of performing the tests exactly as stated in the kit's instructions in order to avoid errors in interpreting results.
Clinical immunology	
Purpose of evaluating immune system function	List the four types of immune function disorders presented in the chapter and provide common examples of each type.
Laboratory tests for immunologic disorders	For each of the four types of immune function explain the diagnostic test recommended.
Failure of passive transfer	Discuss the crucial importance of colostrum for the neonatal and its detection.
Nosocomial infections	
Agents of nosocomial infections	Discuss ways in which these infections are acquired. Distinguish between common reservoir sites and the most frequent locations of nosocomial bacterial infections. Include information regarding the role of antimicrobial resistance in the development of infection.
Recognition of control of nosocomial infections	
Antiseptics, disinfectants, and sterilization	Remind students to always wash their hands between handling patients.
Biologic safety	Show examples of safety manuals from different veterinary hospitals. Ask the students to work in groups to develop their own manual.

ACTIVITIES

1. List the steps for Gram staining a sample out of order. Ask the student to number them in the correct sequence.
2. Provide case examples.

EXAMPLE

A 6-year-old, male, neutered Cocker Spaniel presents for recurrent otitis externa. A colony grown on a blood agar plate is Gram stained and determined to be a positive coccus. It is catalase negative, without hemolysis. This bacterium is probably:
Select one: pathogenic   nonpathogenic

3. Provide several versions of Figure 8-9 (antibiotic disk diffusion on agar) with zones already circled and measured. Ask the student to determine, based on Table 8-9, whether the test organism is susceptible, intermediate, or resistant to the antibiotic.

TROUBLESHOOTING EXERCISES

EXAMPLE

1. Describe the venipuncture, blood/serum processing, and shipment of acute and convalescent serum samples to be tested. Include errors.
2. The lab responds that the sample was contaminated. Ask the students to select possible reasons for the contamination from a list of multiple choice statements.
3. The lab responds that there was no increase in antibody titer in the convalescent sample. The clinician is suspicious that the results are not valid. Ask the students

Copyright © 2006 by Elsevier, Inc. All rights reserved.

to determine possible reasons for the clinician's concern from a list of multiple choice statements.
4. Provide a list of statements that describe the process of serum collection. The student must identify each statement that is wrong and provide a correct answer.

CRITICAL THINKING CHALLENGES

1. Present case histories of animals requiring clinical microbiological testing. Ask the students to determine: the site to sample, how to sample, store and transport the sample, and how to culture and incubate the specimen. Show culture results and ask the students to interpret the results.
2. Provide actual cases of blood or urine culture results that were uninterpretable. Ask the students to troubleshoot and explain potential causes of the results.
3. A DTM plate is red 2 weeks after inoculation. The inoculum was obtained by brushing the patient's coat (a cat) with a new toothbrush. The colonies are predominantly brown and black. Ask the students to interpret these findings. What would they do to confirm their interpretations?
4. A client brings an aborted bovid fetus to your clinic and wants to know the cause of abortion. The cow looks perfectly healthy to him. He is petrified that the rest of the herd will abort soon. He wants the veterinarian to come out and take a blood sample from the cow because that's what he saw done once on television. You discuss the situation with the veterinarian and decide to take paired serum samples. Explain your plan to the owner and why this may be a waste of his money.
5. Clostridial enterocolitis has been isolated as the causative agent in numerous nosocomial infections of patients in your hospital. Work with another student to devise a plan to control the problem and prevent future outbreaks.

QUIZ

Fill in the blank or circle the correct answer for the statements below.

1. Inoculated agar plates must be incubated in the _____ position.
2. *Mycoplasma, Chlamydia, Rickettsia* and viruses should be transported in selective media that contain _____.
3. When performing a slide catalase test, the bacterial colonies must be placed on the slide before/after the hydrogen peroxide.
4. A culture specimen should incubate for ___ days before a negative result is reported.
5. Various types of hemolysis are most commonly seen on _____ agar.
6. Many coagulase-_____ isolates of Staphylococcus produce a double-zone of hemolysis on blood agar.
7. Exudates and pieces of tissues are preferred over swabs for _____ samples.
8. It is a waste of time to try to identify bacterial growth of _____ flora.
9. Gram-_____ bacteria may not be clearly differentiated in the presence of exudates and impression smears because these bacteria may not stain well.
10. Always obtain culture specimens _____ the administration of antibiotics, if possible.
11. Amies transport medium is used to preserve aerobic/anaerobic bacterial specimens on swabs for several days.
12. Blood and _____ agar are the most commonly used primary isolation media.
13. If a sticky strand forms in 20 to 30 seconds on a potassium hydroxide test plate, the sample is gram-_____.
14. Colonies that are smooth, circular, opaque to gray, raised or convex, and have an entire edge are more/less likely to be significant.
15. Should agar plates be labeled on the top, side, or bottom?
16. Red blood cells, mucus, and fibrin may stain gram-_____ and mask gram-____ bacteria.
17. After gram-staining, the color of fungi is _____ or _____.
18. Most cultures are incubated at 35° C and should not fluctuate more than ____° C up or down.
19. Approximately ¼ to ⅓ / ½ to ⅔ of the surface of the agar plate should be inoculated.
20. Urine samples collected for culture should be set up within _____ hours of collection.
21. The two species of mycobacteria that are zoonotic agents of tuberculosis are ____ and ____.
22. *Bordetella bronchiseptica* is associated with atrophic rhinitis in ____ and infectious tracheobronchitis in dogs.
23. When performing susceptibility tests on blood agar plates, false-resistant results may be obtained for _____ and _____ antibiotic activity.
24. The increase (at least twofold) of a serum antibody that would indicate recent antigenic stimulation is called seroconversion/infection.
25. Veterinary clinics should use disinfectants that are registered by the U.S. ___ ___ Agency.

Answers: (1) inverted, (2) antibiotics, (3) hydrogen peroxide, (4) 3 (5) blood, (6) positive, (7) anaerobic, (8) indigenous, (9) negative, (10) before, (11) aerobic, (12) MacConkey, (13) negative, (14) more, (15) bottom, (16) negative, negative, (17) dark-blue, purple, (18) 2° C, (19) ¼ to ⅓, (20) 2, (21) tuberculosis and bovis, (22) pigs, (23) trimethoprim, sulfonamide, (24) seroconversion, (25) Environmental Protection.

# 9

Diagnostic Imaging

TEACHING/LEARNING OBJECTIVES

1. Give the range (in centimeters) of the focal-film distance for large and small animal radiology.
2. Define the roles of the kilovoltage and milliamperage circuits in the x-ray tube.
3. List advantages and disadvantages of large and small filaments.
4. Give indications for stationary and rotating anodes.
5. Explain how the heel effect affects placement of the animal for taking x-rays.
6. Give two disadvantages of scattered radiations and name as many ways as possible to reduce this problem.
7. Compare and contrast the six types of x-ray units including indications, advantages, and disadvantages of each.
8. Compare and contrast digital radiography and computed radiography.
9. Explain why the highest milliamperage and the shortest time is ideal to use.
10. Define the focal-film distance and explain its significance.
11. List the steps required to make a technique chart.
12. Provide five advantages of using intensifying screens.
13. Explain the main disadvantage of using nonscreen films.
14. Briefly describe the function of the developing and fixer solutions used for processing films.
15. Name seven causes of poor radiographic detail and how to prevent each one.
16. Name four causes of compromised radiographic contrast and how to prevent each one.
17. Name three causes of poor radiographic density and how to prevent each one.
18. Define magnification and list its advantages, disadvantages, and indications.
19. Define MPD and give the annual MPD.
20. List three basic principles of positioning.
21. Describe the preparation of a patient for ultrasound imaging and explain the importance of each step.
22. Identify basic ultrasound artifacts and describe their cause.
23. List tissues in order from most to least echogenic and identify basic anatomical structures on ultrasound images.
24. Define radioactive half-life and explain its importance in veterinary medicine.
25. Give the main advantages of teleradiology for the veterinary field.

KEY TERMS

Acoustic enhancement
Acoustic impedance (Z)
  Acoustic shadowing
  Actual focal spot
  Air gap technique
  Amplitude mode
  Anode
  Brightness mode
  Cathode
  Collimator
  Comet tails
  Computed radiography (CR)
  Developer solution
  Digital radiography (DR)
  Direct-exposure cassette
  Dirty shadowing
  Echogenicity
  Effective focal spot
  Film badge
  Film fogging
  Fixer solution
  Fluoroscopy
  Focal-film distance
  Focused grid
  Heel effect
  Hyperechoic
  Hypoechoic
Intensifying screens
Inverse square law

PART TWO CLINICAL SCIENCES

Isoechoic
Kilovoltage
Maximum Permissible Dose (MPD)
Milliamperage
Milliamperage per second (mAs)
Mirror-image artifact
Nonscreen film
Parallel grid
Piezoelectric effect
Potter-Bucky diaphragm
Pulse-echo principle
Rad
Radioactive half-life
Radioactive iodine (^{131}I)
Radiographic contrast
Radiographic density
Radiographic detail
Radionuclide
Rare earth screens

Refraction (edge) artifact
Rem
Reverberation artifact
Rigid cassettes
Roentgen
Safelight
Scale of contrast
Screen craze
Screen film
Slice-thickness artifact
Soft radiation
Sonodense
Sonolucent
Technetium 99m (^{99m}Tc)
Technique chart
Through transmission
Time-motion mode
X-ray tube

Chapter Outline

Radiology
Legal records and film identification
Filing the radiograph
Production of x-rays

Basic principles
The x-ray tube
  Filament and focusing cup
  Focal spot
  Stationary anode
  Rotating anode
  Heel effect
  Tube rating chart

The physics of x-ray production
Scattered radiations

X-ray equipment

Portable unit
Mobile unit
Stationary unit
Fluoroscopy
Digital radiography
Computed radiography
Exposure factors

Milliamperage
Exposure time

Kilovoltage
Focal-film distance
Technique chart

Teaching Strategies

Show films with different types of labels.

Present a diagram of the inside of an x-ray tube and ask the students to label the main parts and to draw arrows representing the flow of electrons and energy.

Explain how the focal spot relates to the size of the filament.

Explain the advantage of the rotating anode versus the stationary anode.

Point out that longer-than-desired exposure times can damage the x-ray tube and repair/replacement is expensive.

Emphasize that their short wavelength makes x-rays invisible and therefore necessitates extra precautions for all personnel.
Show photos of different x-ray units. Present applications of each unit with advantages and disadvantages.

Explain the role of the image intensifier.

Show films and the kilovoltage, milliamperage, and time settings used for each in order to show differences in shades of gray, density, and overall quality.
Explain why milliamperage is a quantity factor.
Show films that illustrate blurring. Describe the relationship between time settings and blurring.
Explain why kilovoltage is a quality factor.
Show a diagram indicating how focal-film distance is measured.
Show several technique charts utilized by different clinics. Stress that each chart is developed uniquely for each machine and that the focal-film distance, film, cassette screen, and development process must remain constant for the chart to be reliable.

Copyright © 2006 by Elsevier, Inc. All rights reserved.

though
CHAPTER 9 Diagnostic Imaging

Chapter outline	Teaching strategies
Formulation of a technique chart	Introduce the importance of grids as they relate to scattered radiations.
Image formation	
X-ray cassette	Bring x-ray cassettes to class and demonstrate placement of screens and film inside.
Intensifying screens	Show films with screen artifacts. Stress the importance of screen cleanliness.
Screen speed	Make a chart of screen speeds and ask the students to include the species for which it might be used and advantages/disadvantages of each.
X-ray film	
Grids	Show films that demonstrate grid cut off.
Potter-Bucky diaphragm	
The darkroom	Discuss film fogging and show sample films that illustrate this artifact.
Equipment	
Hand processing equipment	
Automatic film processors	
Film storage	
Cassette loading and unloading	
Hanging x-ray film	
Developing x-ray film	Explain that the developing solution functions to reduce the exposed silver halides in the x-ray film to metallic silver, which is black. When the film is exposed to the fixer solution, this process is halted.
Silver recovery	Emphasize the importance of recycling silver and the financial advantage it offers.
Radiographic film quality	List causes of poor radiographic contrast, density, and detail as films with evidence of these problems are displayed. The films developed while making the technique charts that are to be discarded can be used.
Detail	
Radiographic contrast	
Radiographic density	
Magnification	
Technical errors and artifacts	Present films representing various types of artifacts caused by technical errors, processing using wet tanks, and the use of automatic processors. Discuss potential causes and ways to prevent this from reoccurring.
Radiation safety	Stress that more rapidly dividing cells are affected most and that all species are susceptible to damage.
Radiation filtration	Discuss aluminum filtration and its effect on soft radiation.
Radiation measurement	Review definitions and practical applications for each of the following five categories.
Roentgen	
Rad	
Rem	
Maximum possible dose	
Personal monitoring	
Protection practices	Show how to detect cracks in the lead of aprons. Ask the students to list as many protection practices as they can and discuss how each way relates to the "time, distance, and shielding" rule.
Radiographic contrast agents	
Common contrast media and applications	Show films that demonstrate the use of radiolucent gases, barium sulfate, soluble radiopaque ionic contrast media, and organic iodides. Discuss indications and contraindications of each, particularly in reference to the body parts being assessed.
Esophagus	
Contrast agents	
Procedure	
Stomach and small bowel	
Contrast agents	
Procedure	
Dosage	
Film sequence	

Chapter outline	Teaching strategies
Large bowel (lower gastrointestinal study, barium enema)	
Contrast agents	
Precautions	
Preparation	
Procedure	
Urinary tract	
Contrast agents	
Complications	
Contraindications	
Procedure	
Urinary bladder	
Contrast agents	
Procedure	
Urethrography	
Contrast agents	
Procedure	
Spinal cord	
Contrast agents	
Contraindications	
Procedure	
Positioning	Present the basic principles of positioning and restraint as they relate to safety of personnel and the patient.
Principles of positioning	
Restraint	
Diagnostic ultrasound	Show images of ultrasound examinations. Compare and contrast images in terms of heterogenicity, hypogenicity, and acoustic impedance.
Ultrasound basics	
Ultrasound-tissue interaction	
Patient preparation	
Ultrasound display modes	Show films of each of the three display modes. Compare and contrast the three display modes. Discuss their indications and limitations.
The ultrasound image	
Ultrasound artifacts	Show images that demonstrate different artifacts. Ask the students to explain the cause of each one. Stress the importance of understanding artifacts for accurate diagnostic interpretation.
Reverberation artifact	
Shadowing	
Acoustic enhancement	
Refraction, or edge artifact	
Mirror-image artifact	
The ultrasound examination	Identify anatomic structures on ultrasound images and point out differences in echogenicity with adjacent tissues. Ask the students to identify structures.
Clinical use	Stress the ever-increasing use of ultrasound imaging in veterinary medicine. Have the students discuss the role of the veterinary technician before, during, and after the ultrasound exam.
Uses of ultrasound in large and small animals	
Nuclear medicine	Differentiate between gamma rays and x-rays. Emphasize the need to understand how electromagnetic radiations behave and thus take appropriate safety precautions. List indications for nuclear medicine studies.
Computed tomography	Highlight major differences between CT and MRI.
Magnetic resonance imaging	
Teleradiology, PACS, and RIS	Discuss implications of this new technology on veterinary medicine.

Copyright © 2006 by Elsevier, Inc. All rights reserved.

CHAPTER 9 Diagnostic Imaging

ACTIVITY

Create a scenario in which the student is asked to train a new assistant who has just been hired in the clinic. The clinician has asked him/her to give a crash course in radiology to the new person. Provide a list of statements that the student (technician) would say and leave some parts blank. The student must select from a list of answers to complete the sentence. The new employee occasionally asks questions to make this exercise more like a conversation.

EXAMPLE

Technician: "X-rays are electromagnetic radiation, just like light rays except that _____."
_____ they are longer than light rays
_____ they are shorter than light rays
New employee: "Does this mean that they have more energy than light rays?"
Technician: "Yes, _____."
_____ but x-rays have a weaker ability to penetrate tissue than light rays
_____ and they have a greater ability to penetrate tissue than light rays

CRITICAL THINKING CHALLENGES

1. Provide approximate costs to purchase and maintain various types of x-ray units. Ask the student to choose the ideal unit for various clinical settings and justify the cost to the veterinarian in charge.
2. Provide old and new mAs settings and ask the students to calculate the new focal-film distance to produce a similar radiographic density.
3. Ask several students to bring in their dogs and to develop technique charts using lateral abdominal films.
4. Present actual cases. Ask the students to design the ideal combination of screen, film, and grid that they would use in order to achieve images of the highest quality while minimizing exposure to scattered radiations.
5. Present films with poor detail, poor contrast, and/or poor radiographic density. Ask the students to identify which of these three qualities is compromised and to list specific steps they would take to improve each one.
6. During an inspection from an Occupational Safety and Health Administration (OSHA) representative you are asked how your team maximizes personal protection in the radiology area. What do you tell her?

QUIZ

Choose the answer for each statement below from the list. Each answer may not be used more than one time.

1. As electrons hit the target in the x-ray tube, approximately _____% of the energy produced is lost as heat.
2. When a perforation in the intestinal tract is suspected, _____ should not be given as a contrast agent because it is not resorbed if it leaks into a body cavity.
3. Within the x-ray tube, electrons travel from the cathode to the _____-charged anode.
4. For thoracic films of dogs or cats, times should be set at _____ to _____ second to prevent blurring as a result of respiratory motion.
5. X-rays are shorter than light waves and therefore have _____ penetrating power.
6. A grid should be used to _____ scattered radiations when the body part being radiographed is _____ than 10 cm.
7. Increased milliamperage _____ the volume of x-rays produced at the target area and _____ film blackness.
8. The thickest part of the body part being x-rayed should be placed toward the _____.
9. Although _____ is expensive, it has the advantage of allowing the user to send images through phone lines; no films, screens, or processing are required.
10. The use of fluorescent intensifying screens allows the use of _____ mAs settings because film is _____ sensitive to light exposure than to radiation exposure.
11. Very homogeneous populations of cells produce few echoes and are generally darker or _____.
12. The mAs dial on x-ray units automatically sets the _____ milliamperage and _____ time to control the photons produced.
13. As more x-rays reach the film (higher mAs), more light is emitted by the screens and the film will be _____, thus _____ film density.
14. Densities that are too high or low may be caused by a problem with the _____ of the developer of an automated system.
15. Two views at _____ angles should be taken in diagnostic studies, if possible.
16. A large _____ in acoustic impedance occurs when sound waves hit gas or air causing a _____ defect.
17. Normal liver tissue appears _____ echogenic than the adjacent gallbladder on ultrasound exam because the liver has _____ attenuation.
18. Radionuclides are primarily administered via the _____ route.
19. Most commonly, computed tomography is used in veterinary medicine to detect neurologic disease in the _____ and _____ areas.
20. Most commonly, magnetic resonance imaging is used in veterinary medicine to detect _____ disease in the head and spinal areas.

A. More
B. Positively
C. Neurologic
D. Lower, more
E. Digital radiography
F. Less
G. Temperature
H. Cathode
I. Anode
J. Decrease, greater
K. Hypoechoic
L. Intravenous
M. Decrease/reverberation
N. 1/20, 1/60
O. 90%
P. Hyperechoic
Q. Decreases
R. More, less
S. Positively
T. Barium sulfate
U. Highest, shortest
V. Darker, increasing
W. Lower, more
X. 90°
Y. Head, spinal
Z. Increases, increases

Answers: (1) O, (2) T, (3) B, (4) N, (5) A, (6) J, (7) Z, (8) H, (9) E, (10) W, (11) K, (12) U, (13) V, (14) G, (15) X, (16) M, (17) R, (18) L, (19) Y, (20) C. ■

10

Veterinary Oncology

TEACHING/LEARNING OBJECTIVES

1. List four ways in which tumor growth can cause clinical signs.
2. Compare benign and malignant tumors.
3. Compare and contrast carcinomas and sarcomas.
4. Compare and contrast low-grade and high-grade tumors in terms of cellular architecture, mitotic figures, and relationship to surrounding structures.
5. List nine factors of carcinogenesis potential.
6. List ten early warning signs of cancer.
7. Discuss the preferred method of obtaining a urine sample in a patient who is suspected of having cancer.
8. List items of a minimum database that the author recommends.
9. Explain the procedure for taking thoracic radiographs for diagnosing and staging cancer.
10. List ways to obtain samples for cytology.
11. Prepare an impression smear for microscopic examination.
12. List three biopsy techniques and explain the advantages and disadvantages of each.
13. List three modalities of cancer treatment. Provide situations in which multiple modalities might be optimal.
14. List four primary indications for chemotherapy in dogs and cats.
15. Briefly explain the mechanism of action of chemotherapeutic agents and the common side effects.
16. Explain why it is important to always ask the client what drug was last administered and when it was given.
17. Describe how chemotherapeutic drugs are handled to prevent inhalation and cutaneous exposure.
18. Describe the mechanism of radiotherapy and why it should not be discontinued because of the development of acute side effects.
19. Describe potential side effects that you might expect to see during radiotherapy treatment and means to prevent further damage.

KEY TERMS

Anaphylaxis
Benign
Bone marrow needle
Bone marrow suppression
Butterfly catheter
Cancer
Carcinogenesis
Carcinoma
Chemotherapy
Cryosurgery
Extravasation
Impression smear
Inhibition
Irritant
Jamshidi bone marrow biopsy needle
Luer lock syringe
Malignant
Mesenchymal tissue
Metastasis
Mitotic figure
Mutagen
Nadir of leukopenia
Oncology
Over-the-needle indwelling intravenous catheter
Paraneoplastic syndrome
Promotion
Radiation sensitizer
Radiotherapy
Sarcoma
Teratogen
TNM system
Transitional cell carcinoma
Vesicant

Chapter Outline	Teaching Strategies
Tumor biology	Explain how a tumor's name, grade, and stage allow prediction of a tumor's behavior. Show histologic slides that illustrate various cellular architectures, mitotic figures, and relationships to surrounding tissues.
Diagnostic approach in the dog or cat with cancer	
History, physical examination, and minimum database	
Radiography	Show radiographs that demonstrate the need for three views instead of two when looking for pulmonary metastases.
Cytology	Show videos of fine needle aspiration and bone marrow aspiration being performed and impression smears being made.
Fine needle aspiration	
Bone marrow aspiration	Bring a bone marrow needle and Jamshidi core biopsy needle to class. Discuss indications and anatomic sites for bone marrow aspirates using a diagram and palpation on a pet.
Histopathology	Show slides of various histopathologic samples. Point out areas of inflammation, necrosis, fibrosis, and neoplasia. Read the pathologist's report and treatment that the patient underwent. Discuss reasons for choosing certain treatments.
Biopsy techniques	Bring a TruCut needle to class. Show videos of biopsy techniques being performed. Have the students determine their role before, during, and after biopsies.
Needle core biopsy Incisional biopsy	
Excisional biopsy	
Biopsy preparation	Review the preparation of buffered neutral formalin solution (see Chapter 6) the ratio of fixative to tissue needed, and the appropriate thickness of slices for penetration.
Therapeutic options	Present case histories, diagnostic reports, photos of cytology and histopathologic lesions, and photos of the patient. Discuss possible treatment options, postoperative care, and prognosis.
Surgery	Discuss indications and contraindications of cryosurgery.
Chemotherapy	Discuss how therapeutic regimens are partly based on the nadir of leukopenia. Present information regarding the stage of gestation that some agents affect and the body systems that are damaged.
Radiotherapy	Discuss indications of radiotherapy. Show pictures of acute side affects and emphasize the importance of continuing therapy despite their development.
Euthanasia	Discuss the technician's role in euthanasia (See Chapter 37.)

CRITICAL THINKING CHALLENGES

1. Ask the students to create handouts for clients that explain the basic concepts of cancer. They should include potential causes, types, diagnoses, prognoses, treatments, and prevention. Students can read each other's handouts and provide critiques. The handout must be written at an appropriate level for the client, must not present an overwhelming amount of information, and can even include contact information for cancer societies.

2. Ask the students to pretend that they are the veterinary technician in charge of the area where chemotherapeutic agents are handled. They are going on vacation and must train a co-worker to take over these responsibilities temporarily. Prepare a list of daily tasks, precautions, and safety procedures for the co-worker to use each day in their absence.

3. Role play. Students can work in pairs with one representing the client and the other representing the veterinary technician. Provide scenarios in which the client is indecisive about euthanasia, has just decided to have his or her pet euthanized after a very long, tormenting treatment plan that failed, etc. The other students in the classroom can provide useful, objective information.

QUIZ

Circle T (true) or F (false) for each statement.

1. T F   Cytology is a more reliable way to obtain a definitive diagnosis of cancer than histopathology.

2. T F The cephalic vein should always be used to obtain blood samples from dogs and cats with cancer.
3. T F The National Cancer Society and the Veterinary Cancer Society are good sources of information regarding cancer and its treatment.
4. T F It is recommended to use Diff-Quik stain to stain all impression smears.
5. T F Paraneoplastic syndromes such as anemia and hypercalcemia are caused by the release of hormones or other substances by the primary tumor.
6. T F As animals age, bone marrow in long bones is replaced by fat making these bones excellent sites for bone marrow aspiration and core biopsies.
7. T F When performing an excisional biopsy, the margins of normal tissue surrounding the tumor must not be disturbed to prevent seeding tumor cells.
8. T F Metastasis is the process by which cancer cells exhibit uncontrolled growth and cause local tissue destruction.
9. T F Preparation for surgical excision requires clipping wide areas around the surgical sites to allow for extensive resections, if necessary.
10. T F Pulmonary metastasis is more commonly seen with carcinomas that with sarcomas.
11. T F An animal's physiologic age is a more important factor for predicting treatment-associated risk.
12. T F Cisplatin and doxorubicin are radiation sensitizers that increase the efficacy of radiotherapy.
13. T F Bone marrow suppression (and thus leukopenia) is a toxic effect of chemotherapeutic agents that is closely monitored to determine the interval between doses.
14. T F Cyclophosphamide and vincristine are highly myelosuppressive chemotherapeutic drugs.
15. T F Radiotherapy, like chemotherapy, targets DNA; therefore, these two modalities must never be used in combination.

Answers: (1) F, (2) F, (3) T, (4) F, (5) T, (6) F, (7) F, (8) F, (9) T, (10) F, (11) T, (12) T, (13) T, (14) F, (15) F. ■

11

Preventive Health Programs

TEACHING/LEARNING OBJECTIVES

1. Explain why the measles virus vaccine is preferred if maternal canine distemper virus antibody is still present in a puppy between 6 and 12 weeks of age.
2. Describe a basic immunization protocol for dogs.
3. Describe the stages of rabies virus infection and include the approximate time frame of each.
4. List the most commonly recognized emerging serovars of *Leptospira* in dogs and the serovars in the currently used leptospirosis vaccine.
5. Describe a basic immunization protocol for cats.
6. List the most important vaccines to administer to cats according to the authors.
7. State the recommended vaccination schedule for feline calicivirus vaccine and feline viral rhinotracheitis vaccine combination.
8. List bodily fluids in which feline leukemia virus may be excreted.
9. Describe the National Vaccine-Associated Sarcoma Task Force's recommendations for the administration of rabies and FeLV vaccines to cats.
10. List the advantages of early spay-neuter programs.
11. Describe a basic immunization protocol for horses.
12. Outline a possible parasite control plan for pastured horses.
13. Describe a basic immunization plan for cattle.
14. List the viruses and bacteria that contribute to bovine respiratory disease complex.
15. Explain the purpose of implants in cattle.
16. List requirements for raising baby calves from birth to weaning including feeding and housing needs.
17. Describe a basic immunization plan for swine.
18. List the most common causes of respiratory disease, chronic pneumonia, and atrophic rhinitis in swine, the approximate ages affected, and common clinical signs.
19. Name the location and route of immunization for a 6-week-old piglet.
20. Describe how ovulations are commonly increased in swine.
21. Describe a basic immunization plan for pet pigs.
22. Describe ways to extend a pet pig's feeding time and why this is important.
23. Describe a protocol to prevent foot rot in sheep and goats.
24. Describe a proper diet for sheep and goats.

KEY TERMS

Active immunization
Acute hemorrhagic diathesis
Acute infectious encephalitis
Adjuvant
Anamnestic response
Ataxia
Attenuated virus vaccine
Azoturia
Bankrupt worm
Barber's pole worm
Bit
Blackleg
Blepharospasm
Blue ear disease
Brown stomach worm
Catarrh
Cell-mediated immunity
Chemosis
Clear, carrier, and affected
Coggins test
Cooper's worm
Cyanosis
Corneal reflex
Cystitis
Dead end host
Deciduous teeth
Diamond skin disease
Dominant gene
Dumb rabies
Dummy lamb
Dyspnea
Endemic
Enzootic

CHAPTER 11 Preventive Health Programs

Epiphora
Epizootic
Excitative stage of rabies
Farrow
Flush
Fomite
Frog
Furious rabies
Gene marker
Gilt
Glossal epithelium
Heifer
Hemibodyectomy
Hepatonephric syndrome
Heterotypic-virus vaccine
Hoof-pastern axis
Humoral immunity
Hyperesthesia
Hyperimmunization
Immunoglobulins
Inactivated virus vaccine
Infectious bovine keratoconjunctivitis (IBK)
Infectious tracheobronchitis
Infectious canine hepatitis
Ivermectin
Kennel cough
Killed virus vaccine
Lacrimation
Laminitis
Lightning strike
Live virus vaccine
Lockjaw
Lymphoreticular neoplasm
Malignant edema
Maternal immunity
Microsatellite
Minute virus of canines
Modified live virus vaccine
Mucopurulent
Mucosal disease
Mutation
Myeloid neoplasm

Mystery pig disease
Orf
Overeating disease
Palatine mucosa
Papules
Paralytic stage of rabies
Passive immunization
Photophobia
Pinkeye
Polyserositis
Polyvalent vaccine
Prodromal stage of rabies
Recessive gene
Red stomach worm
Rooting box
Serous
Serovar
Shaker foal syndrome
Shear mouth
Shipping fever
Slaughter withdrawal time
Sleeper's syndrome
Snaffle
Sole
Sore mouth
Step mouth
Strabismus
Strangles
Subacute icterus
Subacute uremia
Sulci
Thromboembolic meningoencephalitis (TEME)
Thrush
Tissue culture-adapted live-CD virus vaccine
Toxoid
Undulating fever
Urolithiasis
Vaccine-virus shedding
Vesicles
Wave mouth
Wethers
Wolf teeth

Chapter Outline	Teaching Strategies
Tumor biology	Explain how a tumor's name, grade, and stage allow prediction of a tumor's behavior. Show histologic slides that illustrate various cellular architectures, mitotic figures, and relationships to surrounding tissues.
Diagnostic approach in the dog or cat with cancer	
History, physical examination, and minimum database	
Radiography	Show radiographs that demonstrate the need for three views instead of two when looking for pulmonary metastases.

Copyright © 2006 by Elsevier, Inc. All rights reserved.

Chapter Outline	Teaching Strategies
Cytology	Show videos of fine needle aspiration and bone marrow aspiration being performed and impression smears being made.
Fine needle aspiration	
Bone marrow aspiration	Bring a bone marrow needle and Jamshidi core biopsy needle to class. Discuss indications and anatomical sites for bone marrow aspirates using a diagram and palpation on a pet.
Histopathology	Show slides of various histopathologic samples. Point out areas of inflammation, necrosis, fibrosis, and neoplasia. Read the pathologist's report and treatment that the patient underwent. Discuss reasons for choosing certain treatments.
Biopsy techniques	Bring a TruCut needle to class. Show videos of biopsy techniques being performed. Have the students determine their role before, during, and after biopsies.
Needle core biopsy	
Incisional biopsy	
Excisional biopsy	
Biopsy preparation	Review the preparation of buffered neutral formalin solution (see Chapter 6) the ratio of fixative to tissue needed, and the appropriate thickness of slices for penetration.
Therapeutic options	Present case histories, diagnostic reports, photos of cytology and histopathologic lesions, and photos of the patient. Discuss possible treatment options, postoperative care, and prognosis.
Surgery	Discuss indications and contraindications of cryosurgery.
Chemotherapy	Discuss how therapeutic regimens are partly based on the nadir of leukopenia. Present information regarding the stage of gestation that some agents affect and the body systems that are damaged.
Radiotherapy	Discuss indications of radiotherapy. Show pictures of acute side affects and emphasize the importance of continuing therapy despite their development.
Euthanasia	Discuss the technician's role in euthanasia (See Chapter 37.)

CRITICAL THINKING CHALLENGES

1. Students can design a handout for clients that outlines a basic vaccination schedule. The handout can be used beginning with the first visit to the clinic, no matter what the age of the pet. Students can add any other information that they think would be useful for the owners to have. Stress that the sheet should not be too complex because the owners may not be as likely to refer to it as needed.
2. Present various situations in which animals present for vaccinations. Ask the students to select a vaccination schedule for each animal keeping in mind the lifestyle of each pet. In each case, the owners are reluctant to vaccinate at all not only because of the expense but because they may not trust or understand the importance of vaccines. Ask the students to imagine that they are asked the question "Why is this vaccine important?" and have them justify their selections to the owners.
3. Provide scenarios in which the animal presents with a set of clinical signs. Ask the students to create a differential diagnosis list (including the names of the virus, bacterium or other etiologic agent).
4. Have students research alternatives to vaccinations for clients who are leery of them.
5. While vaccinations are essential aspects of any preventive health program, other factors obviously play a role in preventing diseases in animals. Have the students research preventive health programs offered by local clinics and report their findings to the class. Other factors that contribute to health include, but are not limited to, nutrition, dental care, and regular exams.

QUIZ

Fill in each blank.

1. The effective immune periods of licensed rabies vaccines are either ____ or ____ years.
2. In addition to protecting against itself, the current canine adenovirus vaccine-2 (CAV-2) also protects against ____.
3. The intranasal vaccine for infectious tracheobronchitis should be administered to a puppy ____ to ____ weeks before being admitted to a boarding facility or before being shipped.

4. A common source of giardiasis for dogs is _____.
5. The canine parvovirus of cats is known as _____.
6. Oral ulcerations in cats may be seen due to _____ but not due to feline viral rhinotracheitis.
7. The _____ and feline leukemia vaccines have been associated with the development of soft tissue sarcomas at the vaccination site in cats.
8. _____ should always be available to administer immediately if an animal undergoes anaphylaxis after being vaccinated.
9. To reduce the risk of abortions, stillbirths, failure to thrive, and weak neonatal foals associated with rhinopneumonitis, it is recommended that pregnant mares be vaccinated against _____ during the fifth, seventh, and ninth months of gestation.
10. In cattle, no more than ___ ml of any product should be given in an injection site.
11. Common secondary invaders (that are also normal inhabitants of the bovine respiratory tract) in cases of primary viral pneumonia in cattle are _____ and _____.
12. No vaccine currently exists for this disease of cattle that causes infected erythrocytes to be destroyed by the liver and spleen.
13. The most important aspect of successfully rearing calves is to ensure that they ingest _____ soon after birth.
14. Acute rhinitis and destruction of the nasal turbinates in young pigs may likely be caused by either _____ or _____, or both.
15. SMEDI stands for stillbirths, birth of weak piglets, mummified fetuses, embryonic death, and infertility and refers to porcine _____ infection.
16. _____ is the most common nutritional disease of pot-bellied pigs.
17. Urinary acidifiers may help to prevent _____ in pet pigs.
18. Sheep and goats that receive heavy grain rations and nurse from dams with heavy milk production are at increased risk of developing _____.
19. Dehorning, castration, and tail docking of sheep and goats warrant vaccinating against _____.
20. Sheep and goats that consume horse or cattle feeds may develop _____ because its level is so much higher in these diets.

Answers: (1) 1, 3 (2) CAV-1 (3) 2, 4 (4) water, (5) feline panleukopenia, (6) feline calicivirus, (7) rabies, (8) epinephrine, (9) equine herpesvirus-1, (10) 10, (11) *Mannheimia haemolytica, Pasteurella multocida,* (12) *Anaplasma marginale,* (13) colostrum, (14) *Bordetella bronchiseptica, Pasteurella multocida,* (15) parvovirus, (16) obesity, (17) cystitis, (18) enterotoxemia, (19) *Clostridium tetani,* (20) copper toxicity. ■

12

Neonatal Care of Puppy, Kitten, and Foal

TEACHING/LEARNING OBJECTIVES

1. List the following parameters for a healthy neonatal puppy or kitten: age at which eyes are open, age at which ear canals are completely open, heart rate, respiratory rate, age at which umbilical cord drops off, age at which sucking reflex has disappeared.
2. Place a pediatric stethoscope over the areas of the left cardiac base, left cardiac apex, and right cardiac apex.
3. Define BAER, ERG, and VER. Explain what each test measures, how it is measured, and the age at which each is expected to be functionally mature in puppies and kittens.
4. Calculate the volume in milliliters of formula needed for a kitten weighing 90 g and 1 week later when he weighs 150 g. Assume the formula contains 1.0 kcal of energy/ml.
5. List general causes of illness in puppies and kittens.
6. Describe clinical signs that one might expect to see in a malnourished puppy or kitten.
7. Explain what to do if a puppy develops diarrhea while being hand fed a commercial milk replacement formula.
8. Explain what to do to alleviate hypoglycemia and dehydration in a kitten with a decreased sucking reflex with a body temperature of 94° F.
9. Provide reasons why drugs may be poorly distributed in the severely ill neonatal puppy or kitten.
10. List six general conditions that place a mare at high-risk for complications with foaling or the health of the newborn.
11. List four parameters for the fetal foal's heart that can be assessed with transabdominal ultrasonography.
12. For a normal foal, describe the following relative to the time of birth: first urination, passage of meconium, starts to nurse, is able to stand, exhibits suckle reflex, develops a strong bond with the dam, capable of running.
13. On a diagram, point out and describe the boundaries of the foal's lungs.
14. Indicate potential signs of umbilical patency.
15. List the major routes of infection for septicemia in the neonatal foal.
16. Compare the values of packed cell volume, plasma protein, ALP, GGT, SDH, and ALT for foals and adult horses and explain why these differences exist.
17. Describe steps to take immediately with a foal that presents with hypoglycemia, hypothermia, and asphyxia.
18. Describe treatment options of a 20-hour-old foal whose IgG measures 300 mg/dl.

KEY TERMS

Angular limb deformities
Anogenital reflex
Anterior chamber
Arterial blood gas analysis
Asphyxia
Atresia ani
Atresia coli
Borborygmi
Brachial artery
Brainstem
Brainstem auditory-evoked response (BAER)
Capillary refill time (CRT)
Cochlea
Cochlear nerve
Colostrometer
Congenital cataracts
Corneal ulcer
Crackles
Crossed extensor reflex
Cuboidal carpal bones
Decubital ulcers
Desquamative cells
Doppler imaging
Dysmaturity
Ectropion
Electrocardiogram (ECG)
Electroretinography
Empirical treatment

CHAPTER 12 Neonatal Care of Puppy, Kitten, and Foal

Entropion
Euglycemia
Facial artery
Failure of passive transfer
Functional heart murmur
Great metatarsal artery
High-risk foal
Holosystolic murmur
Homeothermic
Hyphema
Hypoglycemia
Hypopyon
Immaturity
Immunoglobulins
Injected mucous membranes
Jaundiced
Jugular pulse
Lacrimation
Laryngotracheal aspiration
Lead II rhythm strip
Left shift
Machinery murmur
Malnutrition
Meconium
Menace reflex
Myocardial hypertrophy
Myoclonus
Neonatal isoerythrolysis
Neutrophilia
Normochromic normocytic anemia
Normothermic
Nosocomial infection

Olecranon
Omphalitis
Osteomyelitis
P wave
Parenteral nutrition
Patellar reflex
Patent ductus arteriosus
Pericardial effusion
Peripheral perfusion
Petechiae
Poikilothermic
Pulse deficit
Pupillary light reflex (PLR)
QRS complex
Ramus of the mandible
Reflex micturition
Regular sinus rhythm
Regurgitation
Right-to-left shunting lesion
Schirmer tear test
Semimembranosus region
Septicemia
Spinal reflexes
Stenotic nares
Thrombocytopenia
Transrectal ballottement
Tuber coxae
Uveitis
Valvular vegetative lesions
Visual evoked response
Wax
Wheezes

Chapter Outline	Teaching Strategies
Puppy and kitten	
Physical and laboratory examination	Review general thoracic, abdominal, and cardiac anatomy. Ask students to bring in their pets and point out the left cardiac base and apex, the right cardiac apex, and the point of maximum auscultation for each landmark. Demonstrate the pupillary light reflex and menace reflex. Discuss these and other reflexes in the neonate in terms of timelines of development. Run a lead II rhythm strip and show examples of normal and abnormal rhythms. Show videos of a BAER, ERG, and VER being performed along with normal and abnormal readings. Discuss the significance of each exam. Emphasize the importance of knowing the age at which eyes and ear canals open, the sucking reflex ends, the pupillary light reflex and menace reflex appear, and they begin to explore the environment. Show radiographs of puppies and kittens that demonstrate poor quality and discuss why this happens and how to improve technique.
Newborn puppies and kittens	Discuss requirements of housing and bedding, temperature control of the newborn and the environment, anogenital stimulation, and what, when, and how to feed kittens and puppies.
Principles of orphan animal care	Show labels from several commercial milk replacers for puppies and kittens. Practice calculating volumes needed to feed animals with various weights. Using diagrams, demonstrate the measurement of tube length and

PART THREE PATIENT MANAGEMENT AND NUTRITION

Chapter Outline	Teaching Strategies
Causes for neonatal care	placement for feeding. Review the protocol for deworming, vaccinating, and starting heartworm preventive medication with puppies and kittens. Look at actual records of neonatal puppies and kittens. Discuss treatments that were performed, results obtained, and ask the students if they agree or disagree with treatment. If they disagree, discuss alternatives.
Malnutrition	
Signs of neonatal illness	
Management of neonatal illness	
Foal	Show a film of a transabdominal ultrasound exam of a pregnant mare and observe the fetal activity and heart rate, aortic diameter, and uteroplacental contact surface.
The high-risk mare	
The high-risk foal	Show a video of the birth of a healthy foal and point out normal behaviors.
Physical examination	On a diagram, point out the arteries used to take the foal's pulse, the outline of the lungs, location of atresia coli and atresia ani, the course of the urachus and umbilical arteries and vein, and umbilical and scrotal hernias. Show a video demonstrating a neurologic exam of a healthy foal. For each body system listed in Table 12-1, discuss the individual diseases in terms of the anatomy affected, etiologies, implications for treatment, and prognosis.
Laboratory examination	
Admitting the critical foal	
Routine perinatal therapy	
Failure of passive transfer	
Nutrition	Discuss ways to determine the nutritional status of foals and ways to meet nutritional needs in the undernourished animal.
Monitoring and nursing care	Emphasize the importance of rigid asepsis when handling the neonatal foal and ask students to list ways that asepsis may inadvertently be broken.

ACTIVITIES

The veterinarian has asked you (the technician) to create posters to hang in various areas in the clinic regarding caring for the neonatal patient. The guidelines are intended to promote efficiency in the clinic and the best care possible for your patients. You have made the following posters. Ask the students to fill in the blanks.

RADIOGRAPHY OF NEONATAL ANIMALS

Reduce kilovoltage to approximately _____ of that used for adult dogs and cats with the same body part thickness because the bones are _____ and soft tissue parts are thinner.

When possible, perform _____ in puppies and kittens to assess the heart because this method is less stressful for the patient and safer for the patient and personnel.

CARING FOR THE SICK FOAL

The three most *immediate, life-threatening* conditions of compromised foals are: asphyxia, hypothermia, and _____.

A foal must ingest its mother's colostrum during the first _____ hours of life in order to promote adequate immunologic protection because _____.

Describe potential, real-life situations and ask the student to fill in the blanks.

EXAMPLE

An orphan puppy has been left at the door of your clinic. The puppy is obviously malnourished. It is thin and crying, the coat is dull, the eyes are open, and the pupillary light reflex is absent. You place the tip of your finger on the pup's muzzle and the suck reflex is extremely weak. You estimate the puppy's age to be approximately _____. The rectal temperature is 96° F. You decide that this body temperature is _____ and you _____. The target temperature is _____.

CRITICAL THINKING STRATEGIES

1. The veterinary technician often receives phone calls from people desperate for help with an orphaned kitten or puppy. Knowledge of normal behavior, physical parameters, and milestones are necessary to be able to ask the right questions and to calm the

nervous caller. Ask the students to generate a list of questions and information to hang by the phone in the clinic so that all personnel can be helpful with these types of calls. You can pretend to be a caller. Determine if their lists are complete and accurate by asking them to pretend to be the technician on the other end of the phone line trying to help you.

2. Box 12-3 provides and excellent list of procedures for the medical management of the severely ill puppy or kitten. Make photocopies of the box and white out key parts such as 20 to 30 minutes, 2.5 mEq/L, and 80 to 200 mg/dl. Ask the students to fill in the blanks.

3. The veterinary technician spends more time with patients than anyone else in the clinic. Their ability to detect changes in patient status is a crucial component of successful treatment. Additionally, the technicians often are the first to observe the patients when they enter the hospital and their initial assessment is especially important for the survival of the emergency patient. Sharpen the students' abilities to detect normal vs. abnormal findings by creating a list of statements to describe a patient's physical status and laboratory results (Table 12-2) and ask the students to check off "normal" or "abnormal."

QUIZ

Circle T (true) or F (false) for each statement.

1. T F Increased ALP in the foal is attributed to greater activity and mass of the liver in the foal compared to the adult horse.
2. T F Membrane color in the foal is an adequate means of assessing peripheral oxygenation in the foal.
3. T F In a healthy puppy or kitten, only the left kidney can be palpated in the abdomen.
4. T F Puppies and kittens generally perform micturition and defecation on their own by 3 months of age.
5. T F The fetal heart rate of a foal generally ranges from 80 to 120 beats/min, is variable during late gestation, and tends to decrease and become more stable during repeat measurements.
6. T F Ideally, fluids and medications should be administered by the intravenous or intraosseous route in sick neonatal puppies and kittens.
7. T F The healthy neonatal foal exhibits a decreased response to visual, auditory, and tactile stimuli until about 4 weeks of age.
8. T F Puppies should gain approximately 1 to 2 g per pound of body weight daily.
9. T F Kittens and puppies should be checked for fecal parasites and dewormed at 3 weeks of age initially.
10. T F When a pregnant mare's cloistral calcium measures 10 to 12 mmol/dl, parturition is likely to occur within the next 2 hours.
11. T F The newborn puppy or kitten is fed by its mother about every 1 to 2 hours during the first week of life.
12. T F A foal is considered premature if born before day 320 of gestation.
13. T F During the first week of life the puppy's or kitten's rectal temperature should be about 97° F to 100° F.
14. T F The ear canals of puppies and kittens should be completely open by 17 or 18 days.
15. T F When tube feeding a puppy, the tube should be inserted only to the distal esophagus to prevent laryngotracheal aspiration.
16. T F Antibiotics should always be administered immediately to any puppy or kitten suspected of having neonatal sepsis before any tests are done.
17. T F About 1% to 2% of most drugs that a lactating bitch or queen is administered is present in her milk, and severely ill neonatal puppies and kittens can be treated this way.
18. T F In the neonatal foal, the normal rectal temperature is approximately 99° F to 102° F.
19. T F All high-risk foals should have thoracic ultrasound performed.
20. T F Ultrasound examination is required to thoroughly examine the umbilical structures in the neonatal foal.

Answers: (1) F (2) F (3) F (4) T (5) T (6) T (7) F (8) T (9) T (10) F (11) T (12) T (13) T (14) T (15) F (16) F (17) F (18) F (19) F (20) T. ■

13

Geriatric Medicine in Companion Animals

TEACHING/LEARNING OBJECTIVES

1. Outline the veterinary technician's role in owner education regarding disease prevention and detection.
2. Explain the importance of organ enlargement in the pet, especially the geriatric animal and what is done to diagnose the cause.
3. Describe the recommended order of events for performing an in-hospital evaluation of a geriatric pet. Begin with scheduling the appointment and end with the owner leaving the clinic.
4. Define the role of the veterinary staff in physical, psychosocial, and spiritual care for the geriatric pet and his/her owner.

KEY TERMS

Ataxia
Autoantibodies
Chemotaxis
Chronic pain
Conscious proprioception
Cortisol-to-creatinine ratio
Crepitus
Diabetes mellitus
Electrocardiography (ECG)
Feline triad disease complex
Gingival hyperplasia
Gingival retraction and atrophy
Hyperadrenocorticism
Hyperextension
Hyperflexion
Hyperkeratinize
Hypermetria
Hypoadrenocorticism
Indirect blood pressure determination
Intramural coronary arteriosclerosis
Keratoconjunctivitis sicca (KCS)
Lameness
Lumbosacral instability
Phagocytosis
Protein-to-creatinine ration
Proteinuria
Schirmer tear test
Secondary hepatic lipidosis
Serum bile acids test
Serum folate/cobalamin test
Serum trypsin-like immunoreactivity test
Stifle joint
Urolithiasis
Valvular fibrosis

Chapter Outline	Teaching Strategies
Life stages guidelines	Differentiate life stages amongst small, large, and giant dog breeds as well as between dogs and cats. Discuss items listed in Boxes 13-1 and 13-3 and explain the clinical signs and laboratory values that might result.
Integrating geriatric care	
Geriatric health care program	
Physical evaluation	Ask a few students to bring in their dog or cat. Perform musculoskeletal and neurologic exams on one limb and ask students to perform the exam on another limb.
Laboratory evaluation	
Healthcare programs	

CHAPTER 13 Geriatric Medicine in Companion Animals

Chapter Outline

Implementation of healthcare programs
Utilizing technical support staff

Relief of suffering
Home care

Physical care
Psychosocial care
Spiritual care

Teaching Strategies

Stress the importance of veterinary technicians in communicating with the owners of geriatric pets. Discuss ways in which the staff helps to make the visit to the clinic less painful for the owner (as well as the pet).

Provide a list of organizations that owners may contact if they need help through the grieving process. Ask the students to contact the organizations and obtain literature so that they are familiar with these groups.

CRITICAL THINKING CHALLENGES

1. Ask the students to create a handout that presents the importance of prevention and early diagnosis of medical disorders in geriatric pets. This handout will be given to all clients. Include strategies that attempt to increase owner compliance.
2. Create scenarios or use actual case histories of geriatric pets with various presentations. The students can role play as they become familiar with the process of effective, tactful communication with owners of geriatric animals.

QUIZ

Fill in each blank below.

1. The first stage of grief is called _____.
2. The term _____ is more owner-friendly than the word *geriatric,* according to marketing information.
3. Organ enlargement can indicate inflammation, infiltrative disease, or _____.
4. The branch of medicine and surgery that treats problems of old age is called _____.
5. The _____ life stage ranges from birth to 6 months of age for dogs and cats.
6. An awkward gait caused by a neurologic problem is called _____.
7. Diminishing function of the _____ system can predispose a geriatric patient to parasitic infections.
8. A clicking sound in joints is known as _____.
9. The mature adult life stage for cats ranges from ___ to _____ years.
10. An awkward gait caused by a musculoskeletal problem is referred to as _____.

Answers: (1) denial, (2) senior, (3) cancer, (4) geriatrics, (5) pediatric, (6) ataxia, (7) immune, (8) crepitus, (9) 4, 12, (10) lameness. ∎

14

Animal Behavior

TEACHING/LEARNING OBJECTIVES

1. Define behavior wellness.
2. List components of a behavior wellness program.
3. List benefits of a behavior wellness program.
4. Explain the disadvantage of the historical emphasis on continuing veterinary education in animal behavior being problem resolution.
5. State the optimum ages for socialization in the dog, cat, and horse.
6. Distinguish between dens used by wild animals and crates.
7. Compare positive and negative punishment and give several examples of each.
8. List steps to crate training a dog and signs that the training is not successful.
9. Describe the cat's behavioral needs for the litter box.
10. Explain the difference between non-leading, open-ended questions and those that lead the client to a particular answer. Give examples.
11. List possible action plans that the veterinary personnel can give to owners of pets with behavioral problems.
12. Describe various agonistic behaviors that animals exhibit at the veterinary clinic and possible actions to take in response in order to promote safety of the pet, personnel, and the client.
13. Define socialization visit and socialization class.
14. List several ways to manage overly excited pets in the waiting room.
15. Describe appropriate ways to approach a dog or cat in the clinic.
16. Describe two ways to get a cat out of the carrier.

KEY TERMS

Agonistic behavior
Anthropomorphic
Behavioral needs
Cat bag
Choke chain
Classical conditioning
Defensive threat
Displacement behaviors
Ethology
Gentle Leader
Interactive punishment
Muzzle
Negative punishment operant conditioning
Offensive threat
Pheromones
Pinch collar
Plexiglas shield
Positive punishment
Problem resolution
Remote punishment
Socialization
Socialization classes

Chapter Outline	Teaching Strategies
Why behavior wellness?	Discuss the advantages of a behavior wellness program for the pet, owner, technician, and veterinarian. Contact a local animal behavior specialist and ask him/her to speak to your class on the subject. Review the requirements to become a certified veterinary behavior technician.
What is behavior wellness? Technicians can play a strategic role in behavior wellness care	

CHAPTER 14 Animal Behavior

Chapter Outline	Teaching Strategies
Behavior education for technicians	Ask the students to go to one of the websites listed in Box 14-3 and research the topic of animal behavior wellness. The students can report back to classmates their findings on the website.
A change in perspective	
Before implementing behavior wellness care	
Components of a behavior wellness program	Obtain a videotape on behavior training from the local Humane Society or animal behavior specialist and show it to the class. Encourage discussion of training techniques and ways to incorporate these into the clinic setting.
Defining the behaviorally healthy pet	
Establishing realistic expectations and helpful attitudes	Review Box 14-4. Have the students prepare questions for each criterion as if they were interviewing a client. The class can determine if the questions are appropriate.
Realistic expectations	
Reinterpreting anthropomorphic interpretations	Discuss the concept of anthropomorphism. Give examples of anthropomorphic statements made by pet owners and ask the students to provide alternative interpretations.
Providing pet selection information	
Importance of socialization	Stress the importance of socializing pets with vaccinated animals. Review diseases that can be transmitted from unvaccinated animals.
Five-Step Plan for Positive Proaction	Obtain or make a video of a pet being trained. Ask the students to identify various techniques mentioned in the Five-Step Plan for Positive Proaction as they occur in the video.
Elicit and reinforce appropriate behavior	
Prevent or minimize inappropriate behavior	
A word about crate training	Emphasize the differences listed in Box 14-5 and discuss the implications for both the pet and owner if owners abide by these misconceptions. Stress that the goal is for the dog to be unconfined in the home when left alone.
Correct size of crate	
How to acclimate the dog to the crate	
How to acclimate the dog to being left alone in the crate	
How and when to make the transition to leaving the dog alone, free in the house	
Warning signs that a dog is not adjusting well to the crate	
Meet the pet's behavioral and developmental needs	Discuss the basic behavioral needs of the dog, cat, horse, and other species as appropriate. Ask the students for ideas regarding ways to meet these needs.
An example of meeting the pet's behavioral needs: elimination	
An example of meeting; the pet's behavioral needs: play Determine individual preferences Use negative punishment (the "take away" method) to discourage inappropriate behavior	
Minimize positive punishment ("discipline") and use it correctly when necessary	
Immediacy	
Consistency	
Appropriate intensity	

Copyright © 2006 by Elsevier, Inc. All rights reserved.

Chapter Outline	Teaching Strategies
Remote punishment is usually preferable to interactive	Show photos of or bring examples of remote punishers to class and discuss how each one works.
Behavior assessments	Review Boxes 14-12 and 14-13. Ask the students to share ideas regarding the importance of each statement/question.
How well the animal meets the criteria for a behaviorally healthy pet	
Family conditions or changes that put pets at risk for surrender	
The pet's daily routine, lifestyle, and whether his behavioral needs are being met	
Identification of early warning signs of problems	
The pet's behavior observed at the veterinary hospital	
Behavior assessment skills	
Interviewing skills: asking good questions	Present questions that might be asked of owners to elicit information about their pet's behavior. Let the students determine if they are appropriately worded? If they are not appropriate, request that they reword the question.
Interview skills: interpersonal communications	
Put clients at ease by sitting down	
Use active listening skills	
Obtain behavioral descriptions, not interpretations	
Using the results of behavior assessments	
Follow-up for behavior assessments	
Making the veterinary clinic a behaviorally friendly place	Stress the importance for all veterinary staff to attend classes, seminars, or other types of continuing education programs on animal behavior. Research local veterinary organizations and their continuing education schedules.
Understanding aggressive behavior	Discuss particular movements and postures that pets exhibit in and out of the clinic and place them into categories listed in the chapter.
Escape, avoidance, or attempts to do so	
Submissive behavior	
Threatening behavior	
Aggressive behavior	
Using puppy and kitten classes to socialize young animals to the veterinary clinic	
Using behavior assessments	
Establish a positive expectation in the waiting area	Without providing names of clinics, ask your students to mention something that establishes a positive expectation in the waiting area of the clinic to which they take their pets. Then ask them to describe something that is negative, if possible. Encourage them to discuss creative ways to improve the negative aspects. Discuss expenses of some changes, space restrictions, and other limitations that can inhibit some types of change.
Manage the environment	
Interactions with staff—greetings	Discuss various ways to greet an animal that is upset.
Interactions with staff—use of treats	Discuss the use of food and toys to calm a patient that is upset.
Fearful or threatening animals	
Unruly dogs	Emphasize the need to ignore undesirable behavior.
Creating a good first impression in the examination room	Remind the students that owners are impressed by the ability of the staff to handle their pets; therefore knowledge of various techniques of approaching unruly pets is essential.
Keeping cats calm	Explain that it often takes longer to calm a cat down enough to be able to perform an exam. This information might help also calm owners down, especially first-time cat owners. Patience is important.

CHAPTER 14 Animal Behavior

Chapter Outline	Teaching Strategies
Removing cats from carriers	
Observe body postures carefully	
Take a preventive (proactive) approach rather than a reactive one	
Create a protocol for handling exercises to be practiced at home	

Dealing with threatening and aggressive animals
  Muzzles
  Gentle leaders
  Cat bags
  Plexiglas shield
  Towels
	Bring each of the following items to class and demonstrate their use on students' pets (except for the Plexiglas shield).

Problem resolution component	Provide examples of cases in which a medical problem was misdiagnosed as a behavioral problem and ask the students what they would have done to prevent this unfortunate situation. Stress the importance of determining if the pet has a medical condition that may be contributing to unwanted behavior.
Dangers of problem solving without adequate preparation	
Owners' frustration	
Technicians' and practice's credibility	
Liability for injuries	
Worsening problem	
Self-assessment	
When to refer	Present common medical conditions that are often incorrectly treated as behavioral problems such as inappropriate use (or none at all) of the litter box.
Type of referral	Compare the role of the behavioral consultant and the obedience trainer. Describe actual case histories and ask the students to categorize them as pets needing behavioral consulting or obedience training. The students will need to ask questions appropriately in order to obtain the information that they need to make the decision.
Evaluating behavioral consultants and dog trainers	
How to make the referral	
Summary	

CRITICAL THINKING CHALLENGES

1. Provide situations in which the Five Step Plan for Positive Proaction can be applied. Ask the students to explain how each step might be applied. Situations might include the foal that bites, the cat that climbs the curtains, the dog that chews table legs, and anything listed in Boxes 14-11 and 14-12.
2. Almost everyone knows someone (or is someone) who has had a pet with behavioral problems. Ask each student to present a pet's behavior problem that they may know from personal experience or second hand. The other students can role-play that they are the veterinary technician, ask behavior assessment questions, and make suggestions for behavior management. If anyone in class has recently acquired a new pet, this conversation can become an ongoing process for the remainder of the semester between the new owner and the rest of the students.
3. Ask the students to contact a local animal behaviorist/consultant and set up an appointment to observe a session. Some animal behaviorist/consultants may not allow this for various reasons. The students can report their experiences to the rest of the class and share information on training techniques. The names of the service and specialist can be kept anonymous.

QUIZ

Circle the appropriate answer for each question. Each statement has only one answer.

1. These animals are typically undersocialized.
   Horses,
   Cats,
   Dogs
2. The ideal time for socialization for horses begins at this age.

Copyright © 2006 by Elsevier, Inc. All rights reserved.

Four weeks,
8 weeks,
Birth

3. The most proactive behavior wellness service one can offer is to educate clients on this topic.
   Pet selection,
   Separation anxiety,
   House soiling

4. Instead of reacting to behavior problems, a behavior wellness program instructs owners how to be more _____ in preventing such problems.
   Tolerant,
   Enthusiastic,
   Proactive

5. These are very powerful tools to use to elicit and reinforce appropriate behavior if used correctly.
   Toys and food,
   Praise and food,
   Toys and praise

6. These stimuli should be presented to pets with a firm, authoritative voice from the beginning of training.
   Aversive,
   Negative,
   Positive

7. This type of punishment is more likely to be immediate and consistent even if the owner is not around at the time of the unwanted behavior.
   Positive,
   Intermittent,
   Remote

8. Doing this during a behavioral assessment interview gives the client an opportunity to provide additional information.
   Stand up,
   Paraphrase the client's description,
   Write down every word

9. Threats can be either offensive or defensive and may overlap with this.
   Acquiescence,
   Submission,
   Aggression

10. These classes are designed specifically to help puppies and kittens become accustomed to the veterinary clinic under enjoyable conditions.
    Socialization,
    Exercise,
    Behavior modification

11. Most cats prefer to have these rubbed than being petted on the head.
    Paws,
    Belly,
    Scent glands

12. It is _____ appropriate to knee a dog who jumps up in the chest.
    Never,
    Always,
    Sometimes

13. Owners can be shown how to place these on their pets before they enter the clinic in order to prevent bites to personnel.
    Plexiglas shields,
    Elizabethan collars,
    Muzzles

14. Technicians can be helpful with problem behavior resolution by:
    Never attempting to help with these situations
    Referring the owners to another veterinarian
    Knowing the correct questions to ask and discussing the case with the veterinarian

Answers: (1) cats, (2) birth, (3) pet selection, (4) proactive, (5) toys and food, (6) aversive, (7) remote, (8) paraphrasing, (9) aggression, (10) socialization, (11) scent glands, (12) never, (13) muzzles or gentle leaders, (14) knowing the correct questions to ask and discussing the case with the veterinarian. ■

15

Companion Animal Clinical Nutrition

TEACHING/LEARNING OBJECTIVES

1. Define ATP and explain its role in energy production.
2. List three energy-producing nutrients and three non–energy-producing nutrients and explain the major difference between the two groups.
3. Describe the appropriate placement of the caged bird's water bowl.
4. Describe the optimum diet for the pet rabbit, the show rabbit, and the production rabbit. Include what to look for on the food label and the appropriate time of day to feed.
5. Explain the necessity of offering a variety of food types to birds.
6. Describe the hazards of feeding diets high in sunflower seeds to gerbils.
7. Explain why stale food should be removed from hamsters' cages.
8. List potential sequelae of decreased fiber in the chinchilla's diet.
9. Name the most common nutritional deficiency in captive turtles, its clinical signs, and how to prevent it.
10. Explain why weight loss and inappetence may be inadvertently overlooked in snakes.
11. Compare the diet of most captive lizards with the diet of the green iguana.
12. Give examples of animals that have higher energy needs.
13. Define fiber and list its functions.
14. Name the fat-soluble and water-soluble vitamins and the major differences between these two groups.
15. Explain the relationship between digestibility and nutritional value.
16. List the functions of water in the body.
17. Describe ways in which excesses of macrominerals can occur and the possible effects on health of each.
18. Define antioxidants and name the vitamins that are called antioxidants.
19. List qualities of a food that pertain to palatability.
20. Compare moisture contents of dry, semi-moist, and moist pet foods.
21. List the benefits of dry food over moist food.
22. Be able to determine if a home-made diet meets a healthy animal's needs using the diet analysis described in the chapter.
23. List components of a nutritional assessment.
24. Explain the differences in diets for small-, medium- to large-, and giant-breed dogs.
25. Describe the changes in food intake in the lactating bitch and include when they begin and end.
26. Outline a program for safely terminating lactation in order to wean puppies.
27. List six reasons for obesity in the small animal.
28. Give reasons for weight loss in the geriatric patient.
29. Name one cause of feline hepatic lipidosis.
30. List patients in whom urinary-acidifying diets are contraindicated and explain why.
31. List indications for clinical nutritional support in small animals.
32. List the various types of enteral feeding tubes and indications for each.
33. Describe clinical signs that might indicate an enteral tube is not positioned properly.
34. Calculate the IER of patients with sepsis and head trauma.
35. Explain why all-seed diets and supplementation of all-seed diets with fruits and vegetables are not recommended as the sole source(s) of nutrition for pet birds.

KEY TERMS

AAFCO Animal Feeding Test statement
Absorptive capability
Active transport
Additives
Adenosine triphosphate (ATP)
Alginates
All-purpose foods
Amino acid
Amino acid composition
Amino group

PART THREE PATIENT MANAGEMENT AND NUTRITION

Anion
Anorexia
Antagonistic interaction
Antioxidant
Arachidonic acid
Assimilation
Atelectasis
Availability
Bacterial translocation
Balanced diet
Biologic quality
Biologic value
Body condition score
Body condition scoring
Cachexia
Carbohydrate
Carboxyl group
Carnivore
Catabolize
Cation
Cellulose
Chelonian
Cholecalciferol
Cognitive dysfunction
Colostrum
Complementary diet
Complete diet
Complex sugar polymer
Coprophagia
Crude protein
Daily energy requirement
Dietary fats
Diurnal
Dystrophic calcification
Electrolyte
Energy-producing nutrient
Essential amino acid
Essential fatty acids
Extrusion
Fats
Fat-soluble vitamin
Fatty acids
Fermentation
Fiber
Formula
Generic food
Gizzard
Gluconeogenesis
Glycogen
Granivore
Grocery brands
Gum
Hemoglobin
Herbivore
Hindgut fermenter
Hip dysplasia

Humectant
Hydrolysis
Hypermetabolic state
Hyperosmotic solution
Hyperplasia
Hypoalbuminemia
Illness energy requirement (IER)
Illness factor
Ingredient
Inorganic
Insoluble fiber
Insoluble mineral grit
Lignins
Lipids
Long-chain fatty acid
Medium-chain fatty acid
Megaesophagus
Metabolic body weight
Monogastric
Monosaccharide
Monosaturated fatty acids
Mucilage
Myoglobin
Non–energy-producing nutrient
Nonessential amino acid
Nonessential fatty acids
Nothing by mouth; non per os (NPO)
Nutrient
Nutrient profile
Nutritional adequacy statement
Nutritional secondary hyperparathyroidism
Oils
Omnivore
Organic
Osteochondritis
Osteochondrosis
Palatability
Panosteitis
Pansteatitis
Parenteral nutrition
Partial parenteral nutrition (PPN)
Passerine
Passive absorption
Pectin
Peptide bond
Phlebitis
Polysaccharide
Polysaturated fatty acids
Preservatives
Production energy requirements
Protein
Protein digestibility
Protein-energy malnutrition (PEM)
Psittacine
Resting energy requirement (RER)
Saturated fatty acids

Copyright © 2006 by Elsevier, Inc. All rights reserved.

Short-chain fatty acid
Simple sugars
Soluble fiber
Soluble mineral grit
Special-purpose foods
Specialty brand food
Starch
Subjective global assessment (SGA)
Substrate
Sugar
Synergistic interaction

Taurine
Total parenteral nutrition (TPN)
Trace element
Triglycerides
True cost of feeding
Urea
Urinary lithiasis
Volume-restricted meal feeding
Water-soluble vitamin
Wobbler's syndrome
Yellow fat disease

Chapter Outline	Teaching Strategies
Overview of nutritional objectives and principles	Discuss major differences between nutritional goals for companion animals versus nutritional goals for food animals.
Energy-producing nutrients	Review basic biochemistry. Show chemical structures of various carbohydrates, proteins, and fatty acids. Discuss the functions of each energy-producing nutrient. Show the chemical structure of ATP and point out the source of energy release. Illustrate the pathways of the intake, utilization, and storage of carbohydrates, fats, and protein. Compare clinical signs seen with deficiencies of each one.
Lipids and fatty acids	Emphasize the dietary need for essential fatty acids.
Amino acids and proteins	Stress the cat's need for taurine.
Protein requirements	Bring pet food labels to class and discuss the concept of crude protein and the problem with quality versus amount (number).
Non–energy-producing nutrients	
Water	Show several chemical reactions in the body that utilize or produce water.
Minerals	
Macrominerals	Show pictures or radiographs of each disease state mentioned.
Microminerals	Emphasize that iron is the micromineral that is found in erythrocytes and can be related to anemia.
Vitamins	Present information on diseases caused by excesses and deficiencies of different vitamins.
Nutrient terms	Ask the students to categorize items on pet food labels as humectants, preservatives, or additives and to infer the function of each. They may need to do research for this activity.
Pet food evaluation	Warn students that foods labeled as all-purpose may be harmful to some pets.
Nutrient content and forms of pet food	Ask the students to perform a cost of feeding analysis for several different animals.
Home-prepared diets	Bring in several recipes for homemade diets and assess them with the class. Discuss potential clinical signs or abnormal laboratory values that might manifest after being on this diet for a while. Contact veterinary nutritionists to see if they would provide input on homemade animal diets in the form of case histories.
Home-prepared diet analysis	
Pet food labels	
Evaluating pet food labels	Contact several food manufacturers and request data on actual analyses of different types of their food. Compare these data with the labels from the products sold in the store or veterinary clinic.
Ingredient percentages	Stress that there is no substitute for patient assessment and feeding performance analysis when trying to determine the quality of a pet food.
Market categories	Review differences amongst grocery, generic, and specialty brand foods.
Companion animal nutrition	
Energy requirements	Review body condition scoring. Practice scoring students' pets if they are brought to class for other activities.
Nutritional assessment	Discuss each component of the nutritional assessment.
Feeding normal dogs	

Chapter Outline	Teaching Strategies
Canine pediatric nutrition	Discuss the role of colostrum in pediatric nutrition, ways to determine if animals are receiving adequate amounts, and the normal growth rate for puppies. Discuss the importance of peak lactation, how to wean puppies, and the importance of not overfeeding during the growing months.
Feeding orphan puppies	
Weaning puppies	
Feeding growing dogs	
Growing concerns for large-breed dogs	Show photos of animals with osteochondritis and hip dysplasia and explain how these diseases relate to nutrition.
Feeding adult dogs	
Feeding adult dogs with increased energy needs	Review insulin function and glucose production, storage, and utilization. Discuss appropriate regimens of carbohydrate and fat intake for working dogs and how to determine if they are appropriate.
Feeding during pregnancy and lactation	
Feeding methods during weaning	
Obesity-prone animals	Discuss ways that technicians can educate owners about the importance of weight control. Ask the students to make an educational poster. Divide the students into groups and ask each group to contribute a separate part of the poster. Parts might include prevention, causes of obesity, diseases related to obesity, dietary recommendations, and feeding through the life stages. Review the pathogenesis of obesity-related diseases such as diabetes mellitus and hepatic lipidosis.
Definition, causes, and health risks of obesity	
Health risks of obesity	
Diagnosis and treatment of obesity	
Feeding the geriatric animal	Burkholder (1999) states that the dietary practices in the first three fourths of an animal's life can affect the nutritional consequences manifested in the last part of its life. Discuss the implications of this statement for veterinary patients and personnel.
Renal disease	Review renal anatomy and physiology and discuss functional changes that occur as animals age.
Feeding cats	List the essential nutrients for cats and discuss clinical signs/disease that result if each is deficient. Explain what foods contain these nutrients for the owner who insists on feeding a homemade diet.
Feline pediatrics	Compare kitten and puppy nutritional requirements.
Adult cats	
Feeding cats in gestation and lactation	Compare nutritional requirements and behavior in the bitch and queen.
Feeding geriatric cats	Stress the importance of oral hygiene in the geriatric pet.
Feline obesity	
Feline urolithiasis and lower urinary tract disease	Review the anatomy and physiology or the lower urinary tract. Discuss factors that contribute to struvite and calcium oxalate crystalluria in cats.
Clinical nutrition	
Nutritional assessment of the hospitalized patient	Discuss the technician's role in performing a continuous nutritional assessment.
Patients at risk for malnutrition	Review physiologic processes that can lead to malnutrition in pediatric, sick, geriatric, or healthy boarding pets.
Feeding hospitalized small animal patients	
Patient selection for assisted feeding	Point out reasons to use enteral feeding tubes. Show photos and/or bring various types of tubes to class.
Routes of feeding	Review anatomy of the gastrointestinal tract and emphasize the placement of each type of enteral tube. Compare advantages and disadvantages of tubes placed for short-term use and those placed for long-term use.
Enteral vs. parenteral	
Tube selection	
Feeding schedules and enteral administration techniques	Discuss enteral tube maintenance techniques. Emphasize the role of water in both nutrition and maintenance.

CHAPTER 15 Companion Animal Clinical Nutrition

Chapter Outline	Teaching Strategies
Food selection	
Calculating nutrient requirements and food selection	Practice calculating RERs and IERs of various patients (either actual or hypothetical patients). Provide labels of different foods and ask the students to determine the amount of food required of each patient and how it might be administered.
Parenteral nutrition	Differentiate between total and partial parenteral nutrition. Review indications for parenteral nutrition. Stress the concept of combining enteral and parenteral nutrition.
Nutritional considerations for the critical patient	Discuss protein utilization in the critically ill patient. Discuss the effects of hypoproteinemia on muscles of respiration and the kidneys.
Case example in small animal nutrition	Review the anatomy and physiology of the pancreas. Point out potential causes of EPI. Discuss reasons for each of the five recommended dietary changes listed in the chapter for the patient with EPI.
Discussion	
Nutrition of small and exotic pets	
Feeding pet birds	Stress the importance of client education. Review the deficiencies of all-seed diets, fruits and vegetables, and homemade diets.
Rabbits	Point out that rabbits have very specific dietary requirements that can be met by commercial pellets supplemented with hay. Explain coprophagia in the rabbit and guinea pig. Discuss the effects on the rabbit and guinea pig's feeding schedule of being nocturnal.
Guinea pigs	Discuss the daily vitamin C requirement of guinea pigs and the need to provide fresh pellets made exclusively for guinea pigs.
Hamsters	Show photos of malocclusions in rabbits, hamsters, and gerbils and review the importance of offering hard food to control this problem.
Gerbils	Emphasize the need to avoid feeding sunflower seeds to gerbils to prevent weight gain.
Rats and mice	
Chinchillas	Outline the mechanism of hindgut fermentation and the ability to easily upset it with diets too low in fiber.
Ferrets	Point out that ferrets' nutritional needs can be met with a high-quality cat food or pelleted commercial ferret diets.
Feeding captive reptiles	
Chelonians	Stress the need to offer a variety of foods and plenty of sunshine. Review the clinical signs of hypovitaminosis A.
Snakes	Review the size requirements for prey and the need to alter the temperature of the environment according to the amount of food digested.
Lizards	Point out that iguanas can be fed alfalfa rabbit pellets and dog food. Lizards need a variety of food and a reptile vitamin 1 to 2 times weekly.
Amphibians	Stress the need to simulate the natural environment as closely as possible and offering live food whenever possible.
Equine nutrition	
Nutrients for horses	Review the basic nutrients required by horses. Show photos demonstrating founder and colic and discuss nutritional causes. Show photos of good-quality grass and legume hay and compare them to poor-quality forage so that the students have an basis for future comparison.
Feeding sick horses	
Assessing forages and grains for horses	

CRITICAL THINKING CHALLENGES

1. Present case histories in which it would be beneficial for the owner to switch to another type of food for the pet. Discuss which type of food would be better and why. Provide the label from the type of food that the owner is currently offering as well as the label from the recommended food. Ask the students to convince the owner that the change is for the best. The students can role-play.

2. Bring in labels from various pet foods. Ask the students to determine if the food is adequate for animals in various states such as lactation, growing giant-breed dog, cat with congestive heart failure, and the geriatric animal by comparing the label with the nutrient guidelines in the chapter.

3. Present situations in which an owner is concerned about a pet with an eating problem. The pet may be over- or underweight, a competitive eater with other pets at home an extremely finicky bird, or a rabbit

Copyright © 2006 by Elsevier, Inc. All rights reserved.

with a decreased appetite and milky-white urine. Ask the students to write down key questions to ask to elicit information needed to make helpful suggestions. Then the students can provide suggestions.

QUIZ

1. Respond to each statement below by placing one letter of the answer on each line. The letters in the boxes spell the answer to the Super Clue.
2. A deficiency of this essential amino acid in the cat can lead to impaired immune function and retinal degeneration.
3. This weight problem in dogs and cats is a growing concern and challenge for the veterinary technician.
4. Carbohydrates may be stored as this molecule.
5. This molecule carries oxygen in muscle cells.
6. With this method of feeding dogs, the pet is fed for 5 to 15 minutes one to three times daily.
7. This is the best type of pellet to feed rabbits.
8. This is defined as the amount of energy needed to raise the temperature of 1 kilogram of water 1° C.
9. Increased amounts of this mineral in the feline diet may contribute to the development of FLUTD.
10. In the United States, methionine and this amino acid are often absent in the pet bird's diet.
11. This oral disorder can be prevented in some small animals by feeding hard foods that promote gnawing and chewing.
12. A deficiency of this mineral may lead to hypothyroidism.

Super Clue: This non–energy-producing nutrient is essential in the guinea pig's diet.

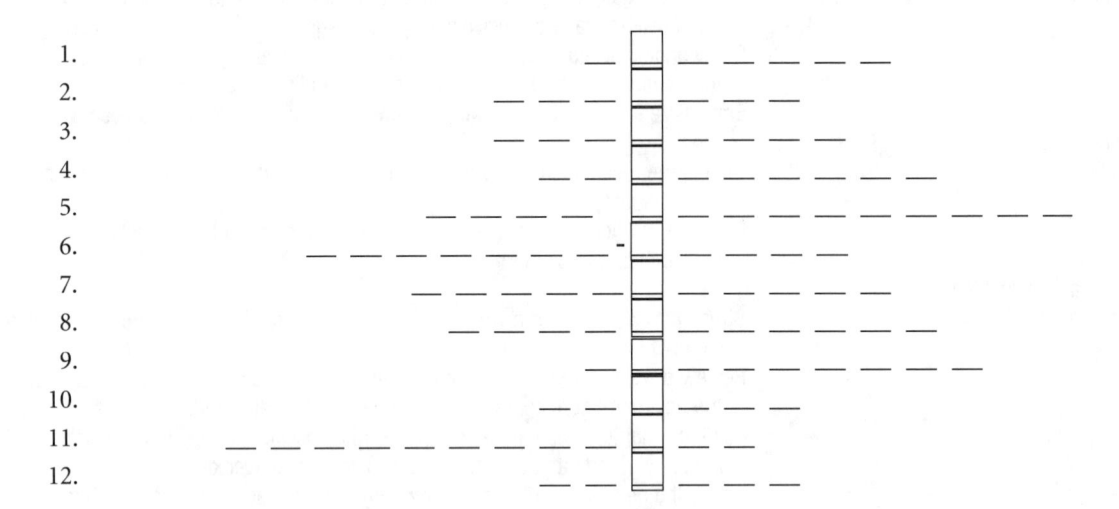

Answers: (1) taurine, (2) obesity, (3) glycogen, (4) myoglobin, (5) time-restricted, (6) alfalfa-based, (7) arachidonic acid, (8) kilocalorie, (9) magnesium, (10) lycine, (11) malocclusion, (12) iodine. Super Clue: ascorbic acid. ■

16

Concepts in Livestock Nutrition

TEACHING/LEARNING OBJECTIVES

1. Define and list maintenance nutrient requirements.
2. Define biologic value and protein efficiency ratio.
3. Describe the fate of protein after it is ingested by ruminants.
4. List the functions of fats and compare their energy content with protein and carbohydrates.
5. Name two ways that carbohydrates are broken down into simple sugars in the ruminant.
6. List three ways that the body obtains water.
7. Compare the total mixed ration feeding program with the forage and grain fed separately diet.
8. Explain why lactating dairy cattle need both concentrate and forage.
9. List vitamins that must be supplemented in the diet of ruminants.
10. Describe the feeding requirements of dairy calves from birth to weaning.
11. Explain when weight gain is preferred in order to increase conception rates.
12. Explain the goal of the finishing feeding program.
13. Explain the feeding requirements of ewes during gestation and the results if these requirements are not met.
14. Define enterotoxemia in lambs and how it can be treated/prevented.
15. List ways to prevent iron-deficiency anemia in pigs.

KEY TERMS

Arachidonic acid
Biologic value
Bovine spongiform encephalopathy (BSE)
Calf starter
Cecum
Cellulose
Concentrates
Creep feeding
Deamination
Digestible energy (DE)
Digestion
Enterotoxemia
Essential amino acid
Essential fatty acids
Feeding standards
Finisher lamb
Finishing cattle
Forages
Founder
Fructose
Glucose
Gross energy (GE)
Grower lamb
Growing-finishing pigs
Hemicellulose
Homeostasis
Ketosis
Lambing paralysis
Linoleic acid
Linolenic acid
Macrominerals
Maintenance nutrient requirements (MNR)
Metabolizable energy (ME)
Microminerals
Milk replacer
Net energy (NE)
Nonessential amino acids
Nonessential fatty acids
Nonprotein nitrogen source
Peptides
Protein efficiency ratio
Roughage
Rumen
Rumen acidosis
Silage
Simple sugars
Starch
Starter pigs
Stored carbohydrates
Structural carbohydrates
Sucrose
Total digestible nutrients (TDN)

Chapter Outline	Teaching Strategies
Nutrients	Compare feeding standards from the National Research Council for different livestock.
Protein	Review the chemical structure of proteins. Discuss factors that compromise protein quality.
Protein use by ruminants	Using diagrams, show the pathway and process of digestion through the ruminant gastrointestinal tract.
Fats	Review the chemical structure of fatty acids, their synthesis, and the pathway to the production of arachidonic, linoleic, and linolenic acid.
Carbohydrates	Point out the differences between concentrates and forages.
Feedstuff energy	Compare TDN, GE, DE, ME, and NE and discuss the usefulness of each one.
Minerals and vitamins	
Water	Explain the effect of water deprivation on different organ systems. Stress the importance of hydration maintenance.
Dairy cattle	Discuss the nutritional needs of dairy cattle and show costs.
Energy	
Protein	Discuss BSE and the impact that it has had on the beef and dairy industry worldwide.
Minerals and vitamins	Review water-soluble and fat-soluble vitamins, their sources, ability to be stored in the body, and the rumen's ability to synthesize them.
Dairy calves	Review the nutritional needs of dairy calves. Give examples of typical milk replacers and calf starters.
Beef cattle	Discuss the nutritional needs of beef cattle and show costs. Compare this information with dairy cattle.
Cow-calf production	Compare the energy, protein, and mineral and vitamin requirements of the breeding herd and finishing cattle.
Breeding herd	Point out the ideal time for a cow to gain weight.
Energy	Review relative costs of high-quality forage, protein, grains, and fats. Explain why energy and protein requirements of cows can usually be met with reasonable expense.
Protein	
Minerals and vitamins	Emphasize the utility of salt blocks to meet some mineral requirements.
Calves	Describe the concept of creep feeding and its advantages.
Finishing cattle	Review the goal of the finishing feeding program.
Energy	Discuss rumen acidosis, founder, and liver abscesses. Explain the disease processes and show photos of animals with these diseases, gross anatomy of an affected organ, and histopathologic images.
Protein	Compare the use of a natural protein source with the use of urea in terms of cost, sources, and performance.
Minerals and vitamins	Discuss ways in which vitamin and mineral requirements of finishing cattle are often met.
Sheep	Review the three most important qualities of feeds that sheep producers want.
Breeding flock	
Energy	Discuss the effects of feeding forages with decreased grain content during the last trimester of pregnancy.
Protein	
Minerals and vitamins	Emphasize the need to carefully monitor copper intake.
Lambs	Stress the importance of colostrum ingestion within the first hour after birth.
Swine	Gather information about historical methods of raising pigs. Compare these methods with current practices in the areas of cost to feed, type of feed, living conditions, and profits. Discuss reasons why changes occurred. Talk about the changes in percentages of nutrients as they relate to the life cycle of the pig.
Breeding herd	Discuss reasons why feed is limited after breeding and during the first two thirds of gestation.
Energy	Describe how methods of feeding lactating sows must be in line with the producer's goal of encouraging as much energy intake as possible.
Protein	Discuss the role of protein in supporting lactation and the effects of inadequate protein intake during this time.
Minerals and vitamins	The ratio of calcium and phosphorus must be carefully maintained throughout the pig's life. Ask the students to give this ratio and describe complications of an upset of this balance.

CHAPTER 16 Concepts in Livestock Nutrition

Chapter Outline	Teaching Strategies
Starter pigs	Explain why feed for starter pigs is expensive.
Growing-finishing pigs	Swine raised today are leaner than in the past. Discuss this fact as it relates to energy and protein composition of feeds.
Energy	
Protein	Compare different sources of protein and their costs.
Minerals and vitamins	

CRITICAL THINKING CHALLENGES

1. Present scenarios in which performance of a herd or certain population within a herd is suffering. Ask the students to list potential causes (in terms of feed).
2. A dairy cattle rancher is considering starting up a small sheep operation. He believes that since he already knows the cattle business, raising sheep will be simple. Ask the students to explain to the person described here the differences between raising dairy cattle and sheep in terms of feeding and cost.
3. Neonatal animals have specific nutritional requirements. The previous chapter addresses this fact in dogs, cats, and horses. The veterinary technician must be ready to meet the challenge of caring for all of these animals. Divide the class into several groups. Give each group a case scenario concerning a neonate. Ask each group to write down a detailed description of how they would meet the animal's nutritional requirements and to share this information with the rest of the class. The rest of the class must determine if each group's treatment is appropriate.
4. Vitamins and minerals should be supplemented during all stages of the pig's life. Ask the students to research the water-soluble and fat-soluble vitamins as well as the minerals calcium, phosphorus, salt, zinc, iron, copper, iodine, selenium, and manganese to determine sources of these for livestock. If time allows, ask them to find out how a deficiency of each vitamin and mineral affects the animal. They can make a chart to be kept in the classroom for reference.

QUIZ

Circle T (true) or F (false) for each statement.

1. T F Finishing cattle fed high levels of grain are more likely to develop digestive problems.
2. T F A mature animal's body is approximately 65% to 85% water.
3. T F There is no minimum or maximum requirement for carbohydrates in livestock feed.
4. T F Fat intake in excess of 5% to 6% in lactating cows can decrease fiber utilization for energy production.
5. T F Lambs can be successfully weaned from their mother after 1 day of age.
6. T F Freezing colostrum for dairy calves destroys immunoglobulins and is not recommended.
7. T F The percentage of true absorbed protein that is available for productive body functions is known as the protein efficiency ratio.
8. T F Proteins are degraded by microbes in the rumen and ammonia, organic acids, and carbon dioxide are released.
9. T F Methionine is the most limiting amino acid for the maturation of wool.
10. T F Feeding determines productivity of lactating dairy cows more than any other factor.
11. T F Protein toxicity may develop in cattle fed a diet consisting of more than 40% protein or nonprotein nitrogen.
12. T F Nonessential amino acids must be supplied in the diet.
13. T F The precursor for vitamin A is thiamin.
14. T F The cow's milk is deficient in iron and calves quickly develop iron-deficient anemia soon after starting to nurse if iron is not supplemented somehow.
15. T F Sheep develop toxicity symptoms to sodium more rapidly than other livestock.

Answers: (1) T, (2) F, (3) T, (4) T, (5) T, (6) F, (7) F, (8) T, (9) T, (10) T, (11) T, (12) F, (13) F, (14) F, (15) F. ■

17

Animal Reproduction

TEACHING/LEARNING OBJECTIVES

1. Describe the stages of parturition in the bitch.
2. Explain the role of GnRH, FSH, LH, progesterone, prostaglandins, cortisol, and corticotropin-releasing hormones in the estrous cycle and pregnancy.
3. Describe the procedure to obtain a canine vaginal cytology sample.
4. Explain the relationship (in days) of the LH surge to ovulation, oocyte maturity, and peak fertility.
5. List four ways to diagnose pregnancy in the bitch.
6. Define pyometra and discuss treatment options.
7. Discuss problems with diagnosing *Brucella canis*.
8. List three possible outcomes of estrus in the queen.
9. Explain how GnRH and HCG are used to control estrus in the queen.
10. Name two sources of estrogen in the queen following ovariohysterectomy.
11. Explain when breeding soundness exams are usually performed in the mare.
12. Explain why it is imperative to perform a cytologic examination in conjunction with a vaginal culture in the mare.
13. Describe three tests used to diagnose pregnancy in the mare.
14. List electrolyte characteristics that must exist before inducing parturition in the mare.
15. Explain the implication of red bag in the mare giving birth.
16. Name a common use of prostaglandin $F_{2\alpha}$ in the mare.
17. Compare the causes and treatment of uterine and vaginal prolapse in cows.
18. List ways to induce puberty in gilts.
19. Name two factors that can initiate estrous cycles in sheep and goats.
20. List four potential periparturient problems in sheep and goats and ways to prevent/treat them.
21. Define polled intersex and explain how this condition can be avoided.
22. Explain the procedure to analyze sperm.
23. Compare ways that semen is collected from different species for analysis.

KEY TERMS

Accessory sex glands
Adrenal gland
Agalactia
Allantois
Altrenogest
Ampullae
Anestrus
Antrum
Aplastic anemia
Arachidonic acid
Artificial insemination
Ballottement
Boar
Broad ligament
Bromocriptine
Bulbourethral gland
Cabergoline
Capacitation
Caruncle
Cesarean section
Chorioallantois
Chorion
Cloprostenol
Cloudburst
Conceptus
Cornified epithelial cells
Corpus hemorrhagicum (CH)
Corpus luteum
Cortisol
Cotyledons
Cria
Cryptorchid animal
Dexamethasone
Diestrus
Doe
Domperidone
Ductus deferens
Dystocia
Eclampsia
Electroejaculator

CHAPTER 17 Animal Reproduction

Embryo
Embryonic disk
Endometrial cysts
Endometrial folds
Epididymis
Equine chorionic gonadotropin (eCG)
Ergovine
Estradiol cypionate (ECP)
Estrogen
Estrone sulfate
Estrous cycle
Estrus
Ewe
Farrowing
Fertilization
Fescue toxicosis
Fetus
Follicle-stimulating hormone (FSH)
Gamete
Genital tubercle
Gilt
Gonadotropin-releasing hormone (GnRH)
Granulosa cell layer
Guanaco
Hematoma
Hemospermia
Hermaphrodite
Heterospermic insemination
Hydrometra
Hypogalactia
Hypophyseal-portal vessels
Induced ovulator
Infundibulum
Inhibin
Interestrus
Interstitial cells
Isthmus
Karyotype
Luteinizing hormone (LH)
LH surge
Lordosis
Mastitis
Megestrol acetate
Melatonin
Metestrus
Metritis
Mibolerone
Milk fever
Müllerian tubular system
Oocyte
Ovarian follicles
Ovariohysterectomy
Oviduct

Ovulation
Oxytocin
Paraphimosis
Pineal gland
Pituitary
Placenta
Placentomas
Polled intersex
Pregnancy toxemia
Pregnant mare serum gonadotropin (PMSG)
Primary uterine inertia
Proestrus
Progesterone
Prostaglandin $F_{2\alpha}$ ($PF_{2\alpha}$)
Prostate gland
Pseudopregnancy
Puberty
Pyknotic nucleus
Pyometra
Queening
Red bag
Relaxin
Ringwomb
Scrotum
Seasonally polyestrous
Semen
Sertoli cells
Sperm cell
Spermiogram
Standing heat
Subinvolution of placental sites (SIPS)
Tease out
Teasing in
Testis
Testosterone
Thecal cell layer
Transimeter
Transition period
Urospermia
Uterine artery
Uterine infusion
Uterine involution
Uterine tube
Vas deferens
Vesicular gland
Vestibule
Vicuna
Whelping
Winking
Wolffian tubular system
Yellow body
Yolk sac

PART THREE PATIENT MANAGEMENT AND NUTRITION

Chapter Outline	Teaching Strategies
General female reproduction	Review Figure 17-1. Ask the students to create timelines for each species that begin with GnRH release from the hypothalamus to pregnancy or the decline in progesterone if pregnancy does not occur.
The estrous cycle	Show photos of vaginal cytology and point out pyknotic nuclei and cornification.
Canine reproduction	
Vaginal cultures	Compare the reliability and cost of vaginal cytology to in-house kits that measure progesterone levels in order to determine insemination or breeding time.
Pregnancy diagnosis	Discuss the difference in gestation lengths depending on whether it is timed from breeding or day 1 of diestrus.
Parturition and dystocia	Review causes of dystocia. Show radiographs as examples.
Postpartum problems	Describe how ergonovine works. Discuss eclampsia and how it is treated.
Pseudopregnancy	Show radiographs of animals with pyometra and compare them to normal abdominal films in which the uterus cannot be visualized. Discuss the life-threatening nature of this disease.
Mismating	Review options for termination of pregnancy in the bitch. Compare side effects, cost, and time requirements.
Brucellosis	Discuss the modes of transmission, difficulty of diagnosis and treatment, and clinical signs associated with *Brucella canis*. Emphasize that this is a zoonotic and reportable disease.
Feline reproduction	
Seasonality	Discuss the implications of queens living in artificial light all year round as they relate to ovulation.
Estrous cycle	Review the three possible outcomes after estrus for the queen: ovulation and pregnancy, ovulation without pregnancy, and no ovulation.
Common reproductive problems	Review signs of dystocia and events related to parturition that warrant treatment from a veterinarian.
Equine reproduction	Explain how lighting is used to control to pregnancy in the mare; explain how pregnancy is diagnosed in the mare. Show ultrasound images.
Breeding soundness examination	Discuss reasons for conducting the breeding soundness exam. Show results from actual cases, including cytology photos and culture results. Ask the students to determine the soundness of each animal.
Breeding management	Discuss the timing of artificial insemination, the use of ultrasonography to assess the uterus after insemination or breeding, the methods used to stimulate uterine clearance, and intrauterine infusion and lavage.
Artificial insemination (uterine infusion)	
Post-breeding treatments	
Pregnancy	
Diagnosis	Review hormonal tests. Show ultrasound photos of equine fetuses.
Vaccinations	Emphasize the importance of vaccinations during pregnancy.
Induction of parturition	Discuss reasons for inducing parturition in the mare and criteria that should be met.
Parturition	
Postpartum problems	Discuss methods of handling the mare with a retained placenta, prolapsed uterus, postpartum hemorrhage, and postpartum metritis.
Hormone use in mares	
Prostaglandin	Emphasize that this hormone must not be used to induce parturition.
Human chorionic gonadotropin	Stress that some mares fail to ovulate after repeated injections.
Deslorelin	List advantages of deslorelin over HCG.
Progestins	Explain how progestins are used to control the estrous cycle.
Oxytocin	Review the two common uses of oxytocin: induction of parturition and uterine clearance.
Domperidone	Discuss fescue toxicosis and the use of domperidone.
Bovine reproduction	Compare the seasonality of the horse and cow. Discuss the metestrus period.
Pregnancy diagnosis	Stress the lack of reliability when using progesterone to diagnose pregnancy.
Breeding/artificial Insemination	Review the importance of synchronization of estrus in cattle and current methods.

CHAPTER 17 Animal Reproduction

Chapter Outline	Teaching Strategies
Abnormalities of the estrous cycle	
Anestrus	Compare treatments of pyometra in the cow and bitch. Compare luteal and follicular cysts and their treatments.
Abnormalities of Pregnancy	
Uterine prolapse	Show photos of uterine and vaginal prolapses. Discuss the implications of each in terms of treatment, causes, and further breeding.
Vaginal prolapse	
Dystocia	
Milk fever	Compare eclampsia in bitches and milk fever in cows.
Swine reproduction	
Puberty	Review methods of inducing puberty in gilts and factors that affect success.
Estrous cycle	
Pregnancy	Discuss the importance of the anatomic shape of the penis and cervix. Stress that at least four embryos must be present in the uterus to cause maternal recognition of pregnancy.
Control of farrowing	
Pharmacologic control of the estrous cycle	
Artificial insemination	Compare artificial insemination and natural mating success rates.
Pregnancy diagnosis	Point out that real-time ultrasound can be used to diagnose pregnancy as early as 20 days 90% of the time.
Postpartum complications and diseases	Since these problems are rare in pigs, emphasize that sows must still be observed closely during and after parturition because, although not common, some problems so still occur.
Ovine and caprine reproduction	
Seasonality	Compare the seasonality of sheep and goats with that of cats.
Estrous cycle	
Breeding management	Discuss different means of insemination.
Pregnancy	Compare the effects of prostaglandin administration in ewes and does during pregnancy. Point out that twinning is common in both species.
Ram/buck effect	Emphasize that a major way to induce cyclicity in ewe and does is with male pheromones.
Pharmacologic control of the estrous cycle	Discuss the use of the hormone-impregnated sponge to synchronize estrus.
Pregnancy diagnosis	Compare the cost-effectiveness of the three methods of determining pregnancy: ballottement, returning to estrus, and ultrasonography.
Periparturient problems	Compare the presentation of a bitch with eclampsia and a ewe or goat with hypocalcemia. Discuss ways to prevent pregnancy toxemia.
Infertility	Discuss the polled intersex phenomenon and how to prevent it.
Camelid reproduction	
Estrous cycles	Discuss the use of HCG to induce ovulation and $PF_{2\alpha}$ to induce parturition. Emphasize that about 90% of crias are born between 7:00 AM and 1:00 PM.
General male reproduction	Review anatomy of the male reproductive system and the pathway from its production to ejaculation. Define cryptorchidism. Discuss the feedback mechanism of testosterone production and the role of FSH, GnRH, and inhibin in maintaining a steady production of sperm cells.
Clinical examination of the male	
Semen analysis	Show photos or films of semen analysis from several different species. Review the anatomy of a healthy sperm cell. Discuss possible normal and abnormal findings of motility, morphology, and concentration.
Bull, ram, and buck	Compare collection methods, common problems with collection, and common reproductive disorders in the following species: stallion, canine, tom, boar, and camelid.
Stallion	
Canine	
Tom	
Boar	
Camelid	

Copyright © 2006 by Elsevier, Inc. All rights reserved.

ACTIVITIES

Provide potential, real-life situations and ask the student to fill in the blanks.

EXAMPLE

A client calls your clinic and is concerned because he found a stray Beagle who is pregnant. Her belly is "big, lumpy, and moves." He has never been present for the birth of puppies and is nervous. He wants to know what to expect. His first question is "How do I know when she will give birth? I may be at work and not be able to help her."

Please fill in the blanks in the conversation below.

Technician: It is great that you want to help your dog so that you can provide the best care possible. When a dog gives birth it is called (*whelping*). The average length of gestation for dogs is (*approximately 57 to 65 days*). Your dog is obviously near the end of her pregnancy.

Client: So, when will she give birth?!!!

Technician: It's difficult to determine the exact whelping date without knowing when she became pregnant; however, there are signs to watch for that will narrow it down. For approximately (*6 to 36 hours*) before whelping your pet may exhibit....

CRITICAL THINKING CHALLENGES

1. Ask students to contact food animal veterinarians in the area and find out the methods of estrous synchronization that they currently use. If the veterinarian is willing, they can discuss advantages and disadvantages of various techniques. Students can present their findings to the class.
2. Students can contact breeders of different species in their area and set up an appointment to visit them to discuss methods that they use, for example, to induce ovulation in cats and rabbits. If possible, they can discuss success rates. Ask the students to present their findings to the class. Zoo veterinarians can be contacted as well.
3. Prepare copies of Figures 17-9, 17-18, and 17-27, and remove labels or days across the bottom of the graph, or both. Ask the students to fill in the blanks. Ask students to create similar charts for feline and swine estrus cycles.
4. Cattle ranchers and owners of commercial swine units are interested in producing as many healthy offspring as possible in the shortest time span possible without risking the health of the offspring, cow, or sow. Ask the students to explain to these owners how this can be accomplished. They can discuss environmental and pharmacologic factors.

QUIZ

Choose the correct answer for each statement from the list below. Only one answer is correct for each statement.

1. In most species, the _____ produces the progesterone that maintains pregnancy.
2. _____ is the period of the estrous cycle after the death of the corpus luteum when follicles are growing.
3. During stage III of parturition, the _____ is expelled.
4. During _____, vaginal epithelial cells are fully cornified.
5. In the canine, the LH peak occurs approximately _____ days before day 1 of diestrus, and ovulation occurs approximately _____ days before day 1 of diestrus.
6. Radiography can be used to diagnose pregnancy in the bitch beginning on day _____ post-D1.
7. No more than _____ hours should elapse between the delivery of each puppy.
8. Postparturient hypocalcemia in the bitch characterized by mastitis, tremors, and excitation is called _____.
9. During the _____ period, mares do not ovulate and this can lead to futile attempts at breeding.
10. Medications used to clear the mare's uterus of fluids include _____ estrus and cloprostenol.
11. If the _____ protrudes from the vulva of the mare during summer parturition, delivery must be assisted.
12. Using ultrasound examination, pregnancy can be diagnosed in metritis the cow as early as _____ days.
13. Female pigs can be sexually stimulated by pheromones released by the boar's _____ glands.
14. The most common postpartum diseases of swine are metritis and _____.
15. Artificial insemination of does and ewes is often done _____.
16. Hydrometra in the pregnant ewe or doe can be treated with _____.
17. A testicle retained in the abdomen is referred to as _____.
18. In stallions, sperm production is typically higher in _____.
19. A dog that is in pain during ejaculation and has white blood cells in the ejaculate might have _____.
20. In the tom, the most common cause of infertility is _____.

Transition
Summer
6, 8.
Laparoscopically
Corpus luteum
24
Cryptorchid

Prostate
8, 6
Eclampsia
Prostatitis
FSH
Domperidone
Corpus luteum
Chorioallantois
4
37
Prostaglandin

Oxytocin
Pregnancy toxemia
Placenta

Answers: (1) corpus luteum, (2) proestrus, (3), (4) estrus, (5) 8, 6, (6) 37, (7) 2, (8) eclampsia, (9) transition, (10) oxytocin, (11) chorioallantois, (12) 24, (13) salivary, (14) mastitis, (15) laparascopically, (16) prostaglandin, (17) cryptorchid, (18) summer, (19) prostaxitis, (20) poor teeth. ∎

18

Care of Birds, Reptiles, and Small Mammals

TEACHING/LEARNING OBJECTIVES

1. List ways to make the bird's visit to the hospital as comfortable as possible.
2. List reasons to perform a cloacal swab in birds.
3. List potential venipuncture sites in birds.
4. Explain how to calculate the basal metabolic rate (BMR) in healthy and ill birds in both passerines and nonpasserines.
5. Describe the ideal hospital environment for avian patients.
6. Explain how to clean the cage of a bird infected with *Chlamydia psittaci*.
7. Explain the procedure for obtaining a fecal sample from reptiles if a fecal sample is not available.
8. List potential sites of bone marrow aspiration in reptiles.
9. List restraint devices for radiographing reptiles.
10. Explain why birds, especially psittacines, should be hospitalized in areas separate from reptiles.
11. List clinical signs of vitamin A deficiency in turtles and tortoises.
12. Explain why reptiles that live in glass aquariums need full-spectrum light during normal daylight hours.
13. Describe how to culture bacterial and fungal organisms on reptile skin.
14. List venipuncture sites for ferrets.
15. Name two agents that can be used to anesthetize ferrets.
16. List clinical signs of estrogen toxicity in ferrets.
17. List clinical signs of adrenal hyperplasia in ferrets and treatment options.
18. Name the potential parasites of ferrets that should be discussed with owners.
19. Name the components of good ferret husbandry.
20. List two defense mechanisms of the rabbit.
21. Explain how to determine the sex of a rabbit.
22. Describe how to induce hypnosis in rabbits and why it is done.
23. List indications that a rabbit is in a suitable plane of anesthesia.
24. List possible causes of anorexia in rabbits.
25. Name the organism that causes snuffles in rabbits and clinical signs.
26. List the antibiotics that should not be given to rodents.
27. List causes of dystocia in guinea pigs.
28. Explain why it is necessary to supplement vitamin C daily and how to do it.
29. Describe how to determine the sex of guinea pigs.
30. Define wet tail and list its causes in the hamster.
31. Describe basic requirements of the hamster's aquarium.
32. Explain how to determine the sex of a hamster.
33. Explain how to determine the sex of a gerbil.
34. Name the most common cause of nasal dermatitis in gerbils.
35. Explain how to determine the sex of a mouse.
36. Describe basic housing requirements of mice.
37. Name the most common geriatric disease condition in mice.
38. Name the type of tumors most commonly diagnosed in rats.
39. Describe how to determine the sex of rats.
40. Define the harderian gland and its function.
41. Explain why deep bedding is important for the prairie dog.
42. Explain how to determine the sex of prairie dogs.
43. List zoonotic diseases that wild prairie dogs may carry.
44. Describe basic husbandry needs of the hedgehog.
45. List diseases commonly diagnosed in the hedgehog.
46. Describe the husbandry needs of the sugar glider.
47. Describe the nutritional requirements of the sugar glider.

KEY TERMS

Atropinesterase
Barbering
Barium sulfate
Basilic vein

Cardiocentesis
Caudal tail vein
Cavy
Cerclage wire
Chelonian
Choana
Cloaca
Coccygeal vein
Cole tube
Crop
Cryptosporidiosis
Dysbiosis
Dystocia
Ecdysis
Glottis
Harderian gland
Heterophil
Iohexol
Lagomorphs

Occipital sinus
Open-rooted teeth
Passerine
Pectoral muscle
Peribulbar plexus
Periorbital sinus
Petechial hemorrhage
Pinna
Poikilothermic
Polyuria
Psittacine
Pterygopalatine sinus
Pubic symphysis
Renal portal system
Retrobulbar plexus
Snuffles
Thrombocytopenia
Ventral abdominal vein

Chapter Outline

Birds
  Taking the clinical history
  Behavior considerations during the examination process
  Sample collections and diagnostic procedures commonly used in birds
    Cloacal swab
    Oral examination and crop wash
    Blood work
    Radiography
  Husbandry and treatment in the hospital
  Zoonoses and common clinical problems
Reptiles
  Taking the clinical history
  Sample collection and diagnostic procedures
    Colonic wash
    Bone marrow
    Stomach lavage
    Urine samples
    Blood samples
    Radiography
  Husbandry in the hospital
  Skin
  Feces

Teaching Strategies

Discuss reasons why birds mask illness.
For each question listed in the chapter, ask the students to explain the relevance of the question in taking a clinical history.
Stress the need to have all diagnostic tools ready before restraining birds in order to reduce the time required to a minimum.
Show photos of normal and abnormal fecal samples and diseases with which they are associated.
Review the anatomy of the gastrointestinal tract from the beak to the cloaca.
Stress the importance of not overfilling the crop.

Discuss the use of the restraint board.
Review the anatomy and function of the renal portal system. Discuss the safest and most effective location to administer medication. Review the feather patterns on wings and emphasize the need to trim feathers symmetrically.
Review the lifecycle of *Chlamydia psittaci* and its mode of transmission to humans.
Review the anatomy of the snake and turtle.

For each question listed in the chapter, ask the students to explain the relevance of the question in taking a clinical history.
Show photos of parasites and eggs diagnosed from a colonic wash.
Indicate the sites commonly used for diagnostic bone marrow aspiration.
Show photos of parasites, especially Cryptosporidium, diagnosed from stomach lavage.
Review anatomy of the reproductive tract, gastrointestinal tract, and urinary tract. Point out sites of cystocentesis.
Review the cardiovascular system and venipuncture sites.
Show radiographs of various reptiles. Explain why it is necessary to take the frontal view when radiographing snakes.
Discuss environmental, temperature, and humidity needs and potential results if these needs are not met. Review the causes of metabolic bone disease and how it can be prevented.
Show pictures of reptiles with dermatologic diseases and discuss causes, treatments, and prevention. Review the process of ecdysis.
Review reasons for collecting fecal samples in reptiles. Show photos

Chapter Outline	Teaching Strategies
	of samples containing bacteria, parasites, and blood. Discuss how pancreatic enzyme levels can be determined from feces.
Sputum	Show photos of sputum samples containing *Rhabdias* spp., *Entamoeba* spp., and *Strongyloides stercoralis*.
Zoonoses and common clinical problems	See Chapter 35.
Small mammals	
Ferrets	Review restraint techniques. Discuss the effects of prolonged release of estrogen on the bone marrow. Discuss ways to diagnose adrenal hyperplasia and its treatment. Review the recommended vaccination protocol for ferrets. Point out the importance of differentiating canine distemper, influenza, and bacterial pneumonia.
Rabbits	Discuss reasons to premedicate a rabbit with extra atropine. Review common parasites of rabbits. Show photos of common parasites, clinical signs, and treatment options for each. Review dental anatomy. Show photos of malocclusions and discuss causes, clinical signs, and treatments.
Rodents	
Antibiotics in rodents	Review the effects of penicillins on rodents.
Anesthetics in rodents	
Antiparasitic agents in rodents	
Zoonotic diseases	See Chapter 35.
Guinea pig	Discuss implications of having open-rooted teeth. Talk about the separation of the pubic symphysis before parturition and how to increase the chances of this occurring. Discuss prevention and treatment of footpad dermatitis and submandibular abscesses. Show photos of animals with these diseases. Review the importance of supplementing vitamin C daily.
Hamster	Show photos of the anatomy of the cheek pouches and flank glands. Review the phenomenon of cannibalism and ways to prevent it.
Gerbil	Discuss how gerbils mark territory. Stress that the tail should never be grabbed. Review Tyzzer disease, the importance of not changing the diet if possible, and nasal dermatitis.
Mouse	Show photos of tumors in mice and discuss the importance of educating owners about this disease. Discuss the importance of not using aromatic shavings in the aquarium.
Rat	Discuss the anatomy and function of the Harderian gland. Review clinical signs of *Mycoplasma* spp. infections and how to treat them.
Prairie dogs	Stress that it is illegal to keep these animals as pets in the United States. Talk about the zoonotic disease that these animals may carry.
Hedgehogs	Discuss the need for hedgehogs to have privacy and burrow. Review dietary requirements. Emphasize the importance of anesthetizing the patient before examination.
Sugar gliders	Stress that nocturnal activity and the need for social interaction are important considerations for owners. Discuss nutritional requirements and explain that malnutrition is the most common disease condition diagnosed.

CRITICAL THINKING CHALLENGES

1. Proper husbandry is crucial to the well-being of birds, reptiles, and small mammals. Owners often depend on technicians to answer their questions on these topics. Ask the students to list highlights of proper husbandry for each group of animals that may be posted in exam rooms. Topics should include, at a minimum, housing (size of housing, humidity, temperature, light requirements), nutrition, clinical signs of illness, and any special needs of each species.

2. For each animal discussed in the chapter, talk about ways to ensure that the physical exam and diagnostic procedures run as quickly and efficiently as possible while causing the least amount of stress to the pet. While these rules are true for all pets, discuss why they are particularly important for birds, reptiles, and small mammals.

Copyright © 2006 by Elsevier, Inc. All rights reserved.

QUIZ

Match each statement with the animal to which it refers. There is one correct answer for each statement.

1. _____ Tumors are a common finding with geriatric animals.
2. _____ Obesity is common in these animals raised in captivity.
3. _____ Hypnosis provides good restraint for injections and radiographic procedures.
4. _____ The sharp spines of this animal necessitate the use of gloves in order to be handled.
5. _____ If tail skin is degloved, the tail must be amputated.
6. _____ A third or frontal radiographic view should always be taken.
7. _____ Full-spectrum light must be available during normal daylight hours.
8. _____ Cardiac puncture is commonly performed to obtain blood.
9. _____ *Psoroptes cuniculi* is the ear mite most commonly diagnosed.
10. _____ A crop wash may be helpful for direct examination of protozoans or yeast.
11. _____ Respiratory infections caused by *Mycoplasma* spp. are common.
12. _____ Males aid in the care of the young.
13. _____ Young may be hidden in cheek pouches.
14. _____ Affected scales may be cultured for bacteria and fungi.
15. _____ The pubic symphysis separates before parturition.
16. _____ A restraint board is essential to obtain high-quality radiographs.
17. _____ A temperature gradient must be provided in the daily environment.
18. _____ Food administered must be a lower temperature than the body temperature.
19. _____ It is illegal to keep these as pets.
20. _____ Wet tail can be caused by cestodiasis, antibiotic administration, and bacterial infection.
21. _____ If ovulation does not occur, estrogen toxicity can be fatal.
22. _____ This animal has only two mammary glands but can raise healthy litters of three or more offspring.
23. _____ The water bowl should be big enough for the animal to completely submerge.
24. _____ These marsupials require tall wire enclosures with fresh branches and places to hide.
25. _____ Some lines have epileptiform seizure activity.
26. _____ Chlamydiosis should always be considered a potential culprit if the patient isn't doing well, no matter what the clinical signs are.
27. _____ Owners should always be asked if the animal is showing any changes in voice.
28. _____ The basilic vein is often used for venipuncture.
29. _____ If not pregnant or lactating, a high-quality cat diet is recommended.
30. _____ Vitamin C must be supplemented daily.
31. _____ Nasal discharge may be tinged with red color due to the pigment of the harderian gland secretions.
32. _____ Canine distemper infection is fatal if the animal is not vaccinated.
33. _____ The pterygopalatine and/or dorsal postoccipital sinuses might be used to obtain a blood sample.
34. _____ Submandibular abscesses commonly result from chewing substrate that splinters in the mouth.
35. _____ Malnutrition is one of the most common diseases diagnosed, especially hypocalcemia and hypoglycemia.
36. _____ The femoral cavity usually yields adequate diagnostic bone marrow.
37. _____ Insulinomas are not uncommon and blood glucose should always be checked if the patient is anorexic.

A. Prairie dog
B. Gerbil
C. Rabbits
D. Rat
E. Bird
F. Sugar glider
G. Snake
H. Guinea pig
I. Mouse
J. Hamster
K. Hedgehog
L. Ferret
M. Hamster

Answers: (1) I, (2) A, (3) C, (4) K, (5) B, (6) G, (7) G, (8) G, (9) C, (10) E, (11) D, (12) B, (13) J, (14) G, (15) H, (16) E, (17) G, (18) E, (19) A, (20) J, (21) L, (22) H, (23) G, (24) F, (25) J, (26) E, (27) E, (28) E, (29) L, (30) H, (31) D, (32) L, (33) G, (34) H, (35) F, (36) G, (37) L. ■

19

Veterinary Anesthesia

TEACHING/LEARNING OBJECTIVES

1. Describe the benefits of the balanced anesthetic technique over the outdated method of administering a large dose of a single drug.
2. List situations in which an endotracheal tube should be placed.
3. Explain situations that require the use of uncuffed endotracheal tubes.
4. In which animals should a laryngoscope always be used to facilitate intubation?
5. List five functions of an anesthetic machine.
6. Name two uses of the oxygen flush valve.
7. Describe the advantage of using a precision vaporizer over a non-precision vaporizer.
8. Explain the purpose of valves in the breathing circuit.
9. Explain when the non-rebreathing breathing circuit should be used and list its advantages and disadvantages.
10. Give the approximate flow rate for induction and maintenance.
11. List the minimum laboratory preanesthetic database for an apparently healthy animal.
12. List reasons for premedicating animals.
13. Name two anticholinergics and list the reasons for using them as premedications.
14. What is the effect of opioids on the respiratory system?
15. For each of the three groups of tranquilizer/sedatives (phenothiazines, benzodiazepines, and alpha$_2$ agonists) name one advantage and disadvantage.
16. List advantages of using guaifenesin as an induction/maintenance agent in large animals.
17. Describe the protocol to treat inadvertent perivascular administration of thiopental.
18. Explain why methoxyflurane is the most commonly used inhalant anesthetic in nonprecision vaporizers.
19. Explain why anesthetic induction is usually accomplished at anesthetic concentrations of 2.0 to 3.0 times the MAC for each anesthetic.
20. Explain how apnea monitors work.
21. List cardiovascular system parameters that should be assessed during anesthesia.
22. What Pao$_2$ is indicative of severe hypoxemia?
23. Compare results of over- and underventilating an anesthetized patient.
24. What signs, other than eye position, are important indicators of the depth of anesthesia?
25. Explain how to determine if an adequate tidal volume has been delivered in small and large animals during assisted ventilation.
26. Define neuroleptanalgesic and list procedures for which this protocol could possibly be used.
27. Describe the site for administration of epidural anesthesia in small animals, small ruminants, swine, cattle, and horses.
28. List five ways to ensure that an endotracheal tube is in the trachea and not the esophagus.
29. Describe fluid administration requirements in small animals, neonates, and birds.
30. Explain the results of ventilating an anesthetized animal too frequently.
31. List ways to prevent hypothermia in smaller animals during anesthesia.
32. List three benefits of continued administration of oxygen in the immediate postoperative period.
33. What is an indication that pharyngeal reflexes have returned after anesthesia?
34. Define ABCs and describe steps taken for each.
35. Explain when internal cardiac massage is warranted.

KEY TERMS

Alpha$_2$ agonist
Ambu bag
Anal reflex
Anesthesia
Anticholinergic
Apnea
Apnea monitor
Arterial blood gas tension

Arterial carbon dioxide pressure ($PaCO_2$)
Arterial oxygen pressure (PaO_2)
Arytenoid cartilages
Assisted ventilation
Atelectasis
Bain non-rebreathing circuit
Balanced anesthetic technique
Barium hydroxide
Benzodiazepines
Brachycephalic
Bradycardia
Butterfly needle
Capnometry
Cardiopulmonary arrest
Cardiopulmonary resuscitation
Carina
Carrier gas
Closed circle system
Costochondral junction
Diastolic blood pressure
End-title carbon dioxide (ET_{CO_2})
Intermittent-positive-pressure ventilation (IPPV)
Eructation
Esophageal stethoscope
Flowmeter
General anesthesia
Hemoglobin saturation with oxygen (SpO_2)
Hypoxemia
Ileus
Inspiratory/expiratory ratio (I/E ratio)
Intubation
Lacrimation
Laryngoscope
Local anesthesia
Mean blood pressure
Mechanical ventilation
Minimum alveolar concentration (MAC)
Myoclonus
Neuroleptanalgesia
Nonprecision vaporizer
Nonrebreathing system
Nystagmus
Oxygen flush valve
Palpebral reflex
Peak inspiratory pressure (PIP)
Phenothiazines
Pop-off valve
Positive inotrope
Precision vaporizer
Pressure regulator
Pulse oximetry
Rebreathing bag
Rebreathing system
Sedative
Soda lime
Solubility
Systolic blood pressure
Tachycardia
Tachypnea
Tidal volume
Tracheostomy
Tranquilizer
Universal F circuit
Vagal tone

Chapter Outline	Teaching Strategies
Definitions	
The concept of balanced anesthesia	Emphasize the safety of the balanced anesthetic technique for the patient and staff. Discuss the importance of having various protocol options for different types of surgical and nonsurgical procedures.
The process of general anesthesia	
Anesthetic equipment	Review the veterinary technician's role in cleaning, maintaining, and ordering equipment and drugs. Present several schedules of maintenance and methods of record keeping.
Catheters	Have a variety of catheters available for demonstration. Review their nomenclature and purposes.
Endotracheal tubes	On an illustration, review the placement of the tube and laryngoscope. Have several sizes available for demonstration. Discuss the use of uncuffed tubes.
Laryngoscopes	Have a laryngoscope available for demonstration in class. Stress the importance of using these on all patients.
Anesthetic machines	Bring an anesthetic machine to class for demonstration. Label/number the parts of the machine and attached an endotracheal tube. Show the pathway of the flow.
Breathing systems	Compare the circle breathing circuit and the non-rebreathing breathing circuits, when they are used, and the advantages and disadvantages of each system. Demonstrate how to check the system for leaks. Stress the importance of minimizing exposure of personnel to gas.

PART FOUR ANESTHESIA AND PHARMACOLOGY

Chapter Outline	Teaching Strategies
Preanesthetic evaluation and stabilization	Review required laboratory tests for apparently healthy animals, animals with cardiovascular and pulmonary disease, and animals that have suffered trauma. Compare fasting times for different animals.
Protocol selection	
Pharmacology of anesthetic drugs	
Premedication	
Anticholinergics	Discuss the vagal effects of working with the gastrointestinal tract. Stress that anticholinergics are not commonly administered to large animals.
Tranquilizers and sedatives	Compare phenothiazines, benzodiazepines, and alpha$_2$ agonists. Differentiate them based on their ability to provide analgesia, effects on the cardiovascular system, availability of a reversal agent, and how they are metabolized. Briefly present the system of alpha and beta receptors.
Opioids	Point out that although opioids generally provide good sedation and analgesia, they have a respiratory depressive effect and pure opioids can produce excitement in horses.
NMDA antagonists (dissociative drugs)	
Induction drugs	
Ultra-short-acting barbiturates	Point out the need to closely monitor respiratory rate and character when administering thiopental.
Propofol	Explain the need to utilize the entire vial of propofol within 6 hours of opening it. Compare thiopental with propofol in terms of respiratory effects and repeating boluses.
Etomidate	
NMDA antagonist (dissociative) combinations	Compare NMDA antagonists, propofol, and thiopental as induction agents.
Guaifenesin	Explain how guaifenesin is used in large animals.
Anesthetic maintenance	
Inhaled anesthetics	Provide situations in which induction with injectable drugs is impossible or contraindicated. Compare isoflurane, sevoflurane, halothane, and methoxyflurane in terms of solubility, MAC, and cardiopulmonary, hepatic, and renal effects.
Monitoring during anesthesia	On illustrations, point out locations of peripheral veins in large and small animals used to monitor pulse rate and character. Bring a blood pressure instrument to class and demonstrate its use. Explain the importance of monitoring Pao$_2$ and PaCO$_2$. Explain how reflective probes work on a pulse oximeter and the reasons for monitoring this parameter. Discuss how to respond to an increase in P$_{ET}$CO$_2$ above 40 mm Hg and why this is important. Review eye positions in small animals, horses, and ruminants that indicate a surgical plane of anesthesia.
Ventilatory support	
Assisted ventilation	Review the procedure to follow to provide assisted ventilation.
Mechanical ventilation	Compare indications for assisted and mechanical ventilation.
Special anesthetic techniques	
Neuroleptanalgesia	Discuss possible drug combinations that could be considered to have neuroleptanalgesic properties.
Epidural analgesia/anesthesia	Discuss indications for the use of epidural analgesia/anesthesia and the effects of these protocols on the respiratory and cardiovascular systems of small animals, ruminants, and horses.
Protocol selection and preparation of equipment	
Protocol selection	See Critical Thinking Challenges.
Equipment preparation	
Endotracheal intubation	Review the positions of animals that best facilitate intubation. On illustrations, point out the placement of the tube in relation to the carina and discuss the negative side effects of dead space. Review the anatomy of the arytenoid cartilages and ways to ensure that the tube is appropriately placed.
Fluid administration during anesthesia	Review the protocols for fluid administration in normovolemic, hypovolemic, and hypervolemic patients. Discuss responses to various plasma protein readings and packed cell volumes during surgery.

Copyright © 2006 by Elsevier, Inc. All rights reserved.

CHAPTER 19 Veterinary Anesthesia

Chapter Outline	Teaching Strategies
Induction and maintenance	Review the need to provide oxygen during procedures using only injectable anesthetics to prevent hypoxia caused by atelectasis and hypoventilation. Discuss methods to assess the depth of the patient.
Padding and positioning of the animal	Compare positioning differences between small animals, horses, and ruminants. Discuss potential postoperative myositis and neuropathies and ways to prevent them.
Recovery	Discuss requirements of small animals, horses, ruminants, and swine during recovery.
Dogs and cats	Stress the importance of leaving the endotracheal tube in place for as long as possible in animals at risk for airway obstruction, including brachycephalic breeds.
Horses	Stress the importance of covering the animal's eyes to minimize external stimulation.
Ruminants Swine	Stress the importance of removing the endotracheal tube with the cuff inflated.
Postoperative analgesia	Compare postoperative analgesia regimens of small and large animals.
Anesthetic emergencies	Stress the importance of scheduling mock drills. Discuss clinical signs that may signal impending cardiopulmonary arrest and how to prevent and/or respond to them.
Readiness and prevention	Discuss the location and contents of the crash cart and the need to check its contents and restock it daily. Endotracheal tubes must be checked for leaks, drugs should be checked for expiration dates, filled saline syringes must be available as well as catheters to administer intratracheal drugs if needed.
Recognition and basic cardiac life support	Review the ABCs of basic cardiac life support. Practice the technique on stuffed animals.
Advanced cardiac life support	Review routes of administration of drugs. Discuss various fluid administration protocols that may be followed during CPR.
Postresuscitative care	Explain why serial neurologic exams are necessary.

ACTIVITY

Exercise utilizing Tables 21-1 and 21-9 in which situations are described giving the protocol used to premedicate, induce, maintain, etc. As complications occur (bradycardia, tachypnea, etc.) ask the student what he or she would do to correct the problem. Have a list of actions from which they must choose. Then ask what the possible causes are.

CRITICAL THINKING CHALLENGES

1. Present signalments, weight, medical histories, and intended surgery of patients. Provide the drugs that will be used for premedication and induction. Ask students to calculate dosages and to determine if the protocol is safe for each animal and justify the answer.
2. Ask the students to choose an appropriate protocol form Boxes 19-1 to 19-5 and Table 19-7 for each animal described in the previous challenge. They should describe the expected effects of each premedication, the volume to give, route of administration, and potential negative side effects. How will they prepare for and respond to such effects?
3. Present case histories in which patients had abnormalities on preanesthetic tests and preexisting medical conditions. Ask the students to discuss what they would do next. Compare their conclusions with the actual records.
4. Ask the students to imagine that one of the above-mentioned animals is undergoing cardiopulmonary arrest during anesthesia. They should be able to explain, in appropriate sequence, the steps to take for cardiopulmonary resuscitation. Alternatively, present clinical signs that occur while a patient is under general anesthesia such as tachypnea or bradycardia and ask the students to explain how they would respond.

QUIZ

Circle T (true) or F (false) for each statement.

1. T F Intravenous access can reliably and safely be gained during surgery by taping a hypodermic needle attached to a syringe to the limb of the animal.
2. T F Uncuffed endotracheal tubes should be used in birds.

Copyright © 2006 by Elsevier, Inc. All rights reserved.

3. T F The most commonly used carrier gas is nitrous oxide.
4. T F Selection of an appropriately sized rebreathing bag is made by multiplying the animal's tidal volume (10 ml/kg) by 5.
5. T F During the maintenance of anesthesia, the flow rate may be reduced to 5 to 10 ml/kg/min from the induction rate of 100 ml/kg/min.
6. T F Cattle should fast for approximately 36 to 48 hours before induction of anesthesia.
7. T F Atropine may cross the placental barrier and therefore is generally not recommended for animals undergoing a cesarean delivery.
8. T F Alpha$_2$ agonists provide analgesia.
9. T F Thiopental is an appropriate, safer alternative to propofol in sight hounds.
10. T F Hyperthermia can usually increase the MAC for an inhaled anesthetic.
11. T F One way to prevent postanesthetic myopathy in horses is to monitor direct blood pressure measurements during surgery.
12. T F An increase in $P_{ET}CO_2$ is a strong indication of hyperventilation.
13. T F The recommended respiratory rate during IPPV for a small animal undergoing the repair of a diaphragmatic hernia is 6 to 12 breaths/min.
14. T F The endotracheal tube's cuff must be inflated before placement to prevent aspiration.
15. T F Blood lost during surgery should be replaced by three times the approximate volume loss in addition to the basic fluid rate.
16. T F Intravenous fluids are generally administered at a rate of 10 or 20 ml/kg/hr during anesthesia in small animals.
17. T F The eyes of animals are always lubricated to protect the corneas during anesthesia.
18. T F The rumen should be on the bottom (closest to the ground or table), if possible, during surgery in ruminants.
19. T F The first thing to do in response to cardiopulmonary arrest in an anesthetized animal is stop delivery of anesthetic to the animal and increase fresh gas flow rate.
20. T F During basic cardiac life support, 20 breaths per minute should be given simultaneously with chest compressions that should be given at a rate of 80 to 120 compressions per minute.

Answers: (1) F, (2) T, (3) F, (4) F, (5) F, (6) T, (7) T, (8) T, (9) F, (10) F, (11) T, (12) F, (13) F, (14) F, (15) T, (16) F, (17) T, (18) F, (19) T, (20) T. ■

20

Pain Management

TEACHING/LEARNING OBJECTIVES

1. List four sequelae of uncontrolled pain in animals.
2. List organs or tissues with high densities of nociceptors.
3. List six examples of NSAIDs used in veterinary medicine.
4. Explain why visceral pain is generally more difficult to localize.
5. Describe the ideal hospital environment for the postoperative patient.
6. Compare the OP_3 (mu) and OP_2 (kappa) receptor subtypes.
7. Explain the relationship among pure agonists, antagonists, and mixed agonist/antagonists as they relate to opioid receptors throughout the body.
8. Describe patients to whom narcotics either should not be administered or should be administered in decreased dosages.
9. Compare the onset of action and duration of lipid-soluble and water-soluble drugs.
10. Discuss the effects on analgesia when using naloxone versus butorphanol to reverse excessive doses of OP_3 (mu) agonists.
11. List three clinical signs of inflammation.
12. Explain how NSAIDs control pain. Include the words *arachidonic acid, gastric ulcers, cyclooxygenase, prostaglandins, inflammation, tissues,* and *cells.*
13. Describe the difference between a COX-1 and a COX-2 inhibitor.
14. List the functions of prostaglandins produced by the stomach.
15. Give the indications for using naproxen in the dog and horse and frequency of administration in each species.
16. Compare the uses of meclofenamic acid and flunixin meglumine in the horse.
17. List drugs commonly used to treat/prevent gastric ulceration associated with the use of NSAIDs and briefly explain the mechanism of each one.
18. Name two alpha$_2$-adrenergic agonists, the species in which they are commonly used, and the reasons for using them.
19. Describe two ways to administer bupivacaine to an animal that has had a thoracotomy.
20. Name two routes of administration for polysulfated glycosaminoglycans.

KEY TERMS

A delta fibers
Adrenal glands
Agranulocytosis
Allodynia
Analgesia
Antiemetic
Antipyretic
Antitussive
Anxiolysis
Arachidonic acid
Ataxia
Autonomic nervous system
Bruxism
C fibers
Catecholamine
Central nervous system
Central sensitization
Cholecystokinin
Controlled Substances Act of 1970
Cortisol
Dorsal horn
Dorsal nerve roots
Dysphoria
Endotoxemia
Epidural
Epinephrine
Euphoria
Fight-or-flight reaction
Glucuronyl transferase
Half-life
Hematemesis
Histamine
Hyperalgesia
Ileus

Interleukins
Isoform
Leukocyte products
Leukotrienes
Lymphocytosis
Lymphokines
Mydriasis
Myelin sheath
Narcotic analgesic
Neuron
Neurotransmitter
Neutrophilia
N-Methyl-D-aspartate (NMDA)
Nociceptive pathway
Nociceptor
Nonsteroidal antiinflammatory drugs (NSAIDs)
Norepinephrine
OP$_2$ (kappa) receptor
OP$_3$ (mu) receptor
Opioid analgesic
Opioid antagonist
Oxygen radicals
Pain
Partial agonist
Peripheral sensitization
Phospholipid
Polycythemia
Prostaglandins
Pure agonist
Serotonin
Somatic pain
Somatostatin
Spinothalamic tract
Substance P
Thalamus
Thromboxane
Vasoactive amines
Visceral pain
Windup
Zone of secondary hyperalgesia

Chapter Outline

Definitions
Organization of nociceptive pathways

Peripheral nervous system
Central nervous system
Pain localization

Recognizing pain in animals
Problems with evaluation

Signs of pain and distress: animal variability
Clinical evaluation of pain
Control of pain in animals
Environment and nursing care

Analgesic drugs
Opioids

  Morphine

  Fentanyl
    Transdermal administration of fentanyl

Teaching Strategies

Using diagrams, show the neural pathways of pain to include the stimulus, peripheral pathway, central nervous system pathway, and the feeling of pain at the site of the stimulus. Point out the spinothalamic tract.

Discuss cases in which patients presented with generalized abdominal or thoracic pain and explain the final diagnosis. Discuss the phenomenon of visceral pain and the challenge of localizing the etiology compared to somatic pain.

Review findings of a physical exam or blood work that one might expect with a painful or anxious patient. Discuss why these occur.
Emphasize that every patient is unique in his or her response to pain. This can be extremely challenging for the veterinary technician.

Ask the students to imagine that they are waking up in a hospital after having had abdominal or orthopedic surgery. They are painful and very uncomfortable. Ask them to list specific things that would help to alleviate the pain and discomfort. Discuss the similarities and differences between human nursing care and veterinary nursing care for the hospitalized patient.

List the opioids used in veterinary medicine and ask the students to categorize them as agonists, antagonists, mixed agonist/antagonists, or partial agonist/antagonists. For each drug, they can describe the expected effects.
Discuss the indications for morphine and include when and how it should be administered. Explain the concept of potency and its implication on the amount of medication to give.

Copyright © 2006 by Elsevier, Inc. All rights reserved.

CHAPTER 20 Pain Management

Chapter Outline	Teaching Strategies
Hydromorphone and oxymorphone	
Epidural administration of opioids	Discuss indications for epidural administration of opioids.
Mixed-action agonist/antagonist	
Narcotic analgesics	
Butorphanol	
Buprenorphine	
Narcotic antagonists	Compare the use of naloxone, nalorphine, and butorphanol as reversal agents. Give examples in which each would be appropriate.
Naloxone	
Nalorphine	
Management of controlled substances	Discuss the purpose of the Controlled Substances Act of 1997. Explain the need to accurately record the use of these drugs and the process of inspections. Point out the legal ramifications of abuse of these drugs by personnel.
Nonsteroidal antiinflammatory drugs (NSAIDs)	
Inflammation	Review the arachidonic acid pathway.
Mechanism of action	Discuss the differences between COX-1 and COX-2 inhibition and the effect on gastric and renal health.
Salicylate analgesics	Explain the gastric and renal effects of these drugs. Stress that cats have lower levels of the enzyme to metabolize these drugs and therefore the dosage regimen is different.
Propionic acid derivatives	Compare these drugs in terms of COX-1 and COX-2 inhibition, potential toxicities, half-lives, indications, and analgesic/antipyretic/antiinflammatory properties.
Carprofen	Stress the need to assess hepatic and renal values before giving this drug to dogs and to continue to monitor these values.
Deracoxib	
Naproxen	Emphasize that this drug is given only once daily in small animals.
Ibuprofen	Point out that this drug is not recommended for use in dogs because of potential to cause gastric irritation.
Ketoprofen	Stress that this drug is not approved for use in dogs and cats in the United States. It is an effective analgesic in horses.
Fenamic acids	Compare the use of these two drugs in the horse.
Meclofenamic acid	
Flunixin meglumine	
Oxicans	
Meloxicam	Emphasize that this drug is not yet approved for use in cattle or pigs in the United States.
Pyrazolone derivatives	
Phenylbutazone	Discuss the concept of margin of safety as it relates to phenylbutazone, flunixin meglumine, and ketoprofen.
Treatment of gastrointestinal ulceration	Review the mechanisms of sucralfate, misoprostol, omeprazole, and H_2 receptor antagonists.
Psychotropic drugs	
Tranquilizers	Review the uses of tranquilizers and emphasize that these drugs offer no analgesia.
Alpha$_2$-adrenergic agonists	Emphasize that these drugs cause both sedation and analgesia.
Xylazine	Review the side effects of stimulating peripheral alpha$_2$-adrenergic receptors.
Detomidine	Discuss the common use of this drug in horses and cattle as a sedative and analgesic.
Corticosteroids	Explain the effects of long-term exogenous administration of corticosteroids as well as the need to taper the dosage when weaning a patient off of these drugs.
Local anesthetics—selective nerve blocks	Review uses of these drugs listed in the chapter and add other common uses including the removal of skin tumors.
Treatment of pain in dogs and cats	
Treatment of pain in horses	Emphasize that the risk to veterinary personnel is decreased when pain and discomfort are controlled in the equine patient.

PART FOUR ANESTHESIA AND PHARMACOLOGY

Chapter Outline	Teaching Strategies
Analgesics in the treatment of colic	Point out that xylazine and butorphanol are generally the most effective drugs for sedation and analgesia.
Analgesics for the treatment of musculoskeletal pain	Review the possible side effects of NSAIDs in the horse and point out that phenylbutazone is a very commonly used antiinflammatory in horses.

ACTIVITY

Provide possible real-life situations in which the student must exercise decision-making skills.

EXAMPLE

1. You work in a mixed animal practice that has the following medications on its shelves: aspirin, carprofen, banamine, ketoprofen, butorphanol, morphine, xylazine, corticosteroids. A 12-year-old, female, spayed mixed-breed dog has been out of surgery (anastomosis and resection) for 2 hours. She is panting, tachycardic, and febrile. Another technician predicts that the clinician will want to administer banamine because of its antipyretic effects. Do you agree? What do you recommend? Why? This can be a multiple choice exercise or matching or both.

CRITICAL THINKING CHALLENGES

1. Side effects of some analgesics can be life-threatening, especially when administered with a sedative or tranquilizer. As the nursing care provider, the veterinary technician is usually the first person to observe effects of any drugs given to the patients. Therefore, he or she must know what to expect, when to alert the veterinarian, and how to respond. Prepare a list of medications and ask the students to indicate potential side effects and actions to take to reverse or treat the effects if they are severe. The list can be expanded as subsequent chapters are studied.
2. Present clinical cases that demonstrate a variety of animals exhibiting pain or that will be undergoing surgery. Ask the students to work in pairs to develop drug regimens for analgesia and explain why they chose each medication. These cases can be used in subsequent chapters as other medications are studied.

QUIZ

Fill in each blank with the appropriate word or phrase.

1. Fentanyl is approximately _____ times more potent than morphine.
2. After giving _____, the animal must be observed for at least 2 hours because this partial agonist of the OP_3 (mu) receptors had delayed effects.
3. The degree of tissue sensitivity to pain is directly related to the density of _____ in that tissue.
4. Carprofen is an example of a _____ antiinflammatory drug.
5. Epinephrine and norepinephrine are categorized as _____ and are released by the _____ glands as a response to pain or stimulation of the autonomic nervous system.
6. The synthetic opioid, _____, is available in transdermal patches and takes about 12 to 16 hours to reach therapeutic plasma levels in the _____ and 24 hours in the _____.
7. The central nervous system consists of the _____ and _____.
8. The _____ opioid receptor subtype causes addiction when a drug stimulates it.
9. An opioid overdose may be reversed with _____ or _____.
10. NSAIDs inhibit the action of an enzyme called _____ at the site of tissue injury and therefore decrease the production of prostaglandins.
11. Carprofen has caused toxic effects on the _____ of some dogs.
12. Aspirin can be administered to the cat no more often than every _____ to _____ hours.
13. Ketoprofen may be administered to _____ for up to 5 days.
14. Flunixin meglumine is an NSAID that is particularly useful to treat _____ pain in the horse.
15. Acetylpromazine is categorized as a _____ and is commonly used as a sedative.
16. After pelvic limb amputation, _____ may be injected around the nerve in the stump to control pain and discomfort after surgery.
17. _____ is a tranquilizer that also provides good control of visceral pain in horses with colic; however, a serious side effect is depression of intestinal motility that can lead to postoperative _____.
18. In the horse, _____ are frequently used to treat musculoskeletal disorders.
19. Polysulfated glycosaminoglycans have been shown to inhibit enzymes involved in _____ degradation.
20. The amount of fentanyl absorbed from the transdermal patch is decreased by hypothermia and _____.

Answers: (1) 100, (2) buprenorphine, (3) nociceptors, (4) nonsteroidal, (5) catecholamines, adrenal, (6) fentanyl, cat, dog, (7) brain, spinal cord, (8) OP_3(mu), (9) naloxone, butorphanol, (10) cyclooxygenase, (11) liver, (12) 36, 48, (13) horses, (14) visceral, (15) phenothiazine, (16) bupivacaine or a local anesthetic, (17) xylazine, ileus, (18) NSAIDs, (19) cartilage, (20) analgesia. ∎

21

Pharmacology and Pharmacy

TEACHING/LEARNING OBJECTIVES

1. Define therapeutic index and explain its importance for the patient receiving digoxin.
2. Explain why digoxin and atropine are ineffective in the ruminant.
3. Compare oral, subcutaneous, and intravenous routes of drug administration and rate of absorption.
4. Define biotransformation and name organs capable of these chemical reactions.
5. Explain how the pH of urine affects excretion of some drugs.
6. Describe the route of a drug taken orally that is excreted through enterohepatic circulation.
7. Describe economical ways to administer medication to large numbers of food animals.
8. List drugs known to be vesicants and explain steps to take to treat extravasation.
9. Name three effector sites.
10. Compare the sympathetic and parasympathetic nervous systems.
11. Define cholinomimetic agent and name one example.
12. Define cholinesterase inhibitor, list three groups of these drugs, and name drugs within each group.
13. List the symptoms of an overdose with anticholinesterase agents.
14. Discuss the classification of atropine and its effects at low, moderate, and high doses.
15. Name as many uses of atropine in veterinary medicine as you can.
16. Name two newer neuromuscular blocking agents used in veterinary medicine and their uses.
17. Describe situations in which epinephrine may be administered and name the route of administration.
18. Explain how loop and osmotic diuretics work. Name one drug from each category.
19. Explain how the heart compensates for aging and weakening myocardium.
20. Discuss care required for a geriatric cat or dog receiving digoxin.
21. List four anticonvulsant drugs and explain situations in which each one might be used.
22. Explain why hydralazine should be given with a diuretic.
23. Explain why it is important to restrict exercise after the administration of malarsomine dihydrochloride to dogs.
24. Describe how resistance to antimicrobials might develop and explain the implications of resistance on healthcare.
25. List clinical signs of hypothyroidism and hyperthyroidism in the dog and cat, respectively, and name the drugs used to treat them.
26. Explain the effects of having too little insulin released by the pancreas and giving too much insulin parenterally.
27. Compare the use of apomorphine and xylazine in dogs and cats to induce emesis.
28. Explain how sucralfate, omeprazole, and misoprostol work to manage ulcers.
29. Explain how to dispose of Schedule II drugs.
30. List as many sources of supplies as possible and discuss advantages and disadvantages of ordering from them, if any.
31. Define nutraceuticals and give reasons that consumers should be very cautious then purchasing them.

KEY TERMS

Absorption
Acetylation
Acetylcholine (Ach)
Acetylcholinesterase
Active metabolites
Afferent fiber
Afterload reducer
Agonist
Albumin
Angiotensin I
Angiotensin II
Angiotensin-converting enzyme inhibitor
Anthelmintic

CHAPTER 21 Pharmacology and Pharmacy

- Antibiotic
- Antiemetic
- Antipyretic
- Aqueous humor
- Arrhythmia
- Atrial fibrillation
- Atrial flutter
- Atrioventricular block
- Autonomic drugs
- Autonomic nervous system
- Avoirdupois system
- Bactericidal
- Belladonna alkaloid
- Biotransformation
- Bradycardia
- Calcium channel blocker
- Cardiac glycoside
- Central nervous system (CNS)
- Chemoreceptor trigger zone (CTZ)
- Chemotherapy
- Cholinomimetic (cholinergic or parasympathomimetic) agent
- Cholinesterase inhibitor
- Ciliary eye muscles
- Congestive heart failure
- Conjugation
- Cross resistance
- Diastolic blood pressure
- Diffusion
- Dimethyl sulfoxide (DMSO)
- Diuretic
- Drug
- Dyspnea
- Effector site
- Efferent fiber
- Emesis
- Empiric treatment
- Endotoxin
- Enterohepatic circulation
- Epaxial muscle
- Epidermis
- Excretion
- Extravasation
- Bacteriostatic
- Free drug
- Glaucoma
- Gut stasis
- Half-life
- Hemostasis
- Hepatic first-bypass effect
- Hepatotoxicity
- Hyaluronidase
- Hydroxylation
- Hyperthyroidism
- Hypertrophic cardiomyopathy
- Hypothyroidism
- Icterus
- Inactive metabolites
- Insulin
- Internuncial neurons
- Intraocular pressure
- Inventory tax
- Inventory turnover
- Inotropic drug
- Lacrimation
- LD_{50}
- Legend drug
- Liposuction device
- Loop diuretic
- Metritis
- Miosis
- Mitral valve insufficiency
- Muscarinic agent
- Myasthenia gravis
- Mydriatic agent
- Myocardium
- Negative inotropy
- Nephrotoxicity
- Neuron
- Neurotransmitter (NT)
- Nutraceutical
- Nicotinic agent
- Norepinephrine (NE)
- Nosocomial infection
- Osmotic diuretic
- P-450 enzyme system
- Parasympathetic nervous system
- Parietal cells
- Pathogen
- Peak serum concentration
- Peristalsis
- Pharmacodynamics
- Pharmacognosy
- Pharmacokinetics
- Pharmacology
- Pharmacotherapeutics
- Pro drug
- Protein binding
- Pulmonary thromboembolism
- Receptor
- Reconstitution
- Reflux esophagitis
- Reverse distribution company
- Ruminal atony
- Rx
- Synaptic cleft
- Somatic (motor) nervous system
- Steady state
- Stroke volume
- Supraventricular tachycardia
- Sympathetic nervous system
- Sympatholytic (adrenergic blocking) agent

Copyright © 2006 by Elsevier, Inc. All rights reserved.

Sympathomimetic (adrenergic) agent
Syncope
Systolic blood pressure
Tachycardia
Target tissue
Therapeutic index

Therapeutic window
Trough serum concentration
Urticarial wheals
Ventricular tachyarrhythmia
Vesicant

Chapter Outline	**Teaching Strategies**
General principles	Review the anatomy of a cell and stress the properties of the lipid bilayer. Explain the phenomenon of lipid solubility.
Definitions	
Drug absorption	Compare rates of absorption of various routes of administration and physical characteristics that affect these rates.
Drug metabolism	Explain that increased protein binding decreases the amount of the drug that is immediately available to cause the desired effect. Review locations of drug accumulation in the body. Give examples of agonists commonly used.
Excretion	Review factors that impact drug biotransformation and excretion such as age, disease states, urine pH, and species idiosyncrasies. Compare renal excretion and excretion via enterohepatic circulation. Review renal and hepatic functions in the healthy animal.
Dosage forms	Review various drug forms. Discuss safety precautions of forms such as handling of fentanyl patches and avoiding touching the surface of the eye with the tube of ophthalmic ointment. Photocopy pages from a veterinary drug reference that contain information on precautions for storage, application, and disposal. Stress the importance of always checking for this information for all drugs, especially new drugs.
Routes of administration	Discuss advantages and disadvantages of each route of administration.
Oral administration	
Parenteral administration	Review anatomy of the skin.
Neuropharmacology	
Autonomic nervous system	Create the outline of a chart titled Autonomic Drugs. Label the columns as Cholinomimetic Agents, Anticholinergic Agents, Neuromuscular Blockers, Sympathomimetic Agents, Sympatholytic Agents, and Alpha- and Beta-Adrenergic Blocking Agents. Label rows as drug name, indications, clinical signs, adverse reactions, etc. Divide the class into groups of three or more students and ask each group to work together to complete a part of the chart. Fill in your own chart with information intentionally misplaced and have students find and correct the errors.
Autonomic drugs	Review basic anatomy and physiology of the eye and point out conditions treated with autonomic drugs. Review the location of alpha and beta receptors in the body. On an illustration ask the students to indicate where these receptors are located.
Cholinomimetic agents	
Anticholinergics	
Neuromuscular blockers	
Sympathomimetics	
Sympatholytics	
Alpha- and beta-adrenergic blocking agents	
Tranquilizers	Teaching strategies for tranquilizers, alpha$_2$ agonists, analgesics, antipyretics, antiinflammatory agents, opioids, corticosteroids, and NSAIDs are found in Chapters 19 and 20.
Phenothiazines	Stress the importance of knowing side effects of phenothiazines: decreased blood pressure, paralysis of retractor penis muscle in horses, and lowering the seizure threshold in dogs.

Copyright © 2006 by Elsevier, Inc. All rights reserved.

CHAPTER 21 Pharmacology and Pharmacy

Chapter Outline	Teaching Strategies
Alpha$_2$ agonists	
Anticonvulsants	Review causes of seizures in animals. Discuss situations in which each anticonvulsant in the chapter might be used.
Barbiturates	
Analgesics, antipyretics, and antiinflammatory agents	
Opioid analgesics	
Opioid antagonists	
Corticosteroids	
Nonsteroidal antiinflammatory drugs (NSAIDs)	
Diuretic and cardiovascular drugs	Emphasize the relationship between the heart and kidneys in regulating blood pressure. Discuss the concepts of preload and afterload.
Diuretics	Review renal anatomy and physiology. Discuss indications for administering diuretics.
Cardiac glycosides	Review anatomy and physiology of the circulatory system. Discuss compensation and the development of congestive heart failure. Explain the effects of digoxin on the heart along with signs of toxicity. Have the students discuss the effects of compromised renal function as it relates to congestive heart failure and the administration of diuretics.
Antiarrhythmia drugs	Briefly present the role of the calcium channel, sinoatrial node, and the atrioventricular node and the ramifications of blocking the influx of calcium through the channels.
Angiotensin-converting enzyme Inhibitors	Briefly explain the enzymatic activity of ACE and the importance of preventing its activation in the dog with congestive heart failure. Discuss the meaning of second-generation drugs.
Agents used to treat parasitism	Stress the need to read package directions before administering anthelmintics to all young and geriatric animals and to any animal with a known or suspected medical condition. Discuss the concept of withdrawal times for food animals and lactating animals. Present manufacturer information on these topics. Bring a variety of new anthelmintics to class to demonstrate that many of the older drugs have been replaced by more broad-spectrum products. Because owners will often ask how much preventive medication costs, prepare a list that compares the cost of currently used products for large and small animals.
Treatment of internal parasitism	
Piperazine	
Benzimidazoles	
Organophosphates	
Tetrahydropyrimidines	
Imidazothiazoles	
Milbemycins	
Ivermectins	
Agents used in heartworm treatment and prevention	Briefly review the life stages of the heartworm. Compare characteristics of heartworm infection in dogs and cats. Review the treatment regimen and discuss the health risks associated with it, particularly pulmonary thromboembolism.
Anticestodal drugs	Briefly review the lifecycle of the tapeworm and emphasize the effectiveness of current treatments.
Drugs used to treat giardiasis	Briefly review the lifecycle of *Giardia*. Discuss signs of metronidazole toxicity.
External parasite treatment	Review common external parasites. Demonstrate the broad-spectrum nature of newer external parasite treatments by bringing products to class and reviewing labels and package inserts with the class.
Chlorinated hydrocarbons	
Organophosphates	
Pyrethrins	
Miscellaneous agents	
Antimicrobial agents	Stress the importance of performing culture and sensitivity testing on tissue/fluid from the site of infection in order to determine proper antibiotic selection and to decrease the chance of resistance developing. Review the

Copyright © 2006 by Elsevier, Inc. All rights reserved.

PART FOUR ANESTHESIA AND PHARMACOLOGY

Chapter Outline	Teaching Strategies
	dangers of indiscriminate use of antibiotics. Divide the class into small groups and have each group research a class of antibiotics regarding spectrum of activity, potential toxicities, indication/contraindications, and the development of resistance. They can consult pharmaceutical companies to determine costs. Then have them contact a local veterinarian to find out what antibiotics are kept in stock. Create a chart for the whole class to fill in as groups report on their findings.
Penicillins	Illustrate the chemical structure of penicillin and explain the activity of penicillinase. Explain why Clavamox is a popular antibiotic.
Aminoglycosides	
Cephalosporins	
Quinolones	
Chloramphenicol	
Tetracyclines	
Miscellaneous antibiotics	
Other antimicrobial agents	
Sulfonamides	
Trimethoprim-sulfonamide combinations	
Nitrofurans	
Antifungal agents	Review the various sites of potential fungal infections and stress the difficulty in treating some of them. Compare costs of these drugs, especially to treat large animals and herds.
Hormones and synthetic substitutes	Explain that altered hormone production can be life threatening. Review the disease states associated with deficiencies and excesses of the hormones listed in the chapter. Also, discuss special handling instructions that affect the efficacy of some of these synthetic products.
Insulin	
Oxytocin	
Prostaglandins	
Gastrointestinal drugs	
Antiemetics	Review situations that might call for the use of antiemetics and emetics. Discuss contraindications for both classes of drugs.
Emetics	Explain how knowledge of the cause of emesis determines the choice of drug and give examples.
Antidiarrheal agents	Emphasize that it is crucial to try to find the cause of diarrhea, if possible, so that the causative agent can be removed (for example, giardiasis or coccidiosis). Review indications of prolonged diarrhea and stress the need to treat these potentially life-threatening problems.
Cathartics (laxatives)	
Ulcer management drugs	Review various causes of ulcers and the different treatment options. Compare the options in terms of cost and frequency of dosing.
Drug laws	
State laws	
Federal laws	
Veterinarian-client-patient relationship	
Label requirements	Prepare labels that are missing required information and have the students determine what is missing.
Controlled substances	Review the nomenclature of scheduled drugs and the reason for this system.
Expiration dates and disposal of drugs	
Expiration dates	Review the purpose of recording the drug's expiration date on the label.
Disposal of drugs	Review the legal requirements of disposing of controlled drugs.
Material safety data sheets	Bring several MSDS to class for the students to read. Discuss the functions of OSHA and talk about inspections.
Calculations	For the following types of calculations, provide practice exercises and have the students work in pairs. Both students in the pair perform the same

Copyright © 2006 by Elsevier, Inc. All rights reserved.

CHAPTER 21 Pharmacology and Pharmacy

Chapter Outline	Teaching Strategies
	calculation. When both are done, they check each other's work. If they arrived at different answers, they must work together to determine the correct answer.
Expression of concentration	
Expression of strength	
Calculating the strength of a drug solution	
Calculating the strength of diluted solutions	
Calculating drug dosages	
Calculating infusion rates	
Inventory control	
Inventory maintenance	Discuss the importance of keeping the number of every item in stock as small as possible without running out between reasonable ordering periods.
Procurement	Discuss advantages and disadvantages of purchasing supplies through veterinary wholesale suppliers and directly from manufacturers.
Veterinary suppliers	Bring in catalogs from various veterinary and human medical suppliers. Ask the students to compare the cost and availability of commonly used items.
Veterinary practices	
Pharmacies and drug wholesalers	Provide examples of human products that veterinarians routinely depend upon in their practices.
Human hospitals and hospital suppliers	Point out that human hospitals may be an important source of some supplies, drugs, and nutritional support (for example, parenteral nutrition).
Other sources of suppliers	
Organizing the pharmacy	
Arrangement of inventory	Compare the methods of arranging drugs mentioned in the chapter and discuss advantages and disadvantages of each one.
Compounding	Explain the reason for the existence of Good Manufacturing Practices (GMPs) and give examples. Give examples of drugs that are commonly compounded.
Nutriceuticals	Bring labels from nutraceuticals to class and ask the students to compare the information provided with the information on labels of over-the-counter and prescription drugs.
What are nutraceuticals?	
Regulations of nutraceuticals	Have the students talk about how they would respond to clients who give nutraceuticals to their pets in different clinical situations.
Matters of public concern	
Internet pharmacy	Have the students discuss advantages and disadvantages of ordering medications over the Internet. If any have actually done this and would like to share information, ask them to do so. Ask students to shop around online for specific drugs and compare prices. Their results can be compared to catalog prices and discussed in class.
Concerns about online sites	
Controlled drugs cannot be sold over the Internet	
Regulations	Bring a picture of the VIPPS seal to class.
Advice for customers	

CRITICAL THINKING CHALLENGES

1. Present medical or surgical cases and describe medication regimens. Have the students determine why those particular drugs were chosen, clinical signs of the drugs' effectiveness and toxicity. Have the students explain how they would monitor the patients. Compare their answers with actual results.
2. Using the cases in the previous Critical Thinking Challenge, ask the students to calculate the amount of drug to give using a veterinary drug reference to obtain dosages.

QUIZ

Fill in the answer to each statement.

1. When injecting a drug into a vein that has recently been punctured, relative to the location of the

puncture, the drug must be injected _____ to the existing puncture site.
2. A drug that mimics acetylcholine to cause muscle constriction is _____.
3. It takes _____ half-lives for a drug to reach steady state after dosing has begun.
4. Enterohepatic circulation involves uptake of the drug by the liver, release into the _____, and elimination in the feces.
5. The predominant neurotransmitter in the sympathetic nervous system is _____, and the predominant neurotransmitter in the parasympathetic nervous system is _____.
6. Intraocular pressure can be reduced by administering _____ agents that lower the resistance to outflow of aqueous humor.
7. In the horse, atropine decreases _____ and can lead to gas and toxin complications.
8. A calcium channel blocker used to treat cardiomyopathy in cats is _____.
9. The anthelmintic _____ is generally not safe for Collies and can cause blindness, ataxia, and death in this breed.
10. In the event of overdosage with melarsomine dihydrochloride, the antidote is _____.
11. Hormones produced by the _____ gland affect metabolism of carbohydrates, protein, and fats.
12. Rodents, rabbits, and _____ are unable to vomit.
13. Apomorphine is not recommended for use as an emetic in cats because it causes extreme excitement; however, _____ is a sedative/analgesic that also acts an excellent emetic agent in cats.
14. If an expiration date on a drug label is 09/05, then the drug expires on the _____ day of the month.
15. To convert a number from grams to milligrams, one must _____ the number by _____.
16. In general, inventory turnover should be approximately ____ to _____ times per year.
17. One publication that offers a complete reference to veterinary pharmaceutical companies and their product lines is _____.
18. Refrigerators that store vaccines and biologicals must be kept at _____° C.
19. A drug that is mixed with legal, obtainable ingredients and/or appropriate vehicles that have not been listed as an unapproved drug for animals by the regulatory action of FDA, USDA, or EPA is said to be _____.
20. Omega 3 fatty acids, antioxidants, and glucosamine/chondroitin sulfate are examples of _____.

Answers: (1) proximal, (2) bethanechol HCl, (3) 5, (4) bile, (5) norepinephrine, acetylcholine, (6) anticholinesterase, (7) peristalsis, (8) diltiazem, (9) ivermectin, (10) dimercaprol (BAL), (11) thyroid, (12) horses, (13) xylazine, (14) thirtieth or last, (15) multiply, 1000, (16) 4 to 6, (17) *Compendium of Veterinary Products,* (18) 40, (19) compounded, (20) nutraceuticals. ∎

22

Surgical Instruments and Aseptic Technique

TEACHING/LEARNING OBJECTIVES

1. Name advantages and disadvantages of incising tissues with a surgical laser.
2. Name two purposes of needle holders.
3. Describe the major differences between thumb forceps, tissue forceps, and hemostatic forceps.
4. What is one advantage of the Roeder towel clamp over the Backhaus towel clamp.
5. Name four ways to attach drapes to a wound edge.
6. Describe the difference in shape between a chisel and osteotome.
7. Name an indication for using Gigli wire and a trephine.
8. Identify the sizes of Steinmann pins and Kirschner wires.
9. Describe the difference between points of bone pins and the reasons for using each one.
10. List uses of the arthroscope in the horse and dog.
11. Explain the importance of using an ultrasonic cleaner for surgical instruments.
12. Name two goals to keep in mind when folding surgical gowns.
13. Name exogenous sources of contamination.
14. Name the factors that determine if contamination will progress to infection at a surgical site.
15. Compare the use of muslin versus nonwoven wrappers to wrap packs to be autoclaved.
16. Compare gravity displacement and prevacuum sterilizers and the implications for autoclave time and temperature requirements of each one.
17. List factors that destroy residual bactericidal activity of povidone-iodine.
18. Describe situations in which cold sterilization is indicated.
19. List methods of sterilizing an arthroscope, light cable, and camera.
20. Describe the method of scrubbing a patient for surgery using povidone-iodine and alcohol.
21. Describe and/or perform the two methods of surgical hand/arm scrubs.
22. Describe the sterile area on a scrubbed-in person.

KEY TERMS

Acetabulum
Adson thumb forceps
Allis tissue forceps
Antisepsis
Army-Navy retractor
Arthroscope
Asepsis
Babcock forceps
Backhaus towel clamps
Balfour retractor
Bard-Parker no. 3 handle
Bard-Parker no. 4 handle
Bipolar electrosurgery
Bone pin
Bone plate
Brown-Adson thumb forceps
Cancellous screws
Cold sterilization
Cortical screws
Crile forceps
Curette
DeBakey thumb forceps
Disinfection
Disinfection time
Double-action rongeurs
Doyen intestinal tissue forceps
Dressing thumb forceps
External fixators
Finochietto rib spreader
Frazier tip
Gelpi retractors
Gigli wire
Hall air drill
Halsted mosquito forceps
Hohmann retractor
Interlocking nails
Intramedullary pins
Iodophor
Kelly forceps
Kern bone-holding forceps

Kernison rongeurs
Kirschner wires (K-wires)
Lister bandage scissors
Littauer suture removal scissors
Malleable retractor
Mayo dissecting scissors
Mayo-Hegar needle holders
Meniscus
Metzenbaum dissecting scissors
Michel skin clips
Monopolar electrosurgery
Olsen-Hegar needle holders
Operating scissors
Orthopedic wire
Osteotome
Periosteal elevator
Periosteum
Poole tip
Rat tooth thumb forceps
Rochester-Ochsner forceps
Rochester-Pean forceps
Roeder towel clamps
Russian thumb forceps
Self-retaining bone-holding forceps
Senn retractor
Single-action rongeurs
Sinuscopy
Snook ovariohysterectomy hook
Steinmann pins
Sterilization
Tenoscopy
Trephine
Triangulation
Weitlaner retractor
Wire suture-cutting scissors
Yankauer tip

Chapter Outline	Teaching Strategies
Instrumentation	Bring instruments to class and have students identify them, state their purpose, and indicate situations in which they should not be used.
General surgery instruments	
Scalpel	
Biomedical lasers	
Electrosurgery	
Scissors	Have students cut different materials with different types of scissors to help clarify how inappropriate use of some scissors will destroy them.
Needle holders	Have the students attempt to clamp various sized needles in different needle holders to help clarify that needle holders are designed to hold specific needle sizes.
Thumb forceps	Have the students provide a situation in which each type of forceps (thumb, tissue, and hemostatic) might be used.
Tissue forceps	
Hemostatic forceps	
Retractors	
Suction tips	
Stapling equipment	Review advantages and disadvantages of using staples versus sutures to close incisions.
Michel skin clips	Demonstrate various ways to attach drapes to wound edges and have students provide advantages and disadvantages of each method.
Ophthalmic instruments	
Orthopedic instruments	
Rongeurs	
Bone-holding forceps	Demonstrate the use of these on chicken, ham, and turkey bones or pet toys.
Curettes	
Periosteal elevators	Review the anatomy and function of periosteum. Discuss possible reasons for the use of a periosteal elevator. Have the students determine anatomical structures for which they must be on the lookout when using these instruments.
Osteotomes and chisels	Demonstrate the use of osteotomes on ham, turkey, and chicken bones. Have the students discuss indications for the use of osteotomes, Gigli wire, and trephines.
Gigli wire	
Trephines	
Power equipment	

CHAPTER 22 Surgical Instruments and Aseptic Technique

Chapter Outline	Teaching Strategies
Orthopedic implants	For each type of implant, discuss the role of the veterinary technician in postoperative care of the patient. Review instructions to give owners caring for the pet at home. Show radiographs of the placement of each type of implant.
Bone pins	Explain how to determine the size of a bone pin to use and explain why different points exist. Remind student that they should have several pin sizes available intraoperatively.
Interlocking nails	Provide situations that require the use of interlocking pins instead of intramedullary pins.
Orthopedic wire	
External fixators	Provide indications for external fixators.
Bone screws	Point out the differences between cortical and cancellous screws.
Bone plates	
Total hip prosthesis	
Arthroscopic instruments and equipment	Show a video of this procedure being performed and point out the instruments as they are used.
Arthroscope	
Ancillary arthroscopic equipment	
Sharp trocar and sleeve	
Blunt obturator	
Light cable, light projector, and television camera	
Fluid delivery systems	Review reasons for inflating the joint with fluid during arthroscopy.
Pressurized bag system	
Automated pump system	
Hand instruments for arthroscopic surgery	Ask the students to provide reasons to use the instruments listed during arthroscopic surgery as you point to them.
Blunt probe	
Rongeurs and grasping forceps	
Elevators and osteotomes	
Curettes	
Motorized burrs	
Instrument packs	Set up instrument packs in class. As you set them up, have the student name the instrument and its purpose.
Instrument care	Bring containers of common detergents and lubricants to class. Have students read the labels and/or MSDS for them. Stress the need to allow instruments to completely dry before autoclaving.
Drapes and gowns	Demonstrate ways to fold gowns that allow easy unfolding without contaminating the exterior surface. Have the students demonstrate proficiency with at least one method.
Aseptic technique	Compare sterilization and disinfection and ask the students to provide indications for each method.
Physical methods of sterilization	
Filtration	
Radiation	
Thermal energy	
Autoclave sterilization	Show students how to wrap packs and place sterilization indicators.
Sterilization quality control	Emphasize the need to have regular maintenance performed on autoclaves. Some form of quality control assurance should be a daily duty.
Care and handling of sterile packs	
Chemical methods of sterilization	Give examples of items that might be sterilized with ethylene oxide or hydrogen peroxide gas plasma.
Ethylene oxide	
Hydrogen peroxide gas plasma	
Chemical disinfection	Compare the terms *disinfection, asepsis, antisepsis,* and *sterilization.* Ask the students to provide situations that would require each one.
Antiseptic and disinfectant compounds	Discuss the differences between aqueous, tincture, and detergent formulations of antiseptics.
Iodine	Discuss advantages and disadvantages of iodine-containing compounds for disinfection/antisepsis.

Chapter Outline	Teaching Strategies
Chlorhexidine	Emphasize that this compound has a more rapid onset and longer residual activity than povidone-iodine. Explain how to prepare chlorhexidine to produce a 0.05% solution.
Alcohol	Point out that alcohol has no residual effect and is painful in open wounds.
Phenols	Explain that these compounds are not generally used because they have been replaced by safer, more effective agents.
Quaternary ammonium Chloride	Stress that this is a popular disinfectant, particularly benzalkonium. Emphasize that bleach is commonly used as a disinfectant in many hospitals.
Aldehyde	Point out that formaldehyde and glutaraldehyde are commonly used aldehydes for tissue preservation and chemical sterilization in cold trays, respectively.
Cold sterilization	Stress that cold sterilization does not guarantee complete sterilization.
Sterilization of arthroscopic equipment	Compare advantages and disadvantages of gas and chemical sterilization for arthroscopic equipment.
Operating room preparation	Have the students describe the agents that they would use to clean the operating room and the schedule that they would follow.
Patient preparation	
Surgical clip	Describe common procedures (spay, tracheostomy, celiotomy, chest tube placement, cranial cruciate repair, femoral head and neck excision, etc.) and have the students draw the incision and area to be clipped on an outline of an animal.
Surgical scrub	Compare the use of chlorhexidine gluconate and povidone-iodine as surgical scrubs.
Patient positioning	Review methods of maintaining the patient's position on the surgery table. Have the students describe patient positioning for different procedures.
Surgical team preparation	Scrub, gown, and glove as if you are going to perform surgery. Demonstrate closed, open, and assisted gloving. As you make mistakes, have the students point them out.
Attire	
Hand scrub	
Gowning and gloving	
Maintaining sterility	Once gowned and gloved, outline the sterile area on your body and demonstrate acceptable ways to hold your hands.
Scrubbed-in personnel	On a stuffed animal, demonstrate how to drape the patient for different surgeries.
The patient	
Opening sterile items	Have the nonsterile students open packs for you and demonstrate how to maintain sterility of the unpacked items as they are handed to you.

CRITICAL THINKING CHALLENGES

1. Make a video of a surgical team preparing for surgery. The sterile members scrub, gown, and glove. The nonsterile members open packs and pour saline. Ask the actors to occasionally make intentional breaks in sterility. Have the students find all instances of these breaks and any other inappropriate actions. Alternatively, have several students enact this scene for the class while students raise their hands as mistakes are made.
2. Have students determine what instruments are needed in a spay/neuter, orthopedic, and laparotomy pack and prepare the packs. A list of instruments with pictures can be provided from which the students may choose.
3. Bring instrument catalogs to class and ask the students to pretend to purchase instruments to stock a mixed, large, or small animal clinic. Give them a budget.

QUIZ

Match the statement with the instrument that it describes. Each choice is used only once.
1. ____ These instruments achieve sterilization by producing steam under pressure.
2. ____ These scissors are used to cut more delicate tissue such as fat or thin muscle.
3. ____ Repeated contact with this surgical scrub may rarely lead to the development of thyroid dysfunction.

4. ____ These are named by the number of screw holes in them and the screw diameter that best fits.
5. ____ If left on the arthroscope, residues of this chemical sterilization agent can cause chemical synovitis.
6. ____ These tissue forceps are considered to be traumatic and should only be used on tissue to be removed.
7. ____ This procedure destroys all organisms and spores on an object.
8. ____ This method of sterilization has replaced ethylene oxide sterilization because it is safer for the environment and personnel.
9. ____ These are often used to obtain cancellous bone grafts.
10. ____ This chemical disinfectant is commonly used to preserve tissues for histopathologic assessment.
11. ____ If this happens to a gown or drape, it is no longer sterile.
12. ____ In this type of electrosurgery, no ground plate is needed.
13. ____ These are often placed in the intramedullary canal of long bones to repair fractures.
14. ____ Before the large surgical drape is placed over the patient, these are placed around the area to be incised.
15. ____ These thumb forceps have a broad curved surface that is good for needle handling but traumatic for tissues.
16. ____ Instruments "sterilized" with this method should only be used for minor procedures, and they must be cleaned for at least 3 hours.
17. ____ The contact time for this surgical scrub solution is not as critical as with povidone-iodine.
18. ____ Special glasses must be worn by everyone in the room when this method is used to cut tissue.
19. ____ These forceps are commonly used to crush the ovarian pedicle and body of the uterus during spays and have both longitudinal and cross grooves at the tip.
20. ____ This method of gloving decreases the chance of contamination.

A. Allis tissue forceps
B. Steinmann pins
C. Formaldehyde
D. Metzenbaum scissors
E. Russian thumb forceps
F. Cold sterilization
G. Bipolar
H. Chlorhexidine
I. Hydrogen peroxide gas plasma
J. Quarter drapes
K. Biomedical lasers
L. Glutaraldehyde
M. Povidone-iodine
N. Closed gloving
O. Rochester-Carmalt forceps
P. Bone plate
Q. Sterilization
R. Strike-through
S. Autoclave
T. Curette

Answers: (1) S, (2) D, (3) M, (4) P, (5) L, (6) A, (7) Q, (8) I, (9) T, (10) C, (11) R, (12) G, (13) B, (14) J, (15) E, (16) F, (17) H, (18) K, (19) O, (20) N. ■

23

Surgical Assistance and Suture Material

TEACHING/LEARNING OBJECTIVES

1. List the presurgical duties of the surgical technician.
2. List the intraoperative duties of the surgical technician.
3. List the postsurgical duties of the surgical technician.
4. Drape a patient for abdominal or orthopedic surgery.
5. Set up an instrument table for surgery.
6. Describe the borders of a sterile field.
7. Compare effects of scissors, blades, and high-energy cutting instruments when used to cut skin.
8. Name two ways to prevent leakage of luminal contents during intestinal resection.
9. Describe situations requiring the use of stay sutures.
10. Explain the changes that occur in tissues as a result of leakage of luminal contents from hollow organs and iatrogenic tissue trauma during surgery.
11. Explain why muscles adjacent to fractured bones must be handled as delicately as possible during orthopedic surgery.
12. List three reasons for hemostasis during surgery.
13. Describe one method of ensuring that sponges are not left in the thoracic or abdominal cavity.
14. Demonstrate proper use of hemostatic clamps.
15. List four reasons for incision irrigation and lavage.
16. Describe the ideal lavage fluid.
17. List five functions of suture material.
18. List qualities of ideal suture material.
19. Name two suture materials recommended for use with bladder closure and explain why they are used in this environment.
20. List five synthetic nonabsorbable suture materials and describe advantages and disadvantages of each one.
21. List seven synthetic absorbable suture materials and describe advantages and disadvantages of each one.
22. List three ways in which knots can weaken suture material.
23. Describe how to sterilize suture material that is purchased in bulk.
24. Describe a needle that would be recommended for use to close a hollow viscus.

KEY TERMS

Active drain
Allis tissue forceps
Aseptic
Autoclaving
Backhaus towel clamp
Bipolar electrosurgery
Cutting needle
Cyclopropane
Doyen intestinal forceps
Electrosurgical scalpel
Enterotomy
French-eyed needle
Hemostasis
Hemostats
Holding layers
Iatrogenic
Ischiatic nerve
Knot security
Laparotomy sponges
Mayo scissors
Mayo stand
Memory
Mesocolon
Mesoduodenum
Metzenbaum scissors
Michel clips
Monopolar electrosurgery
Needle holders

Ovarian pedicle
Passive drain
Penrose drain
Phagocytosis
Plasma scalpel
Radial nerve
Retraction
Reverse cutting needle
Scalpel
Seroma
Silver nitrate

Single-eyed needle
Spring needle
Stay sutures
Sterile
Strike-through
Swaged needle
Taper needles
Throw
Ulnar nerve
Viscus

Chapter Outline	Teaching Strategies
Role of the veterinary technician in surgical assistance	Stress the importance of preparing the surgery suite, including having instrument packs and towels ready the day before surgery. Explain that being prepared may help to decrease the time the patient is anesthetized thus making the procedure safer for both the patient and the veterinary team.
Setup of patient and instrument tables	
Positioning the patient	
Draping	Show pictures or a video of a patient being prepared for orthopedic or abdominal surgery. Discuss various methods of draping and types of drapes.
Instrument setup and handling	Demonstrate several ways to set up an instrument tray. Review instrument names and functions.
Sterility in the operating room	Review the boundaries of the sterile field and how to clean an operating room.
Proper tissue handling techniques	
Skin	Give examples of situations in which scissors or instruments other than blades are used to incise skin.
Hollow organ surgery	Emphasize the goals of preventing contamination with luminal contents and gentle tissue handling to prevent iatrogenic trauma and delayed healing.
Musculoskeletal surgery	Review the course of the radial, ulnar, and ischiatic nerves and abdominal anatomy. Show photos of nerves, blood vessels, and abdominal organs being retracted. Stress the reasons for keeping gloves and sponges moistened during retraction.
Retraction techniques	
Hemostasis	Review the blood clotting mechanism.
Sponge hemostasis	Demonstrate the use of a sponge forceps and laboratory sponges. Discuss sequelae of inadvertently leaving surgical sponges in the abdomen or thoracic cavity and how this is diagnosed and treated.
Sponge complications	
Hemostatic forceps	Have different types of hemostatic forceps in the classroom and discuss situations requiring the use of each one.
Suture ligation	Practice using hemostatic forceps with shoestrings (representing blood vessels) and suture material. Tie ligatures as students control the clamps.
Electrosurgery	Compare monopolar and bipolar electrocautery. Discuss advantages and disadvantages of each method.
Electrocoagulation and cutting function	
Monopolar and bipolar electrosurgical modes	
Battery-powered cautery units	
Safety with electrosurgery	Review safety precautions that must be taken when using electrosurgery.
Hemostatic agents	Bring gelatin sponges, bone wax, bovine dermal collagen, and cellulose gauze to class and demonstrate the use of each one. Discuss benefits and drawbacks of each one.

Copyright © 2006 by Elsevier, Inc. All rights reserved.

108 PART FIVE SURGICAL AND MEDICAL NURSING

Chapter Outline	Teaching Strategies
Chemical cauterization	
Vascular clips	
Incision irrigation and suction	Review the reasons for irrigating and suctioning incisions and surgical sites.
Lavage fluid	Ask the students to list characteristics of an ideal lavage solution and to describe the results of using hypertonic, hypotonic, and excessively acidic or basic solutions.
Lavage technique	Bring single- and multifenestrated suction tips to class and discuss uses of each. Demonstrate how to unplug the tips.
Surgical drains	Define active and passive drain and bring examples of each to class. Provide examples of situations calling for each kind of drain to be used.
Passive drains	
Active drains	
Suture material	Bring a variety of suture material to class and ask the students to observe their memory and knot security.
Qualities of ideal suture material	
Suture nomenclature	Compare absorbable and nonabsorbable, mono- and multifilament suture materials. Discuss advantages and disadvantages of each.
Absorbable suture material	
Synthetic absorbable suture material	
Nonabsorbable suture material	
Synthetic nonabsorbable suture material	
Suture size and strength	Stress that the knot is the strength-limiting area of most suture material. Discuss this fact as it relates to characteristics of coefficient of friction, changes in longitudinal tensile force, and abrading suture material as knots are made.
Suture reaction	Discuss the effects of infection and inflammation on reactive sutures.
Preparation of suture material	Stress that expiration dates must be respected. Demonstrate methods of opening suture packs. Review the process of autoclaving and discuss its effects on some suture materials.
Suture needles	Bring various needles to class and demonstrate their use on different materials. Discuss the shape, point design, method of attachment to the suture, and size as they relate to trauma, air-tight and water-tight seals, and hemorrhage.

ACTIVITY

Describe possible real-life situations and ask students to fill in the blanks.

EXAMPLE

While you are assisting with a long surgery to remove a string foreign body from a cat's intestine, the surgeon becomes concerned that the tissues are desiccating. He asks you to lavage the abdomen. You have prepared a 10% solution of povidone-iodine and physiologic saline by adding _____ ml of povidone-iodine to _____ ml of saline. Because the intestines were so inflamed, the surgeon chooses a(n) _____ suture.

CRITICAL THINKING CHALLENGES

1. Present various surgical scenarios. Ask the students to anticipate the suture material and needle that the surgeon will use and justify the selections. Alternatively, provide a suture material and ask the students to determine if it is an appropriate choice. If not, ask them to explain why not.
2. List surgeries that are scheduled on a typical day at a veterinary clinic. Ask the students to make a checklist of their duties before, during, and after surgery. It is Monday and surgeries will be performed on Wednesday.
3. Role-play. One student is the surgeon, one is the surgical assistant, and one is the assistant who runs

Copyright © 2006 by Elsevier, Inc. All rights reserved.

for items and who enters and leaves the operating room as needed. The students must demonstrate knowledge of gowning, gloving, boundaries of the sterile field, draping the patient, setting up and placement of an instrument tray, passing instruments to the surgeon, opening suture material, and instrument identification and their uses.

QUIZ

Circle T (true) or F (false) for each statement.

1. T F Low-pressure bleeding from small vessels can usually be controlled with gentle wiping motion of a moist sponge.
2. T F Instruments should not be soaked in saline solution because this can cause corrosion.
3. T F Monofilament nylon suture material should not be used for skin sutures that are to be removed.
4. T F 7-0 suture material is more likely to be used in orthopedic surgery than ophthalmic surgery.
5. T F Polyglyconate and polydioxanone sutures take approximately 180 days to be completely absorbed.
6. T F Once a sterile drape is placed on a patient it can only be moved toward the sterile site if it needs to be adjusted.
7. T F Enzymatic hydrolysis of surgical suture material tends to induce a more significant inflammatory reaction than phagocytosis induced by surgical gut.
8. T F Incision of skin with high-energy cutting instruments such as an electrosurgical scalpel usually causes less hemorrhage than use of blades.
9. T F 3/8 curved needles are commonly used in ophthalmic surgery.
10. T F Synthetic multifilament suture is more reactive than synthetic monofilament suture.
11. T F Stay sutures are sutures placed in a simple interrupted pattern in order to avoid leakage of contaminated organ contents.
12. T F Hypotonic lavage solutions decrease edema in tissues.
13. T F The sterile field extends from 5 cm above the shoulder to the level of the cuff of the sleeve.
14. T F Knot security increases as suture size increases.
15. T F Silver nitrate is commonly used to control bleeding from nail beds during nail trimmings.
16. T F Passive drains such as Penrose drains depend on the application of negative pressure or suction.
17. T F Taper needles should not be used when closing a urinary bladder.
18. T F The spring needle is the most atraumatic needle one can use.
19. T F Antibiotics diminish a cancellous bone graft's biologic activity.
20. T F Cloth drapes that become damp during surgery can wick bacteria onto the surgical site.

Answers: (1) F, (2) T, (3) F, (4) F, (5) T, (6) F, (7) F, (8) T, (9) F, (10) T, (11) F, (12) F, (13) F, (14) F, (15) T, (16) F, (17) F, (18) F, (19) T, (20) T. ■

24

Small Animal Surgical Nursing

TEACHING/LEARNING OBJECTIVES

1. List indications for prophylactic antibiotics.
2. Describe methods of keeping patients warm during surgery.
3. List clinical signs of pain in small animals.
4. List means to prevent animals from licking and chewing surgical incisions.
5. Explain causes of wound dehiscence.
6. Explain potential sequelae of thoracic or abdominal complete dehiscence.
7. List indications that a bandage has been placed too tightly.
8. When are drains typically removed?
9. List potential complications of feline onychectomy in the immediate postoperative period and later.
10. Explain how to clip a small animal for an exploratory celiotomy.
11. Describe how to handle abdominal viscera during a celiotomy.
12. Explain the role of omentum in abdominal surgery.
13. Describe the duties of the surgical assistant during intestinal anastomosis and resection.
14. Explain why trocharization may need to be performed on a pet with gastric dilatation-volvulus and how it is done.
15. List potential postoperative complications that the veterinary technician must monitor carefully.
16. List reasons to perform ovariohysterectomy in an adult dog or cat.
17. Explain how to treat scrotal hemorrhage or seromas after castration.
18. List indications for feline castration.
19. Describe common postoperative observations after cystotomy to remove calculi.
20. Explain ways to stimulate respiration in neonates during a cesarean delivery.
21. Explain why mechanical ventilation or intermittent manual respiration is necessary during diaphragmatic hernia repair.
22. List potential postoperative complications of neurologic patients and describe methods of preventing each one.
23. List the duties of the surgical assistant during the reduction of long bone fractures.
24. Explain why articular cartilage should never be in direct contact with retractors during joint surgery.

KEY TERMS

Anastomosis
Arteriovenous fistula
Atlantoaxial subluxation
Broad ligament
Carpometacarpal joint
Cauda equina
Celiotomy
Cellulitis
Dorsal laminectomy
Doxapram
Dystocia
Electrocautery
Endotoxemia
Eunuchoid syndrome
Evisceration
Exploratory celiotomy
Falciform fat
Flank incision
Gravid uterus
Hematoma
Hemilaminectomy
Hydrometra
Inguinal canal
Intervertebral disk fenestration
Intestinal ileus
Intussusception
Laparotomy
Linea alba
Manubrium sterni

CHAPTER 24 Small Animal Surgical Nursing

Mastectomy
Metastasis
Mucometra
Nymphomania
Oxytocin
Paracostal incision
Paramedian incision
Parapreputial incision
Pedicles
Pneumothorax
Pseudocyesis

Radical mastectomy
Scrotal ablation
Seroma
Splenectomy
Strike-through
Tarsometatarsal joint
Trocharization
Ventral slot
Wound dehiscence

Chapter Outline	Teaching Strategies
General principles of surgical nursing	
Preoperative patient assessment	Review the preoperative role of the veterinary technician regarding various situations including the pet that has eaten shortly before surgery, the febrile animal, the dehydrated animal, and the fractious animal.
Surgical preparation and animal positioning	Discuss methods of preparing a surgery suite for surgery (include cleaning, sterility/disinfection, heating pad, instrument tray, lights, etc.). For each surgical procedure in the chapter, have diagrams showing the appropriate clipping (include a description of landmarks) and positioning. Emphasize that each patient may have slightly different requirements and that some surgeons have specific preferences.
Perioperative antibiotics	See Chapter 21.
Monitoring	See Chapter 19.
Blood loss	Review potential sites of blood loss during and after surgery and associated clinical signs. Review normal blood parameters for cats, dogs, and other small animals. Have the students describe methods of keeping pets warm during and after surgery.
Hypothermia	
Pain	Review the role of preanesthetic medications in controlling pain. Have the students discuss their role in preventing and managing their patients' pain.
Incision evaluation	Review indications of infection around any incision. Show photos of infected incisions. Have the students discuss treatment options for infections and associated clinical signs to anticipate. Have students discuss their role in preventing incision infections, includes strategies to prevent licking and chewing at incisions postoperatively.
Bandage care	See Chapter 4. Show photos of complications arising from bandages placed too tightly. Have the students practice giving instructions to owners regarding incision and bandage care at home.
Drain care	Discuss nursing care implications in the event of strike-through with incisions or drains.
Restraint	See Chapters 1 and 19.
Common surgical procedures	For all surgical procedures, obtain photos and/or diagrams that illustrate the pertinent anatomy, restraint, surgical site preparation, and patient positioning. Students can practice some restraint techniques with stuffed animals.
Elective versus nonelective surgery	For all surgical procedures, have the students list instruments and equipment that will or may be needed and any special postoperative care that should be anticipated.
Tail docking on puppies	Stress the importance of performing this procedure during the first week of age along with dewclaw removal, if desired.
Dewclaw removal	Stress the importance of performing this procedure during the first week of age along with tail docking, if desired.
Tail docking and dewclaw removal in the adult	Compare indications for these procedures between adults and puppies, particularly postoperative care.
Feline onychectomy	Emphasize that this is a painful procedure for which analgesics should always be administered.

Copyright © 2006 by Elsevier, Inc. All rights reserved.

Chapter Outline	Teaching Strategies
Celiotomy	Review the intraoperative implications of preparing a surgical area that is neither wide nor long enough.
Gastrointestinal surgery	Review ways in which the veterinary surgical assistant can help (for example, counting sponges, traction, keeping structures moist, and suctioning). Have the students determine the possible effects if any of these activities are performed inappropriately.
Gastric dilatation and volvulus	Emphasize that mortality is 100% with this disease if it is not treated early. Review critical roles of the veterinary technician during treatment of dogs with GDV such as immediate catheter placement and fluid administration, setting up a selection of stomach tubes and bucket with warm water, trocharization, obtaining appropriate radiographs, and preparing the animal for surgery. Present various clinical scenarios of postoperative complications and ask the students how they would respond, including pulse deficits, arrhythmias, inappetence, vomiting, and fever.
Ovariohysterectomy in the dog and cat	Review the potential sequelae of incomplete removal of an ovary. Ask the students to explain the most common postoperative complication, clinical signs, how it is treated, and how it might have been prevented.
Pyometra	Stress the need to make the surgical site long and wide for patients with pyometra to avoid rupturing a potentially friable uterus as it is removed from the abdomen.
Canine castration	Remind students that clipping the scrotum is not recommended unless scrotal ablation is to be performed.
Feline castration	Stress the importance of substituting shredded paper for gravel litter after this procedure and declawing.
Cesarean delivery	Emphasize the important role of the veterinary technician in helping to stimulate neonates to breathe. Review various techniques.
Cystotomy	Review methods of flushing the lower urinary tract and have the students describe the equipment that will be needed.
Urethrostomy	Stress the importance of substituting shredded paper for gravel litter postsurgically.
Hernias	
Umbilical hernias	Explain that breeding pets with congenital umbilical hernias is not recommended.
Inguinal hernias	Emphasize that although the hernia may be unilateral, herniation may occur through the opposite ring at a later point in time.
Diaphragmatic hernia	Show radiographs of diaphragmatic hernias. Review the procedure of induction for the patient undergoing surgery to correct a diaphragmatic hernia.
Lumpectomy	Remind students that a wide area around the lesion should be prepared presurgically because the surgeon may want to remove up to 3 cm of surrounding skin.
Removal of mammary neoplasia	Compare the behavior and required treatment of mammary neoplasia in cats and dogs. Remind students that it is important to have containers of formalin ready during surgery in order to submit sections for histopathology interpretations.
Amputation	Remind students that considerable blood can be lost during this surgery; therefore, all supplies needed for a blood transfusion should be on hand. Have the students compare postoperative care of patients with an amputation, intervertebral disk disease, and long bone fracture.
Neurologic patient care	Stress the importance of minimizing trauma when moving or handling the patient. Review ways to prevent decubitus sores, gastrointestinal ulceration, pneumonia, joint stiffness, and urinary bladder infections.
Orthopedic surgery	
Long-bone fractures	Emphasize that preparation of the surgical area is time-consuming and that the veterinary technician must manage time wisely before these surgeries. In addition to preparing the patient, the technician often assists during long bone fracture reduction.
Joints	Review the various types of cartilage and how they tend to respond to trauma. Stress the importance of avoiding direct contact with articular cartilage during surgery. Have the students research the developmental physiology of hyaline cartilage.
Client education	Bring examples of client handouts to class from several local veterinary clinics. Have the students compare and discuss them.

CHAPTER 24 Small Animal Surgical Nursing

CRITICAL THINKING CHALLENGES

1. Divide the students into pairs and give each pair the name of a surgery mentioned in the chapter and the signalment of a pet on a piece of paper. Have them role-play. One student is the veterinary technician and one is the owner. The owners have just been told by the veterinarian that their pet must have a certain operation, or the owner has questions regarding an elective surgery and the veterinarian is not available to speak with him or her. The owner has many questions. The students should be able to describe the reason for surgery, potential intraoperative and postoperative complications and what the technician (with instructions from the veterinarian) will do to prevent and/or treat them, how the owner will handle the pet at home, and various scenarios if the surgery is not performed. Provide questions for the students who play the role of the owners if their questions are not thorough.
2. Have the students develop premedication, induction, general anesthetic, and postoperative pain control protocols for each surgery in the chapter. With each drug, ask them to describe the side effects to be anticipated and how they will respond if the side effects occur.

QUIZ

Match each statement with the surgical procedure to which it refers. Each choice is used only once.

1. _____ Gastropexy is usually performed to treat this disease in order to prevent rotation, but bloating can still occur.
2. _____ The contents of the abdomen, fat or intestines, is excised or replaced, respectively, and the incision is closed.
3. _____ This procedure should be performed when the animal is approximately 3 to 5 days old, at the time of the dewclaw removal.
4. _____ All germinal epithelium must be removed and pain medication is recommended for at least 4 to 5 days postoperatively.
5. _____ The veterinary technician must be ready to help stimulate neonates' respiration during this procedure and prepare for ovariohysterectomy in some cases.
6. _____ The uterus, intestines, broad ligament, or other abdominal organ can protrude through the rent.
7. _____ This procedure may be performed to remove a large foreign object from the stomach.
8. _____ This disease typically occurs 4 to 6 weeks following estrus and is usually treated with ovariohysterectomy.
9. _____ The patient is placed under general anesthesia and the transection is made at the carpometacarpal joint and/or tarsometatarsal joint.
10. _____ If a section of intestines must be removed, this procedure is performed to recreate a continuous flow of ingesta in the intestines.
11. _____ If the procedure is performed to remove cystoliths, the entire lower urinary tract must be flushed with sterile saline solution until all calculi are removed and before closure.
12. _____ The patient is placed under general anesthesia, a tourniquet may be used, and the skin incision is made 1 to 2 cm distal to the expected disarticulation.
13. _____ This procedure may be done to help determine the cause of abdominal pain.
14. _____ This procedure should be performed when the animal is approximately 3 to 5 days old at the time of the tail docking.
15. _____ If scrotal ablation is also to be performed, the scrotum is clipped and prepared aseptically with the rest of the surgical field.
16. _____ Indications for this procedure include irresolvable osteomyelitis, nonunion fractures that will not result in limb function with orthopedic repair, and arteriovenous fistulas.
17. _____ Movement of these patients must be minimized as much as possible especially after they are anesthetized.
18. _____ If this procedure is performed before the first estrus, the chance of mammary neoplasia is greatly reduced.
19. _____ Thoracic radiographs should always be performed before this surgery to check for metastasis.
20. _____ Scrotal hairs are gently plucked with the thumb and forefingers.
21. _____ An indwelling chest tube may be placed before this surgery to allow periodic aspiration of air from the pleural space.
22. _____ Sections from these tissues should always be submitted for histologic evaluation; the surgical assistant should have formalin ready during these procedures.
23. _____ The surgical assistant helps with retraction and to cause muscle fatigue so that alignment and reduction can be performed.
24. _____ Stricture is a common postoperative complication and can manifest as stranguria.
25. _____ A foreign body lodged in the intestines can be removed via this procedure.
26. _____ Retractors should never be placed directly on articular cartilage and the cartilage must be kept moist.

A. Mammary neoplasia removal
B. Tail dock of puppy
C. Cystotomy

D. Gastrotomy
E. Diaphragmatic hernia
F. Canine castration
G. Dewclaw removal
H. Cesarean delivery
I. Onychectomy
J. Urethrostostomy
K. Gastric dilatation volvulus
L. Lumpectomy
M. Enterotomy
N. Inguinal hernia
O. Tail Dock of adult
P. Declaw of adult
Q. Joint surgery
R. Feline castration
S. Pyometra
T. Umbilical hernia
U. Long bone fracture
V. Celiotomy
W. Amputation
X. Surgery for neurologic disorders
Y. Anastomosis
Z. Ovariohysterectomy

Answers: (1) K, (2) T, (3) B, (4) I, (5) H, (6) N, (7) D, (8) S, (9) P, (10) Y, (11) C, (12) O, (13) V, (14) G, (15) F, (16) W, (17) X, (18) Z, (19) A, (20) R, (21) E, (22) L, (23) U, (24) J, (25) M, (26) Q. ■

25

Small Animal Medical Nursing

TEACHING/LEARNING OBJECTIVES

1. List four reasons for the veterinary technician to apply knowledge of good grooming and bathing care to patients.
2. Describe a systematic method of bathing dogs.
3. Explain how to force-feed a hospitalized pet.
4. Name three reasons for regular nail trimmings.
5. Explain specific concerns regarding nail trimmings in pets with dark, pigmented nails and pets whose nails are not trimmed regularly.
6. Explain what products to use to clean a pet's ears if the integrity of the tympanum is not known.
7. Describe ways to prevent decubital sores from developing.
8. What is a disadvantage of taking a patient's temperature only once daily?
9. Describe a normal sinus arrhythmia.
10. What are the normal systolic and diastolic blood pressures in dogs and cats?
11. Explain why a urine specific gravity of >1.035 in dogs and >1.040 in cats with normal renal concentrating ability is an indication of dehydration.
12. Describe how to give subcutaneous fluids to a 30-lb dog over the course of 24 hours.
13. Give reasons for falsely elevated central venous pressure.
14. List the diagnostic tests that must be performed on each dog or cat donating blood and explain why this information is essential to have on file.
15. List reasons for giving plasma transfusions.
16. To help prevent transfusion reactions, what can be done before starting the transfusion?
17. Describe how to use superficial heat and cold packs as physical therapy modalities.
18. Name two factors that can alter arterial blood gas values.
19. Describe ideal positioning of the patient with pulmonary problems and explain your answer.
20. Explain why measles virus vaccine is commonly used to protect puppies against distemper virus.
21. Differentiate diagnostic procedures used to diagnose dermatophytosis and demodicosis.
22. Describe clinical signs associated with right-sided and left-sided heart failure.
23. Compare the causes, typical signalment, clinical signs, diagnostic tests, and treatments for hyperadrenocorticism and hypoadrenocorticism in the dog.
24. Name the treatments for hyperthyroidism in cats and briefly explain how each works.
25. What sodium/potassium ratio is expected in a dog with hypoadrenocorticism?
26. Describe basic factors to assess and treat for a patient with acute gastroenteritis.
27. Describe the best way to prevent parvovirus in a dog.
28. List the most frequently prescribed preventive measures for feline lower urinary tract disease.
29. List the different etiologies of canine hip dysplasia.
30. List several preventive measures for canine uroliths.

KEY TERMS

Acetabulum
Acute moist dermatitis
Addison disease
Anal gland
Anal sac
Anaphylaxis
Anestrus
Annulus fibrosus
Ascites
Azotemia
Bedsores
Blepharospasm
Burrow solution
Cardiomegaly
Central venous pressure
Cerumen
Chemosis
Colostrum
Complement system

Copyright © 2006 by Elsevier, Inc. All rights reserved.   115

Contemporary fluid losses
Coupage
Cushing disease
Decubital sores
Demodicosis
Dermatophytosis
Diastolic blood pressure
Diathermy
Dilated cardiomyopathy
Disseminated intravascular coagulation (DIC)
Distichiasis
Districhiasis
Diurnal
Dyspnea
Entropion
Episcleral blood vessels
Feline lower urinary tract disease (FLUTD)
Feline urologic syndrome (FUS)
Force feeding
Gastric gavage
Glucocorticoid
Glucosuria
Hemoconcentration
Hemoptysis
Hot spot
Hyperadrenocorticism
Hyperpnea
Hypertrophic cardiomyopathy
Hyperventilation
Hypoadrenocorticism
Hypoxia
Insensible fluid losses
Isotonic fluids
Keratoconjunctivitis sicca (KCS)
Ketonemia
Ketonuria
Labored breathing
Left-sided heart failure
Mineralocorticoid
Mitotane
Mitral valve
Mitral valvular fibrosis
Nuclear sclerosis
Nucleus pulposus
Occult heartworm disease
Orthopnea
Otitis externa
Otodectes
Paroxysmal coughing
Pitting edema
Pleural effusion
Poikilothermic
Point of maximal intensity
Polydipsia
Polyphagia
Polyuria
Pulmonary edema
Pulse deficit
Pulse oximeter
Rales
Restrictive cardiomyopathy
Right-sided heart failure
Saprophyte
Schiøtz tonometer
Sensible fluid losses
Sinus arrhythmia
Skin turgor
Syncope
Systolic blood pressure
Tachycardia
Tachypnea
Thromboembolism
Tonopen
Tricuspid valve
Tympanum
Urine scald
Urticaria
Valvular insufficiency
Zoonosis

Chapter Outline	Teaching Strategies
General care	In this chapter, have the students determine drug regimens based on information from Chapters 19 to 21.
Bathing	Stress the need to protect the eyes and ears every time a pet is bathed.
Exercise	
Feeding	See Chapter 15.
Nail trimming	Bring different types of nail trimmers to class and demonstrate their appropriate use. Bring various products that are used to stop bleeding nails to class.
Ear cleaning	Review the anatomy of the ear. Show photos of healthy ears and ears with bacterial and yeast infections and mite infestations. Have the students discuss potential sequelae of using inappropriate agents to clean ears if the tympanic membrane is ruptured.
Anal sacs	Stress that regular expressions are discouraged. Review clinical signs of anal sac disease.

CHAPTER 25 Small Animal Medical Nursing

Chapter Outline	Teaching Strategies
Bedding	Review the potential negative effects of using gravel litter with cats that have undergone common surgical procedures.
Decubital sores	Show photos of animals with decubital sores. Stress that prevention can be achieved with attentive nursing care, proper bedding, and regular patient rotations.
Geriatric nursing	Have the students discuss ways that they can help to make the geriatric pet's visit or hospitalization less stressful.
Pediatric nursing	See Chapter 12.
Practical nursing procedures	
Temperature	Have the students convert several temperatures form Fahrenheit to Celsius and vice versa.
Pulse	On a diagram or a student's pet, point out the sites commonly used to monitor pulse rate and character and point of maximal intensity. Bring a blood pressure machine to class and have the students take readings on their own pets. Review basic interpretation of an EKG tracing and point out a normal sinus arrhythmia. Discuss various pulse characters and their potential causes. Have the students give reasons for pulse deficits to exist.
Respiration	Have the students bring their pets to class and monitor their respiratory rates and character.
Administration of medications	See Chapter 21.
Fluid therapy	Have the students practice calculating fluid requirements of different animals.
Routes of administration	Have students discuss the safest way to administer fluids to a patient with renal disease, cardiac disease, or hypoproteinemia.
Central venous pressure	Have the students give reasons for repeating a central venous pressure measurement.
Blood transfusion	Have the students discuss reasons for determining the blood type of the donor and recipient before transfusion in cats and dogs. Students can bring their dogs to class and perform blood typing and cross-matches. Ask them to decide from whose pet they would allow their own pet to receive blood.
Blood donors	Compare reasons for giving plasma transfusions, packed red blood cell, and whole blood. Have the students research acellular oxygen-carrying replacement fluids and explain why they would or would not prefer to uses these systems for red blood cell replacement.
Blood collection	
Transfusion reactions	Compare the causes and clinical signs associated with various types of transfusion reactions. Have the students discuss steps that they can take before the procedure begins that may help to prevent these reactions.
Delayed hemolytic reactions	
Transfusion-induced fever	
Nonimmunologic	
Transfusion reactions	
Physical therapy	Have the students describe injuries or diseases that they think would respond positively to physical therapy and explain why. Discuss reasons why some modalities would be indicated and others contraindicated.
Oxygen therapy	Stress that oxygen toxicity is possible with an inspired oxygen concentration greater than 40%. Discuss the advantages and disadvantages of each method of oxygen delivery.
Oxygen cage	
Mask induction	
Intratracheal catheter Induction	
Nasal catheter Induction	
Respiratory physical therapy	Have the students describe the role of the veterinary technician in treating the patient with or at risk of developing pulmonary disease.
Topical therapy	Bring various topical products to class and have the class compare the ingredients and indications. Emphasize that some topical therapy may help cleanse and heal the lesions but the cause of the problem should be determined and treated, if possible. Describe dermatologic conditions in different animals and ask the students to choose the best topical therapy and explain their answers.

Copyright © 2006 by Elsevier, Inc. All rights reserved.

Chapter Outline	Teaching Strategies
Soaks	
Astringents	
Baths	
Dips and rinses	
Powders	
Creams and ointments	
Otic preparations	
Infectious diseases	Have the students create nursing plans for an animal diagnosed with each of the infectious diseases mentioned. The plan should include clinical parameters to assess, methods of transmission prevention, and how to disinfect the area where the animal has stayed after discharge.
Canine respiratory disease complex	
Feline respiratory disease complex	
Canine distemper	
Feline panleukopenia	
Feline leukemia virus and feline immunodeficiency virus infection	
Routine immunization program for dogs and cats	See Chapter 11.
Colostral antibodies	Explain the role of colostrum in the neonate's defense system and how it interferes with vaccinations.
Type of vaccine	Bring copies of package inserts from various vaccines to class. Discuss differences in their reconstitution, storage, handling, and frequency and route of administration. Emphasize the need to strictly adhere to the manufacturers' recommendations to achieve maximum efficacy of vaccination protocols.
Route of administration	
Age of patient	
Nutritional status	
Concurrent disease or therapy	
Program guidelines	
Vaccine reactions	Review various clinical signs associated with vaccine reactions and how to prevent and treat them.
Pet-associated zoonoses	See Chapter 35.
Canine brucellosis	
Toxoplasmosis	
Campylobacter and *Salmonella*	
Leptospirosis	
Plague	
Cat scratch disease	
Rabies	
Ophthalmology	Review anatomy and physiology of the eye.
Glaucoma	Explain the mechanisms of fluid inflow and outflow balance.
Cataracts	Review the differences between true cataracts and nuclear sclerosis. Bring photos of each to class and explain how they are differentiated.
Corneal ulcers	Show photos of different ulcers along with varying degrees of fluorescein stain retention. Review proper methods of administering ophthalmic medications.
Dermatology	Show photos of skin lesions and their associated microscopic diagnostic pictures. Ask the students to describe how they would collect a sample for testing if demodicosis or dermatophytosis is suspected.
Skin scraping	
Cardiology	Review the anatomy and physiology of the circulatory system.
Congestive heart failure	Have the students determine clinical signs to look for with patients diagnosed with right- or left-sided heart failure. How will they prepare for these signs and what will they do if they present?
Mitral insufficiency	
Heartworm disease	Bring different heartworm preventative products to class and stress the importance of prevention versus treatment. Contact a few local veterinary clinics to find out how much it costs to treat an infected adult dog and compare this amount with the cost of giving preventives.

Copyright © 2006 by Elsevier, Inc. All rights reserved.

Chapter Outline	Teaching Strategies
Canine heartworm disease	
Feline heartworm disease	
Cardiomyopathy	Compare the functional heart changes and resulting clinical signs of hypertrophic, dilated, and restrictive cardiomyopathy. Show ECG tracings of each and ask students to identify the patterns. Have the students imagine that they are parts of the circulatory system and organs (atria, ventricles, valves, pulmonary arteries, aorta, cranial and caudal vena cava, liver, lungs, etc.). Describe the pathology occurring in a valve or chamber and ask the students to explain what they would experience as this disease became chronic.
Feline cardiomyopathy	
Canine cardiomyopathy	
Endocrinology	Review the anatomy and functions of the adrenal glands, hypothalamus, pituitary gland, pancreas, and thyroid, and parathyroid glands.
Canine hyperadrenocorticism	For all endocrine disorders, ask the students to list the clinical signs that a patient might demonstrate and to explain how the veterinary technician can help to treat the patient and promote a more comfortable hospital stay. Review the hypothalamic-pituitary-adrenal axis and provide examples of various abnormal responses within this axis. Because diagnosing adrenal diseases might be difficult, present different tests and ask the students to imagine what results would indicate an abnormality. For example, if ACTH is administered, what response is expected and what might be an abnormal response?
Canine hypoadrenocorticism	
Hypoglycemia	Review the metabolism of glucose, including its production, storage, and catabolism. Discuss normal values and the variety of potential presentations of animals with hypoglycemia. Have the students review means of restoring glucose to a normal level (foods, fluids, insulin, etc.)
Hypothyroidism and hyperthyroidism	Review the anatomy and functions of the thyroid and parathyroid glands. Have the students correlate an excess or deficiency of hormones to expected clinical signs.
Diabetes mellitus	Have the students write out step-by-step owner instructions for storage, handling, and administration of insulin, when *not* to give it, and clinical signs to be aware of that indicate that the pet might be under- or overdosed.
Theriogenology	See Chapter 17.
Postpartum disorders in the bitch	
Canine brucellosis	
Pyometritis (Pyometra)	
Canine prostatic disease	
Gastroenterology	
Acute gastroenteritis	Discuss the three key elements of treating acute gastroenteritis: dietary restriction, medication administration, and fluid therapy. Ask the students to practice taking a dietary history from an owner. Provide several case scenarios of animals with varying degrees of gastroenteritis and have the students explain how they would determine the hydration status, the fluids and medications they would give, and how they would give them.
Canine viral enteritis	Compare and contrast coronavirus and parvovirus infections in dogs. Ask the students to describe how these pets should be hospitalized and handled and why.
Nephrology and urology	Review the anatomy and function of the urinary tract.
Canine uroliths	Show radiographs of different types and locations of stones. Review diets intended to control the production of stones. Have the students develop client handouts that present the topic of urolith prevention and treatment.
Feline lower urinary tract disease	Review preventive measures. Emphasize the potentially life-threatening nature of this disease.
Chronic renal failure	Discuss the components of supportive therapy for chronic renal failure patients, including reasons for each one and potential reasons to not do them.
Orthopedics	
Canine hip dysplasia	Review the anatomy of the coxofemoral joint and show radiographs of different degrees of severity. Discuss medical management versus surgical management and have the students interpret their role in each method.

Chapter Outline	Teaching Strategies
Intervertebral disk disease	Define chondrodystrophied and nonchondrodystrophied. Review the anatomy and function of intervertebral disks and causes of diseases. Discuss the veterinary technician's role in patient management after intervertebral disk surgery and surgery to correct canine hip dysplasia.

CRITICAL THINKING CHALLENGES

1. Present case histories and have the students describe how they would provide the best possible nursing care. For example, the geriatric canine patient with congestive heart failure requires quite different care than the adult dog that has undergone surgery to treat intervertebral disk disease.
2. A client's dog (or cat) has been diagnosed with heartworm disease. Have the student explain the cause of this disease to the owner, the treatment, potential side effects of treatment, lifestyle requirements after treatment, and prevention. Include pretreatment of the pet before admission to the hospital.
3. As a patient's clinical signs resolve during hospitalization, indications of other problems may be exposed. It is important for the veterinary technician to be able to anticipate these challenges. For example, as hyperthyroidism is treated, signs of underlying renal disease may manifest. Ask the students to predict what to expect as animals are treated for different disorders and explain what should be on hand for treatment, diagnosis, and nursing care.
4. Invite representatives from different pet nutrition companies to speak to your class. Ask them to focus on diets formulated specifically for disease states such as renal and liver diseases and cardiomyopathies. Students should be able to explain reasons for the inclusion of various ingredients. Have them role-play and explain to an owner in basic terms why a particular diet is recommended. Ask the students to compare similar diets marketed by different companies.

QUIZ

Circle T (true) or F (false) for each statement below.

1. T F Canine blood donors that weigh 50 lb can theoretically have 500 to 1000 ml of blood drawn every 3 weeks.
2. T F If dextrose solution of more that 2.5% is given subcutaneously, skin may slough and abscesses may form.
3. T F Dogs receiving dexamethasone for intervertebral disk disease may develop secondary problems such as anorexia, abdominal pain, acute pancreatitis, and gastrointestinal hemorrhaging.
4. T F Modified live virus vaccines are not recommended in dogs and cats receiving immunosuppressive agents as with cancer or autoimmune disease.
5. T F If serial readings of central venous pressure on a dog are 10 cm, 8 cm, and 9 cm, then intravenous fluid administration rate should be increased.
6. T F Appetite stimulants may increase interest in eating but do not assure adequate intake by the patient.
7. T F Sensible and insensible fluid loss can be calculated as approximately 60 ml/lb/ day.
8. T F All transfusion reactions occur within 1 hour of beginning the procedure.
9. T F The pulse oximeter measures hemoglobin saturation in peripheral blood vessels.
10. T F It is recommended that anal sacs be expressed regularly.
11. T F Urinary acidifiers are often given to cats with FLUTD in order to kill microbial infections in the urine.
12. T F Hypothermia partially contributes to a puppy's or kitten's inability to mount a good immune response during the first 2 weeks of life.
13. T F Glaucoma results from a decreased production of aqueous fluid or excess drainage of it from the eye.
14. T F Feline heartworm disease is more difficult to diagnose than canine heartworm disease, partially because the worm burden in the cat is so much lower than in the dog.
15. T F The deficiency of taurine commonly found in most commercial cat foods today contributes to the increased incidence of dilated cardiomyopathy in this species.
16. T F Diabetes mellitus is diagnosed by documenting polydipsia, polyuria, and cataracts in an older animal.

Copyright © 2006 by Elsevier, Inc. All rights reserved.

17. T F Pepto-Bismol can cause an animal's stools to be black and appear as melena.
18. T F Urethral obstructions in cats can be fatal because severe metabolic derangements can result.
19. T F Clinical signs of hip dysplasia almost always correlate with the severity of the disease detected radiographically.
20. T F The overall recurrence rate for bladder stones is high in dogs, approximately 25%.

Answers: (1) F, (2) T, (3) T, (4) T, (5) F, (6) T, (7) F, (8) F, (9) T, (10) F, (11) F, (12) T, (13) F, (14) T, (15) F, (16) F, (17) T, (18) T, (19) T, (20) T. ∎

26

Emergency and Critical Care Medicine

TEACHING/LEARNING OBJECTIVES

1. What equipment is needed in a crash cart for airway maintenance and oxygen delivery?
2. What equipment is needed in a crash cart for intravenous catheter placement and fluid administration?
3. What drugs should be kept in a crash cart and why?
4. List basic laboratory data that are typically determined in emergency situations and the importance of each value.
5. Discuss the coagulation process. Review the reasons for obtaining PT, PTT, ACT, and buccal mucosal bleeding time. How are these tests performed?
6. When is blood typing and cross-matching required? Explain how to perform each test.
7. List seven reasons for fluid support for the critically ill patient.
8. Calculate replacement fluids volume required for a 70-lb dog and a 10-lb cat.
9. Explain two ways to calculate the maintenance fluid volume.
10. List clinical signs related to overhydration.
11. What is normal urine output (volume)?
12. What objective parameters can be used to assess a patient's response to fluid therapy?
13. Define triage.
14. Explain methods to control arterial bleeding.
15. List four clinical signs of hemodynamic instability in the veterinary patient.
16. List four signs of upper airway trauma.
17. Explain the potential benefits of thoracocentesis.
18. Define flail chest and describe the patient with this condition.
19. List as many ways as possible to quickly assess blood loss in the trauma patient.
20. Name two potential sites of internal hemorrhage and how to determine if the patient is bleeding into either of these places.
21. Explain what changes in mentation, consciousness, pupillary light response, and pupillary size might be expected in the patient with head trauma.
22. List three causes of increased intracranial pressure.
23. What is mannitol?
24. Discuss why mannitol is contraindicated in animals with active intracranial bleeding.
25. Explain the challenge of treating the patient with intracranial bleed and hypotension.
26. Define "spinal shock" and explain how trauma patients might exhibit this phenomenon.
27. List clinical signs associated with pain in animals.
28. Which major body systems must be monitored in patients receiving opioids?
29. Describe clinical changes that occur during the hypercoagulable stage of disseminated intravascular coagulation.
30. Describe clinical changes that occur during the hypocoagulable stage of disseminated intravascular coagulation.
31. Explain how the body attempts to compensate for impaired perfusion in the early stage of shock and the resulting clinical signs.
32. Describe what happens to blood during the hypodynamic phase of shock and the resulting clinical signs.
33. List four categories of shock that are based on causes, and provide the causes.
34. Explain the number one priority in treating patients in shock and how this priority is carried out.
35. What are the shock doses of crystalloids for dogs and cats?
36. What systemic disorders may result from reperfusion injuries?
37. Describe actions to take to address the "A" in basic life support.
38. Describe methods of providing oxygen to a patient who has stopped breathing.
39. Define cardiac pump and thoracic pump and describe how to optimize each one.
40. List, in order of preference, the routes of drug administration during advanced life support.
41. List physical parameters that must be monitored during the postresuscitation period and describe how each one is done.
42. Describe how mannitol works, when it might be effective, and when it is contraindicated.

43. Explain the purpose of pulse oximetry and capnography.
44. Describe the procedure of drawing an arterial blood sample and explain the importance of an arterial blood gas analysis.
45. How is ventilation determined on a blood gas analysis?
46. How is oxygenation determined on a blood gas analysis?
47. What parameters must be monitored to assess hydration status?
48. Describe physical signs of overhydration.
49. What is the normal average range of systolic blood pressure in cats and dogs.
50. What is the normal average range of mean arterial blood pressure in cats and dogs.
51. Select an appropriately sized blood pressure cuff and determine the blood pressure of a cat and a dog using an oscillometric blood pressure monitor.
52. Using a Doppler probe and sphygmomanometer, determine the systolic blood pressure of a cat and dog.
53. Describe the procedure required to assess central venous pressure in a cat or dog.
54. Why is it important to measure central venous pressure?
55. Estimate the platelet count from a blood smear. Evaluate the result.
56. What is the normal platelet count in cats and dogs?
57. Perform an activated clotting time (ACT) test on a cat or dog. Evaluate the result.
58. What does the buccal mucosal bleeding time (BMBT) represent?
59. When should a urinalysis be performed on animals in an emergency/critical care setting?
60. What is the normal urine production for cats and dogs?
61. What parameters should be assessed to determine the neurologic status of a patient and when should this assessment be performed?
62. When is abdominocentesis indicated and how is it performed?
63. When is diagnostic peritoneal lavage indicated and how is it performed?
64. When is thoracocentesis indicated and how is it performed?

KEY TERMS

Activated clotting time (ACT)
Alveolar oxygenation
Ambu bag
Anisocoria
Apnea
Arterial oxygenation
Asystole
Baroreceptor reflexes
Buccal mucosal bleeding time
Capnography
Cardiac pump
Cardiogenic shock
Central venous pressure
Chemosis
Colloid fluid
Crash cart
Crystalloid fluid
Decerebellate rigidity
Decerebrate posture
Decerebrate rigidity
Diagnostic peritoneal lavage
Disseminated intravascular coagulation
Distributive shock
Dyspnea
Ecchymoses
Echinocytes
Electrical defibrillation
Electrical defibrillation
Electromechanical dissociation (EMD)
Flail chest
Hemothorax
Hyperdynamic phase of shock
Hypodynamic phase of shock
Hypovolemic shock
Obtunded
Opisthotonus
Partial thromboplastin time (PTT)
Petechiae
Pneumothorax
Polytrauma
Prothrombin time (PT)
Pulse deficit
Pulse oximeter
Pulseless electrical activity
Reperfusion injury
Schiff-Sherrington
Septic shock
Shock
Spherocytes
Sphygmometer
Spinal shock
Syndrome of multiple organ dysfunction (MODS)
Systemic inflammatory response syndrome (SIRS)
Thoracic pump
Triage
Vagal tone
Vagus nerve
Ventricular fibrillation

Copyright © 2006 by Elsevier, Inc. All rights reserved.

PART FIVE SURGICAL AND MEDICAL NURSING

Chapter Outline	Teaching Strategies
Introduction	Emphasize that the veterinary technician is the team member most directly involved with patient care and with maintaining accurate patient records. Ask students to discuss reasons why this is true.
The emergency care station and resuscitation area	Review basic components of the emergency care and resuscitation area.
Crash cart	Discuss the contents of the crash cart and include the reason for each item. Ask students to include all accessory items needed for each procedure. For example, to gain venous access what items are needed in addition to an intravenous catheter? (Answer: clippers, antiseptic scrub, tape, saline flush.)
Laboratory	Review normal values for temperature, pulse rate, respiratory rate, blood pressure, and oxygen saturation, blood glucose, blood urea nitrogen, urine specific gravity. Ask the students to describe methods of obtaining these data and the reason for them. Review canine and feline blood types and situations in which blood typing and cross-matching are required. Bring card tests and kits to class for demonstration.
Fluid therapy	Compare and contrast indications for crystalloid and colloid fluids. Provide real examples of cost differences. Provide lists of the contents of a variety of crystalloid and colloid fluids. Practice calculating replacement and maintenance fluid volumes. Ask students to describe signs of overhydration and how to address these problems.
Standards of care and emergency protocol	Discuss the benefits of having clearly documented approaches for treating patients in crisis situations.
Triage of the trauma patient	**Respiratory Evaluation:** Review clinical signs of hemodynamic instability, upper airway trauma, and hemo/pneumothorax. Discuss causes of upper airway trauma/rupture, hemo/pneumothorax, pulmonary contusions, diaphragmatic hernia, and flail chest. Show radiographs of patients with these conditions. Review indications for various methods of oxygen administration. Review other diagnostic modalities, including thoracocentesis, radiographs, pulse oximetry, and arterial blood gas analysis. **Cardiovascular Evaluation:** Review methods of quickly assessing the cardiovascular status and potential blood loss. Demonstrate on a stuffed animal how to place an abdominal pressure bandage. **Neurologic Evaluation:** Review clinical signs of head trauma. Discuss how and which drugs and fluids are used to treat secondary effects of head trauma; stress the controversial nature of corticosteroids. Define "shock patient" and show videos of patients exhibiting clinical signs of Schiff-Sherrington, and decerebrate/decerebellate rigidity. Discuss ways to handle the patient with potential spinal cord injuries.
Triage of the critical care patient	Stress the importance of a systematic and team-oriented approach to triage.
Secondary complications	Emphasize that while it is not the role of the veterinary technician to diagnose, the technician plays a vital role in anticipating and recognizing clinical signs of secondary complications.
Pain	Review clinical signs of pain. Stress that if a human is likely to experience pain in a similar situation, then so is the animal.
Disseminated intravascular coagulation (DIC)	Review the process of coagulation and the clinical signs that may be observed during early and later stages of DIC. Stress that DIC is not a primary disease. Review the standard tests of clotting function, including protocols for venipuncture, tubes to use, and storage/handling protocols.
Shock and the systemic inflammatory response syndrome	Review physiologic changes that occur during the hyperdynamic and hypodynamic stages of shock and ask the students to describe clinical changes that they might expect to see as a result of these changes.
Treatment of shock	Explain that underlying causes must be treated but circulatory collapse must be prevented immediately. Review methods of administering shock volumes of fluids and physical parameters to be monitored during their administration. Discuss the role of vasopressors in treating patients with shock.
Perfusion failure and reperfusion injury	Stress the role of the technician in monitoring specific parameters during reperfusion.

Copyright © 2006 by Elsevier, Inc. All rights reserved.

Chapter Outline	Teaching Strategies
Cardiopulmonary arrest	Review the anatomy and function of the vagus nerve. Stress that respirations, pulse rate/character, mucous membrane color, body temperature, and unexplained changes in anesthetic depth must be monitored in high-risk patients.
Cardiopulmonary cerebrovascular resuscitation	
Basic life support	Discuss ways to clear an obstructed airway, provide oxygen and assisted ventilation, and perform chest compressions. Students can work in pairs and practice on stuffed animals.
Advanced life support	Review the procedure to follow to attach ECG leads to a patient. Bring rhythm strips to class that demonstrate ventricular fibrillation, asystole, and electromechanical dissociation. Review methods and routes of drug administration.
Prolonged life support	Review the neurologic, respiratory, and cardiovascular parameters that should be monitored during prolonged life support. Emphasize that conditions that existed before resuscitation still require treatment.
Medical treatments in the postarrest period	Discuss indications and contraindications for the use of mannitol, furosemide, glucocorticoids, dobutamine, dopamine, sodium bicarbonate, and lidocaine during the postarrest period.
Patient monitoring	Review subjective and objective parameters that are monitored during the postarrest period. Ask the students to discuss their role as technicians during this period.
Respiratory system	Review the meaning of crackles, wheezes, and muffled heart and lung sounds, including conditions that might cause them. Ask the students to explain what to do if any of these characteristics is detected. Bring actual blood gas results to class and discuss the concepts of ventilation, oxygenation, acid/base balance, and alveolar-arterial gradient.
Cardiovascular system and perfusion/hydration	Discuss changes in cardiac auscultation and pulse palpation caused by various diseases. Review the causes of pulse deficits. Ask the students to determine physical signs that must be monitored to assess hydration status.
Blood pressure	Ask several students to bring their pets to class. Compare systolic blood pressure measurements obtained an oscillometric monitor and Doppler/sphygmometer. Ask the students what they should do if a patient's mean arterial blood pressure is dropping to 60 mm Hg.
Central venous pressure	Discuss reasons for measuring central venous pressure.
Coagulation status	Review indications for performing platelet counts, activated clotting time, and buccal mucosal bleeding time tests. Ask the students to discuss potential clinical signs that might be seen and treatments to anticipate in patients with abnormal results of these tests.
Renal/urinary system	Review how urine specific gravity is assessed and its significance. Stress that it is ideal to obtain a urine sample for analysis before administering drugs and fluids, but that this is not always possible. Ask the students to explain the effects of diuretics on urinalysis interpretation and sample collection.
Central nervous system	Emphasize the importance of performing serial neurologic exams. Review clinical signs of increased intracranial pressure.
Abdominal cavity	Bring actual abdominocentesis and diagnostic peritoneal lavage results to class and discuss final diagnoses. Emphasize that, when performing abdominocentesis and the needle is in the abdomen, it must not be redirected. Discuss potential complications if this should happen. Students can practice this procedure on plastic bags filled with water.
Thoracic cavity	Discuss ways to differentiate respiratory from cardiac disease. On a diagram, demonstrate the appropriate place to perform thoracocentesis and to place a chest tube. Review indications for thoracocentesis.

PART FIVE SURGICAL AND MEDICAL NURSING

CRITICAL THINKING CHALLENGES

1. Describe the presentation of a patient in an emergency hospital. List diagnostic tests and treatments and ask the students to explain how they would perform each one. They should include anatomical locations for blood draw and venous access and all equipment required. Examples are: a puppy with parvovirus infection, a tomcat with feline urologic syndrome, or a patient with autoimmune hemolytic anemia.
2. Ask the students to explain the role of the veterinary technician for the dehydrated patient. They can discuss initial assessment, replacement, maintenance, and means of monitoring fluid therapy.
3. Create an imaginary scenario in a veterinary emergency clinic. Describe several patients that arrive at the clinic within minutes of each other. Include signalment, case histories, vital signs, and the animals' presentation. Ask the students to perform triage in order to determine the order in which patients will be treated and what can be done for other patients in the meantime. Have the students explain their choices.
4. Describe specific situations in which an animal has stopped breathing or has no pulse. Have the students describe what actions to take and explain their choices.

QUIZ

Match each statement with the word/phrase that it defines.

1. ____ These analgesics have little effect on the cardiovascular system, but they can affect the gastrointestinal and renal systems.
2. ____ In small animals and animals with narrow chests, this model of forward motion of blood during cardiopulmonary cerebrovascular resuscitation states that chest compressions apply force to the heart that mimic normal heart mechanics.
3. ____ The diuretic effect of this drug increases urine output and may enhance the effects of mannitol.
4. ____ This is the presence of ECG complexes with no cardiac contractions to generate a pulse, also known as pulseless electrical activity.
5. ____ It is difficult to palpate an animal's pulse if this value is less than 60 mm Hg.
6. ____ In patients with this condition, air becomes trapped between the body wall and lung.
7. ____ Endotracheal intubation and ventilation with an Ambu bag in room air provides this percentage of oxygen to the animal.
8. ____ During this disease, massive activation of coagulation overwhelms the boy's clot prevention and clot dissolution functions; instead of controlled clot formation confined to sites of injury, systemic clot formation begins on a widespread basis.
9. ____ To perform the activated clotting time test (ACT) this amount of whole blood is needed.
10. In dogs and cats, an ideal mean blood pressure range is ____.
11. ____ Severe brainstem injury with a grave prognosis may be indicated by this posture.
12. ____ These fluids are used to expand vascular volume and contain large-molecular-weight particles, which remain intravascularly for long periods of time.
13. ____ The dosage for emergency drugs administered via this route is twice that of drugs administered intravenously.
14. ____ Cyanosis, or blue mucous membranes, is a sign of this problem.
15. ____ When inserting a needle for thoracocentesis, the needle should be placed here to avoid damaging vessels and nerves.

A. Cardiac pump
B. On the rib's caudal border
C. von Willebrand disease
D. 2 ml
E. Electromechanical dissociation
F. 105 to 120 mm Hg
G. Opisthotonus with limb rigidity
H. Colloids
I. Intraosseous
J. Hypoxemia
K. On the rib's cranial border
L. 75 to 90 mm Hg
M. 3 ml
N. Hemoabdomen
O. 40%
P. Head Pressing
Q. 21%
R. Nonsteroidal antiinflammatory drugs
S. Disseminated intravascular coagulation
T. Flaccid paralysis
U. Asystole
V. 30 to 110 mm Hg
W. Crystalloids
X. Thoracic pump
Y. Dobutamine
Z. Furosemide
AA. Pneumothorax
BB. Mean arterial blood pressure
CC. Diastolic blood pressure
DD. Subcutaneous emphysema
EE. Opioids

Copyright © 2006 by Elsevier, Inc. All rights reserved.

FF. Endotracheal
GG. Intracardiac
HH. Kidney failure
II. Thromboembolism
JJ. 21%

Answers: (1) R, (2) A, (3) Z, (4) E, (5) BB, (6) AA, (7) JJ, (8) S, (9) D, (10) L, (11) G, (12) H, (13) FF, (14) J, (15) K. ∎

27

Toxicology

TEACHING/LEARNING OBJECTIVES

1. Describe the procedure required to flush a patient's eyes.
2. Explain the procedure to dilute the ingestion of a corrosive agent.
3. List contraindications of emesis induction.
4. Explain why an inflated, cuffed endotracheal tube must be placed when giving activated charcoal to a sedated patient or when performing gastric lavage.
5. List ways to prevent absorption of toxicants.
6. Explain how to treat an animal with dermal exposure to a corrosive agent.
7. Name three things that can cause a false positive test result for propylene glycol.
8. Describe the treatment protocols for dogs and cats that have ingested ethylene glycol within 1 hour and later.
9. List three main types of rat or mouse baits, clinical signs seen with each, and recommended treatment for each one.
10. Explain the effects of methomyl on acetylcholinesterase and pseudocholinesterase.
11. Identify the dangerous plants presented in the chapter, name the toxic principal of each (if known), list clinical signs, and describe the treatment recommended for poisoning with each one.
12. List safe dosages for dogs of acetaminophen, ibuprofen, and aspirin.
13. List anticipated clinical signs of an animal that ingests a sympathomimetic agent such as ma huang.
14. Name the agonist of isoniazid.
15. Explain how hypercalcemia affects the body?
16. Explain the toxic effects of anticancer agents such as 5-fluorouracil.

KEY TERMS

Acetylcholinesterase
Adsorbent
Amphetamines
Anticoagulant
Anuria
ASPCA
Azotemia
Biotoxin
Blood urea nitrogen (BUN)
Capillary refill time
Cardiac glycosides
Central nervous system
Chemoreceptor trigger zone
Clotting factors
Cyanotic
Cycasin
Demulcents
Dialysis
Disulfoton
Disyston
Dyspneic
Emesis
Enterohepatic circulation
Extensor rigidity
Grayanotoxins
Heinz bodies
Hypernatremia
Hyperosmolality
Hypokalemia
Icterus
Lacrimation
Metabolic acidosis
Metaldehyde
Methemoglobinemia
Methomyl
Muscarinic central nervous system effects
Mydriasis
Myelin sheath
Nicotinic central nervous system effects
n-Propyl disulfide
Oliguria
Organophosphate
Osteoclastic bone resorption
Oxidative phosphorylation
Paresis

Phosphide gas
Polydipsia
Polyuria
Prothrombin time (PT)
Pseudocholinesterase
Ricin
Rodenticide
Sinus tachycardia

SLUDGE syndrome
Sodium/potassium ion channel pump
Sympathomimetic
Through and through lavage
Toxicant
Toxin
Vitamin K epoxide reductase
Zinc phosphide

Chapter Outline	Teaching Strategies
Managing poison emergencies	Photocopy pages from a veterinary drug formulary and the *Physician's Desk Reference* and familiarize the students with the formats of these publications. Emphasize that appropriate initial communication with owners is essential. Technicians should ask owners to bring in any information that may help treatment such as the plant or part of the plant if they don't know the name of it, labels or containers of the product that the animal ingested, and names or containers of anything that the owners have already used to treat their pet.
Assessment of the animal's condition	Review normal parameters and ranges for respiratory rate, capillary refill time, mucous membrane color, heart rate, and core body temperatures. Discuss causes of and treatments for abnormal values.
Stabilization of vital functions	Introduce/review the ABCs of basic life support.
Decontamination	
External exposures	
Ocular irrigation	Stress that ocular exposure to a corrosive agent is an emergency and the implications of this fact for the technician communicating with the owner.
Bathing	Stress that the patient's body temperature must be monitored closely during and after bathing.
Dilution	
Emesis	
Oral ingestion	
Dilution	
Emesis	
Emetic agents	Ask students to begin a list of emergency medications, dosages, routes of administration, and important notes regarding each drug. Alternatively, the class can create a chart together that is developed during the course of the semester. Box 27-1 can be used for this activity. Emphasize the use of xylazine in cats. Discuss instructions for owners at home.
Activated charcoal	Discuss enterohepatic circulation and toxicants that are metabolized this way. Sress that activated charcoal is contraindicated after ingestion of caustic agents.
Cathartics	
Enemas	
Gastric lavage	
Enterogastric lavage	
Supportive care	Present toxicants in terms of the primary organs that they affect and biochemical changes expected such as liver damage and changes in liver enzymes. Emphasize the importance of nutrition as a basic component of supportive care.
Household hazards	
Household cleaning agents	Ask the students to bring in labels or containers of household cleaning agents. Alternatively, ask the students to go to the store and write down toxic components of a few of these agents. Discuss instructions that technicians could give to owners whose pets have ingested them, clinical signs to anticipate, and what to do when the animal arrives at the clinic.
Acids	
Alkali	
Bleaches	
Detergents	

130 PART FIVE SURGICAL AND MEDICAL NURSING

Chapter Outline	Teaching Strategies
First aid treatment of exposures to corrosive agents	
Miscellaneous household items	Stress that the owners may not know the cause of their pet's illness. In this case, the symptoms are treated. The age, preexisting medical conditions, and immune status of the patient are important factors to address when treating patients that have been exposed to toxins.
Ant baits	
Silica gel packs	
Toilet water with tank cleaning drop-in tablets	
Glow necklaces	
Liquid potpourri	Emphasize that some of these products can be harmful if ingested or through dermal exposure.
Batteries	Remind students that emesis induction is contraindicated for animals that have ingested corrosives.
Cigarettes and other nicotine products	
Pennies	Review the mechanism and signs of zinc toxicosis.
Mothballs	
Moldy food (tremorogenic mycotoxins)	
Ice or snow melts	
Dangerous plants	Show pictures of the plants discussed in the chapter. Expand the list to include other plants that are common in your area. Bring some plants to class and discuss which parts are poisonous. Ask students to print pictures of toxic plants from the Internet and begin an emergency reference guide.
Rhododendron spp.	
Cardiac gycoside-containing plants	
Castor beans *(Ricinus communis)*	
Cycad Palms (Cycas, Zamia)	
Lilies	
Raisins/grapes	
Onions and garlic (*Allium* spp.)	
Calcium oxalate containing plants	
Pesticides	Emphasize the importance of immediate veterinary treatment for intoxication with fly bait, snail/slug bait, and gopher/mole bait.
Fly bait	Review the effects of acetylcholine accumulation and increased parasympathetic activity. Compare the clinical signs of muscarinic and nicotinic receptor stimulation and the clinical signs that are controlled by current treatments.
Snail or slug bait	
Gopher or mole bait	
Systemic insecticides (disulfoton or disyston)	Point out that animals may be poisoned by ingesting the insecticide or the soil and plant to which it was applied and that recovery can take weeks.
Rat and mouse baits	Point out the importance of knowing the name of the rodenticide that owners use. Each one causes different clinical signs and new products are being developed as rodents develop resistance.
Anticoagulants	
Bromethalin	
Cholecalciferol	
Antifreeze products	Compare the three forms of antifreeze. Discuss the importance of knowing the time of ingestion.
Methanol	
Propylene glycol	
Ethylene glycol	
Dangerous human medications	Stress that many human drugs have different dosages for animals and that some should not be given to animals at all.
Acetaminophen	Point out that cats can present with brown or cyanotic mucous membranes and facial swelling.
Ibuprofen	Emphasize that cats should not be given ibuprofen because of their limited glucuronyl-conjugating capacity.
Aspirin	Compare strengths of baby aspirin and regular aspirin. Discuss the use of coated aspirin.

Copyright © 2006 by Elsevier, Inc. All rights reserved.

CHAPTER 27 Toxicology

Chapter Outline

Sympathomimetic alkaloids
  Ma huang (pseudoephedrine/ephedrine)
Isoniazid
Calcipotriene (vitamin D derivatives)
5-Fluorouracil (antimetabolites)

Teaching Strategies

CRITICAL THINKING CHALLENGES

1. Veterinary technicians usually have the first contact with owners of animals exposed to toxins. Therefore, it is imperative that technicians know what questions to ask of the owners as soon as the animal presents or as soon as the owner calls. Present scenarios of (potential) animal intoxications and ask the students to ask the questions needed to determine if the pet should be brought to the clinic or to an emergency clinic, what the owner should and should not do at home, or how to begin treatment at the clinic.
2. It can be a challenge to figure out if clinical signs such as lethargy, vomiting, hyperexcitability, seizures, and ataxia are related to intoxication, infection, foreign body ingestion, trauma, or other etiologies. Ask the students to prepare a list of questions to ask owners that will help to rule out causes of clinical signs.
3. Ask students to prepare a patient education pamphlet entitled Pet-Proofing Your Home. Students can work in groups and critique each other's work. Contact the ASPCA and request information that they normally mail to the public or go to their website and print their educational materials. Compare their information to the students' work.

QUIZ

Circle the correct answer for each question or statement. There is only one correct answer for each one.

1. This drug is commonly used to control seizures.
   Apomorphine
   Furosemide
   Diazepam
2. How long should eyes be flushed if they have been exposed to (potential) toxins?
   10 to 20 minutes
   20 to 30 minutes
   5 to 10 minutes
3. Emesis is contraindicated in rabbits, horses, rodents, ruminants, and this species.
   Birds
   Cats
   Dogs
4. What should an animal be given after ingestion of a corrosive agent?
   Diluted milk/water
   Hydrogen peroxide
   Antibiotics
5. Glow-in-the-dark necklaces can cause this clinical sign if they are bitten or chewed.
   Urticaria
   Seizures
   Foaming at the mouth
6. What procedure is beneficial for exposures to toxicants that can cause kidney damage?
   Emesis
   Diuresis
   Peritoneal lavage
7. Anemia resulting from intravascular hemolysis can result from the release of this element from pennies.
   Magnesium
   Copper
   Nitrogen
8. This bean contains one of the most potent plant toxins known.
   Castor
   Cocoa
   Soy
9. Easter lilies can cause this in cats.
   Liver failure
   Respiratory paralysis
   Renal failure
10. In what animal can commercial baby food be toxic?
    Cats
    Birds
    Dogs
11. What is the most obvious clinical sign seen with SLUDGE syndrome?
    Vomiting
    Diarrhea
    Seizures
12. Anticoagulant rodenticides may be treated by giving this with fatty meals.
    Blood transfusion
    Vitamin K_1
    Activated charcoal

Copyright © 2006 by Elsevier, Inc. All rights reserved.

13. Facial and paw edema occurs as a result of an overdose of this common human medication.
    Ibuprofen
    Aspirin
    Acetaminophen
14. Ma huang, a human weight loss aid, can cause elevated blood pressure, tachycardia, seizures, and this ocular sign in animals.
    Mydriasis
    Chemosis
    Miosis
15. What can be released when peace lilies, pathos, and philodendron plants are chewed, causing oropharyngeal edema?
    Cycasin
    Grayanotoxins
    Calcium oxalate crystals

Answers: (1) diazepam, (2) 20 to 30 minutes, (3) birds, (4) diluted milk/water, (5) foaming at the mouth, (6) diuresis, (7) copper, (8) castor, (9) renal failure, (10) cats, (11) seizures, (12) vitamin K$_1$, (13) acetaminophen, (14) mydriasis, (15) calcium oxalate crystals. ■

28

Veterinary Dentistry

TEACHING/LEARNING OBJECTIVES

1. List the ancillary dental services for which the AVDC supports training of veterinary technicians.
2. List the dental services for which the AVDC supports training of veterinary assistants.
3. Name the four types of brachydont teeth in dogs and cats and their primary function.
4. Explain how the care of horses' teeth and ruminants' cheek teeth might differ from dogs', cats', and pigs' teeth.
5. Describe the location of the canines in a normal scissors occlusion.
6. Describe the location of the carnassial teeth in relation to the mandibular first molar tooth in a normal scissors bite.
7. Describe neutroclusion and name one sequela.
8. Describe a class I malocclusion with a posterior crossbite.
9. Describe a class II malocclusion and give possible causes.
10. Describe a class III malocclusion and give possible causes.
11. Explain why brachycephalic breeds can be considered as having a normal class III occlusion (breed normal).
12. Describe a wry bite.
13. Compare the healthy gingival sulcus of a cat and a dog.
14. Explain the progression from plaque to periodontitis.
15. Compare open and closed root debridement.
16. Explain why root planing is no longer recommended.
17. Explain the significance of the VOHC seal on pet food.
18. Why must the person performing a dental cleaning wear eye protection and a mask?
19. Explain why felids have no teeth numbered 305, 306, 405, and 406 according to the Modified Triadan System.
20. What benefits does fluoride provide in a polishing paste?
21. Explain the benefits of using an intraoral technique to radiograph a pet's teeth.
22. What are the advantages of a shorter film focal distance (FFD) when taking dental radiographs?
23. Explain the SLOB phenomenon using the upper fourth premolar as an example.
24. Explain the purpose of the bisecting angle technique.
25. Describe how to position a dog or cat to radiograph the mandibular incisors.
26. Describe how to position a dog or cat to radiograph the maxillary incisors.
27. Describe how to radiograph the maxillary canines of a dog or cat.
28. Explain how to radiographically isolate the tooth roots of the fourth premolar.
29. List the constituents of the tooth pulp.
30. List signs of endodontic disease.
31. Explain why hypochlorite is commonly used as an irrigating solution when cleaning out root canals.
32. List the contents of a surgical pack to be used for a tooth extraction.
33. What is the purpose of a cervical bulge?

KEY TERMS

Adontia
Alveolar bone
Anterior crossbite
Apical delta
Base narrow canines
Bisecting angle technique
Brachycephalic
Brachydont teeth
Brachygnathic
Buccal object rule
Buccal surface
Carnassial teeth
Cementoenamel junction
Cementum
Cingulum
Clark's rule

Class I malocclusion
Closed root debridement
Coronal
Crown
Cusp
Deciduous teeth
Dental arcade
Dental calculus
Dental caries
Dental explorer
Dentin
Diphyodonts
Distoclusion
Dolichocephalic
Endodontics
Eugenol
Exodontia
Feline odontoclastic resorptive lesions (FORLs)
Frenulum of the tongue
Furcation
Gingiva
Gingival sulcus
Gingivitis
Gutta-percha
Hypodontia
Hypsodont teeth
Interdental
Interradicular
Labial
Lingual surface
Mandible
Maxilla
Mesaticephalic
Mesioclusion
Neutroclusion
Obturation

Occlusal surface
Odontoblast
Oligodontia
Open root debridement
Oroantral fistula
Oronasal fistula
Palatal
Periapical abscess
Periapical tissue
Periodontal ligament
Periodontal probe
Periodontitis
Periodontium
Periodontosis
Phosphor storage plates (PSPs)
Plaque
Posterior crossbite
Prognathic
Pulp
Pulp canal
Pulp chamber
Root
Root debridement
Root planing
Root-tip forceps
Root-tip picks
Same-lingual, opposite-buccal (SLOB)
Scaler
Subgingival curettage
Tertiary dentin
Tooth socket
Vital pulpotomy
Wry bite
Zygomatic arch

Chapter Outline	Teaching Strategies
Ethical and legal aspects	Obtain a copy of the AVDC's statement in the Journal of the American Veterinary Medical Association regarding veterinary dental health care providers and make copies for the class. Review tasks that the veterinary technician and veterinary assistant can perform with supervision.
Veterinary dental organizations	Obtain literature that describes requirements of the 2-year training program and discuss requirements with the students. Invite a veterinary technical specialist in dentistry to talk to your class about the program and opportunities that the specialty offers.
Dental morphology and occlusion	Review the dental formulas of cats and dogs. On a diagram, point out the normal location of incisors, canines, premolars, carnassial teeth, and molars on a scissors bite. Have students identify on line drawings or actual photos the type of malocclusion present.
Periodontics and periodontal disease	Ask the students to label the anatomy on a line drawing of teeth and to explain the function of each part of the periodontium. Bring dental instruments to class and explain the purpose of each. Show pictures of animals with various grades of periodontal disease and ask the students what procedures might be required for each pet and what the owners can do at home.

Chapter Outline	Teaching Strategies
Advanced periodontal procedures	Discuss splinting and situations in which this is and is not recommended.
Proper diet	Bring different diets to class that have the claim of preventing plaque and calculus buildup and have the students examine the ingredients.
Dental scaling and polishing	Have the students determine an antibiotic, preanesthetic, induction, anesthetic, and postanesthetic analgesic regimen for different pets. Emphasize that these may differ depending on the veterinarian's preference. Have the students practice holding the instruments and a scaling movement using the wrist.
Dental home care	Bring various pet toothpastes and toothbrushes to class for demonstration purposes.
Sharpening dental scalers	Demonstrate different methods of sharpening scalers and stress the importance of regular sharpening to prevent damage to patients' teeth.
Dental radiography	
Intraoral radiography in the dog and cat	Discuss the bisecting angle technique and have students practice drawing these angles on paper. Show intraoral and extraoral radiographs to compare image quality. Review the anatomy and nomenclature of tooth roots and apply the buccal object rule to different situations. Using a stuffed animal, cardboard (intraoral film), and a box or can (PID), have the students position the animal and place the film as if they were going to take actual radiographs of various teeth.
Endodontics	Review the process of tooth formation in the young animal. Show photos of different manifestations of endodontic disease.
Conventional root canal therapy	Set up a table with stations of the root canal process. At each station, have the instruments used and a brief description of the stage on the table. Then, remove the instruments and have the students replace them to the appropriate stages.
Exodontics	Review potential complications associated with tooth extractions. Have the students discuss how these complications might occur and ways to prevent them.
Orthodontics	Show photos of retained deciduous teeth and the resulting malocclusions.
Impressions and models	Obtain negative and positive impressions from local specialists. Have the students research this topic to find out more information regarding maintenance that is required by the owner, price, and length of treatment time generally required.
Restorative dentistry	Discuss reasons for performing restorative dentistry in cats and dogs.

CRITICAL THINKING CHALLENGES

1. An owner is told that his pet must switch to a dry diet for the health of the pet's teeth. The owner is reluctant because she doesn't believe that this will make a difference and because she doesn't know how to make the change. Ask the students to prepare statements to educate such owners on these issues.
2. Have the students create owner educational flyers regarding dental care. The information must include the approximate dates of eruption, common problems, proper diet, preventive home care, treatment, and the importance of regular cleanings.

QUIZ

Fill in the blank with the correct word, phrase, or number.

1. The fourth maxillary premolar of dogs and cats is known as the _____ tooth and it usually has _____ roots.
2. Cats and dogs have a bite described as a(n) _____ bite.
3. A mandible that is short in relation to the maxilla is described as _____.
4. Whippets' skulls have a(n) _____ shape and Persian cats' skulls have a(n) _____ shape.
5. The _____ is defined as the supporting structures of the tooth.
6. Plaque that mineralizes on the teeth is called _____.
7. The procedure in which the gingiva is cleaned of foreign debris and granulation tissue is called _____.
8. According to the Modified Triadan System of numbering mammalian teeth, the first mandibular molar on the right is numbered _____.
9. In addition to 0.1% chlorhexidine, _____ or _____ can be used to rinse the mouth after polishing is completed.
10. _____ fistulas usually occur near the maxillary fourth premolar.
11. The amount of gingival attachment loss for a tooth is equal to clinical probing depth plus _____.

12. The film-focal distance (FFD) for a dental radiograph machine is _____ inches or less.
13. In brachycephalic dogs and cats, the _____ can be superimposed over the maxillary premolar tooth roots; to prevent this problem, the PID can be placed in a(n) _____ oblique position.
14. The most commonly fractured teeth in dogs are the _____ and _____.
15. All teeth with exposed pulp should be treated either with endodontic treatment or _____.
16. The most common irrigant solution used during root canal therapy is _____.
17. The bulk of the filling material used to fill a root canal is _____.
18. When extracting a tooth, the goal is to fatigue the _____ and avoid tooth root fracture.
19. Premolars and molars have a(n) _____ that naturally deflects food away from the gingival sulcus and helps to prevent periodontal disease.
20. The most commonly capped teeth in cats are _____.

Answers: (1) carnassial, 3, (2) scissors, (3) brachygnathic, (4) dolichocephalic, brachycephalic, (5) periodontium, (6) dental calculus, (7) subgingival curettage, (8) 307, (9) 3% hydrogen peroxide, physiologic saline, or zinc ascorbate, (10) oroantral, (11) gingival recession, (12) 16, (13) zygomatic arch, rostrocaudal, (14) canines, maxillary fourth premolar, (15) extraction, (16) hypochlorite, (17) gutta-percha, (18) periodontal ligament, (19) cervical bulge, (20) canines. ■

29

Equine Medical and Surgical Nursing

TEACHING/LEARNING OBJECTIVES

1. List behaviors that might indicate that a horse is experiencing abdominal pain.
2. Describe the stance that horses with laminitis and navicular disease commonly assume and explain why they do this.
3. Identify atrial fibrillation and atrioventricular blockage on electrocardiogram tracings.
4. Other than observation, describe a method of measuring abdominal distention in a horse.
5. List the normal pulse rate, respiratory rate, and temperature of an adult horse.
6. Explain the significance of an elevated digital pulse and hoof heat.
7. Describe how to prime a nasogastric tube placed in a horse.
8. Explain how a twitch is used?
9. Explain why a recumbent horse's head should be above the level of the stomach.
10. List feeds appropriate for horses with diarrhea, allergic airway disease, and after colic resolution.
11. Name three medications that should never be administered intramuscularly.
12. Explain the purpose of a fistulogram, arthrogram, cystogram, and myelogram.
13. Explain why the serum of horses is yellow.
14. List causes of moderate elevations of creatine phosphokinase in horses.
15. Explain why packed cell volume readings are not reliable indicators to use to determine the amount of blood loss during the first 24 hours after massive hemorrhage in horses.
16. Describe the normal appearance and pH of horse urine.
17. Name three processes that abnormalities in cell counts and protein in cerebrospinal fluid can identify.
18. Name the required vaccines for all horses.
19. Describe seasonal deworming programs for horses in the northern United States and Canada and in the southern United States.
20. Describe the dentition of a healthy male horse.
21. Explain how guttural pouch tympany may develop in foals and how guttural pouch empyema might be related to strangles.
22. List factors that predispose horses to gastrointestinal ulcers.
23. Name the five most common equine neurologic diseases and describe the most common treatment of each one.
24. List indications that a foal is premature.
25. Explain causes and clinical signs of hypoxic-ischemic syndrome in foals.
26. Describe patent urachus and explain one sign of its presence.
27. List potential causes of dystocia in the mare.
28. Explain how to keep mares' stools soft after performing caudal reproductive tract surgery.
29. What is the purpose of Caslick surgery?
30. What are potential complications after castration?
31. What are reasons for performing ovariectomy in mares?
32. Describe causes of umbilical, inguinal, abdominal, and incisional hernias.
33. Describe the medical treatments for laminitis.
34. Explain how the presence of a core lesion might affect the treatment of tendinitis.
35. Compare the causes of septic arthritis in adult horses and foals.
36. Describe various behavior of horses with colic.
37. Name as many causes of colic related to the gastrointestinal tract as possible.
38. Describe the cause and anatomy of epiglottic entrapment.
39. How are most horses with dorsal displacement of the epiglottis initially treated?
40. What drugs most commonly cause skin wheals in horses?

KEY TERMS

Abaxial
Abduction

Adduction
Adventitious lung sounds
Ampullae
Anaphylaxis
Angioedema
Anhidrotic horse
Arthrocentesis
Arthrogram
Aryepiglottic membrane
Arytenoid cartilages
Arytenoid chondritis
Ataxia
Atlantooccipital space
Axial
Azoturia
Bagging up
Barium swallow
Barker
Basioccipital bone
Basisphenoid bone
Bastard strangles
Bile acid concentration
Blepharospasm
Blood urea nitrogen (BUN)
Brood mare
Bruxism
Buccal surface
Callus
Cheek tooth
Choke
Chondroids
Chronic obstructive pulmonary disease (COPD)
Closed herniorrhaphy
Clostridial myonecrosis
Coffin bone
Coggins test
Colpotomy
Core lesion
Coronary band
Crackles
Cremaster muscle
Cricoarytaenoideus dorsalis muscle
Cryptorchid testicle
Cryptorchidectomy
Cutaneous colli muscle
Cystogram
Decubital ulcers
Deep digital flexor
Digital pulse
Diverticulum
Dorsal displacement of the soft palate
Dummy foal
Dysphagia
Endotoxemia
Epiglottic entrapment
Epiglottis

Epiphora
Epistaxis
Esmarch bandage
Ethmoid turbinates
Eustachian tube
Fetlock
Fetotomy
Fibroblastic sarcoid
Fistulogram
Floating
Founder
Frog
Frontal bones
Gamma glutamyltransferase (GGT)
Granulosa thecal cell tumor
Gravel
Guttural pouch
Guttural pouch empyema
Guttural pouch mycosis
Guttural pouch tympany
Heave line
Hemoglobinemia
Hemoglobinuria
High flanker
High ringbone
Hypsodontic dentition
Hooks
Hot spot
Hyoid apparatus
Hypopyon
Hypoxia-ischemia syndrome (HI)
Iatrogenic
Icterus
Insensitive laminae
Laminitis
Left laryngeal hemiplegia
Linguofacial vein
Low ringbone
Lumbosacral space
Malignant edema
Meconium
Melena
Modified Whitehouse technique
Moldy corn toxicity
Monday morning sickness
Moon blindness
Myelogram
Myositis
Nasopharynx
Navicular disease
Neonatal isoerythrolysis
Neonatal maladjustment syndrome
Nuchal ligament
Nystagmus
Obtunded
Open herniorrhaphy

CHAPTER 29 Equine Medical and Surgical Nursing

Osteochondritis dissecans
Paraphimosis
Parietal bones
Parrot mouth
Patent urachus
Periodic ophthalmia
Periosteum
Peritoneal cavity
Persistent urachal remnants
Petechiae
Phthisis bulbi
Pinnae
Pleural effusion
Pneumouterus
Pneumovagina
Points
Poll
Pollakiuria
Primiparous mare
Quidding
Rain rot
Rain scald
Recurrent airway obstruction (RAO)
Retained deciduous caps
Ringworm
Robert Jones bandage
Semimembranosus muscle
Semitendinosus muscle
Sensitive laminae
Septic thrombophlebitis
Sequestrum
Sesamoid bones
Sinkers
Sorbitol dehydrogenase (SDH)
Spur vein
Staphylectomy
Sternothyrohyoideus muscle
Strangles
Stranguria
Subchondral bone cysts
Subepiglottic cysts
Superficial digital flexor
Surfactant dysfunction
Synechiae
Teratoma
Throat-latch region
Thrombophlebitis
Tieback
Tuber coxae
Twitch
Tying up
Verrucous sarcoid
Vesicovaginal reflux
Vyborg's triangle
Waxing
Wheals
Wheezes
Wobbler's syndrome
Wolf teeth

Chapter Outline	Teaching Strategies
Physical examination of the equine patient	Show photos that illustrate a heave line, facial crest, and the transverse and linguofacial arteries. Stress that the handler and examiner should always stand on the left side of the animal. Review a normal ECG tracing and show some that demonstrate atrial fibrillation and atrioventricular block. Review the significance of wheezes, crackles, and muffled lung sounds. Obtain thoracic radiographs that demonstrate diseases corresponding with various sounds heard on auscultation. Discuss implications of mucous membranes that are pink and moist, dark pink to bright red, whitish blue, and dry and tacky. Have the students explain the possible treatments and disease processes occurring with different types of gastric fluid. Review methods of determining if a nasogastric tube is in place.
Restraint of the equine patient	Bring a halter to class and demonstrate various ways to place the chain. Show videos of physical restraint techniques during lameness examinations and other procedures. Have the students create sedative/analgesic protocols for various problems and procedures.
Care of the hospitalized patient	Have the students list the four life-threatening complications that can develop in the recumbent horse and describe prevention and treatment methods.
Patient monitoring	Have the students list the four life-threatening complications that can develop in the recumbent horse and describe prevention and treatment methods.
Feeding	Have the students describe nutritional requirements in horses with diarrhea, medical or surgical colic, inappetence, and allergic airway disease and how these requirements can be met.

Copyright © 2006 by Elsevier, Inc. All rights reserved.

PART FIVE SURGICAL AND MEDICAL NURSING

Chapter Outline	Teaching Strategies
Therapeutics	On a diagram, review the muscles into which IM injections are given and veins into which IV drugs are given. See Chapters 19 to 21.
Endoscopy	Obtain endoscopic images of various parts of the body. Bring an endoscope to class and label its parts. Discuss the importance of this technique in preventing the need for surgery and formulating diagnoses.

Imaging techniques
  Plain film radiography
  Contrast radiography
  Ultrasound
  Nuclear scintigraphy
  Clinical pathology
	See Chapter 9. Bring radiographs to class to demonstrate different techniques.

Serum chemistry	Review functions of the liver and kidneys and explain why the indicators of liver and kidney dysfunction develop as they do in horses. Discuss why excessive loss of electrolytes into the gut lumen leads to diarrhea. Have the students predict subsequent clinical signs and explain steps that they can take to prevent the development of these signs. Have the students research tying up, azoturia, and Monday morning sickness and explain why CK is elevated in horses with these diseases.
Hematology	See Chapter 6. Review the functions of the spleen and emphasize its increased capacity to contain erythrocytes. Explain sequestration and margination.
Urinalysis	Emphasize that normal equine urine is thick and mucoid, may give a false positive protein reading on urine dipstick because of its normally alkaline pH, and may appear red. Present causes of hemoglobinemia and hemoglobinuria.
Evaluation of body fluids	Review indications for CSF analysis, arthrocentesis, and abdominocentesis. On diagrams, point out centesis sites. Show photos (gross and microscopic) of normal and abnormal fluids. Have the students explain how they can help to prevent iatrogenically induced disease in patients before and during the procedures.
Bacterial culture and sensitivity Testing	See Chapter 8.
Preventive health care	Obtain shipment requirements from several states to show examples of what students might expect to experience when they begin working.
Vaccination	Have the students create vaccination programs for various horses (brood mares, show horses, etc.). They should describe the route and frequency of administration.
Deworming	See Chapter 8.
Dental care	Obtain a mold of equine teeth and indicate the areas where points and hooks develop. Bring a dental float to class. Have the students select a drug protocol for a rasping procedure. On radiographs show the relationship between the maxillary sinuses and roots of the teeth on the upper arcade.
Equine infectious anemia	Ask the students to explain how the veterinary technician assists in the control of this disease. Explain how a Coggins test works.
Selected medical diseases	For each disease mentioned in the chapter, have the students describe characteristics (clinical signs, behavior, environmental clues) that help distinguish them. Some disease processes can be demonstrated on radiographs.
Equine respiratory diseases	On a diagram and radiographs, show the anatomic relationship of the guttural pouch to surrounding structures.
Gastrointestinal disease	
Neurologic disease	Show a video of a horse undergoing a neurologic exam and explain each step.
Dermatologic disease	Have the students describe the lesions for each disease mentioned in the chapter. Show photos of each lesion.
Ophthalmologic disease	Review the anatomy and physiology of the eye. Discuss tests to determine intraocular pressure and the presence of corneal ulcers.
Neonatal care	Review neonatal isoerythrolysis and primary and secondary surfactant dysfunction. Have the students discuss the role of the technician in caring for the recumbent foal in terms of the respiratory, gastrointestinal, ophthalmologic, musculoskeletal, dermatologic, and cardiovascular systems.

Copyright © 2006 by Elsevier, Inc. All rights reserved.

CHAPTER 29 Equine Medical and Surgical Nursing

Chapter Outline	Teaching Strategies
Dystocia	Have the students explain how to prepare for the delivery of a foal. Review methods of stimulating respirations in the newborn foal.
Surgery of the female caudal reproductive tract	Have the students research the causes and treatments for pneumovagina, pneumouterus, and vesicovaginal reflux. On a diagram, show the result of Caslick surgery.
Urogenital tract surgery	Discuss methods to prevent and treat urinary calculi. Review the potential locations of the nondescended testicle in high flankers. Compare closed and open castration techniques. Have the students discuss how the veterinary technician helps to prevent complications of castration and ovariectomy procedures postsurgically. Show videos of castrations and ovariectomies being performed.
Hernia repair	Review the anatomy of various hernias. Have the students explain how long-term incarceration of intestines in a hernia may affect the technician's role in hernia repair.
Musculoskeletal diseases	On a diagram, review anatomy of the foot. Point out structures involved in laminitis and sole abscess.
Surgery of the equine patient	Review the medical treatments of laminitis and have the students explain long-term effects of these drugs. Discuss the pathogenesis of osteoarthritis and point out on a diagram the location of bog spavin, bone spavin, high ringbone, and low ringbone. Show radiographs of osteochondritis dissecans, osteochondral fragments, cartilage erosion, and subchondral bone cysts. Review requirements of radiographic positioning for these diseases. Demonstrate the use of hoof testers.
Preoperative preparation of the equine patient	Have the students describe their future preoperative duties as veterinary technicians in terms of patient positioning, foot care, preparation of the surgical site, preoperative blood work, fluid and drug administration, and anesthetic monitoring. Review the use of an Esmarch bandage and signs of infection at the surgical site.
Intraoperative nursing	
Postoperative nursing	
Colic	Review the anatomy of the intestinal tract. Discuss methods to differentiate the many causes of colic. For each cause of colic mentioned in the chapter, ask the students to anticipate the veterinarian's requests for medical and/or surgical treatment.
Abdominal surgery	
Arthroscopic surgery	Obtain a video of an arthroscopic surgery. Explain the procedure as it is being performed. Have the students describe what they would do to prepare the patient and surgery suite for this procedure.
Orthopedic surgery	Using diagrams, review various surgical implants used to correct orthopedic problems. Discuss the importance of asepsis during these procedures.
Upper respiratory tract surgery	On diagrams, review the anatomy of the pharynx and larynx (including innervation). Point out structures that are affected in the diseases mentioned in the chapter and the landmarks of Vyborg's triangle. Describe the modified Whitehouse procedure. Obtain endoscopic videos of these disease processes. Have the students describe the role of the veterinary technician postoperatively.
Surgical musculoskeletal diseases	Review the basic physiology of bone growth. Explain how a superior or inferior check ligament desmotomy may help with flexural limb deformities.
Emergency situations and procedures	Review the contents of a tracheotomy pack and the role of the veterinary technician in caring for the tracheotomy site after placement. Point out the relationship between the carotid artery and jugular vein and discuss the effects of injecting drugs into the carotid artery inadvertently.
Anesthesia for the equine patient	See Chapter 21.

ACTIVITY

Provide a conversation between a technician and owner. Every time the owner asks a question, a list of possible answers can be brought up and the student must choose.

EXAMPLE

An owner has left his mare at your clinic because he is going out of town. She is a very valuable animal and the owner is concerned. This will be his first foal.

2:00 AM

Owner: I'm just calling to check in.
Technician: Hello, Mr. Smith. She started to get restless and began pacing a few hours ago. She's even sweating quite a bit.
Owner: What?!
Technician:
- A. This is an indication of infection. We're going to take a blood sample to culture
- B. Please relax. It's normal behavior. She's repositioning her baby. Contractions may have begun. This is considered the first stage of labor.
- C. This is a strong indication of fetal distress.

5:00 AM

Owner: Do you have any news?
Technician: It's a boy. Her water broke at about 4:10 am and the foal was born at 4:40 am.
Owner: That's great! How is her appetite?
Technician:
1. She isn't interested in food yet so we started to feed her a calf milk replacer.
2. She should start to suckle in about 2 hours.
3. She probably won't be hungry until tomorrow night.

CRITICAL THINKING CHALLENGES

1. For each of the abnormal findings mentioned in the Physical Examination of the Equine Patient section of this chapter, have the students anticipate the next step of treatment. They can explain equipment, drugs, and restraint requirements that the veterinarian might call for. For example, the horse in the field with dry, tacky mucous membranes will probably need to have a blood sample drawn to measure the packed cell volume and total plasma protein. A 5-ml syringe and a 25-gauge needle will be needed.
2. Hand out clinical pathology results from different cases and ask the students to identify abnormal readings and write differential diagnosis lists. Have them discuss possible situations that could cause the values to be artificially abnormal.
3. Provide clinical signs of colic, respiratory disease, dermatologic disease, or musculoskeletal disease. Have the students develop a differential diagnosis list and explain methods of diagnosing and treating the disease.

QUIZ

Circle the correct answer for each question. There is only one correct answer for each question.

1. To what level should a nasogastric tube should be inserted in foals?
   A. Stomach
   B. Middle/distal esophagus
   C. Proximal esophagus
2. Where should the examiner and handler stand when examining a horse?
   A. On the horse's left side
   B. On the horse's right side
   C. In front of the horse
3. What is a commonly used tranquilizer in horses?
   A. Buprenorphine
   B. Fentanylc
   C. Acepromazine
4. What feeds can a horse with diarrhea be offered?
   A. Corn and grass hay
   B. Oats and grass hay
   C. Alfalfa and bran mash
5. When giving an intramuscular injection, what should be done immediately after attaching the syringe to the placed needle?
   A. Wipe the site with alcohol
   B. Draw back to ensure that the needle is not in a vein
   C. Place a tourniquet
6. What does a white blood cell scan commonly help to diagnose/determine?
   A. Osteomyelitis
   B. Stage of gestation
   C. Urolithiasis
7. What artificial serum chemistry results are seen in a blood sample that is not submitted right away?
   A. Hypoglycemia and hyperkalemia
   B. Hyperglycemia and hyperkalemia
   C. Hyperbilirubinemia and hypokalemia
8. What vaccines are required for horses other than Eastern, Western, and West Nile encephalitis?
   A. Tetanus
   B. Rabies
   C. Equine herpesvirus
9. What is the name of the remnant of the upper first premolar?
   A. Upper first canine tooth
   B. Wolf tooth
   C. Upper first premolar

10. If a horse has a positive result on a Coggins test, for how long must the animal be quarantined?
    A. 6 months
    B. For life
    C. Until it tests negative
11. What is the most common treatment for equine protozoal myelitis (EPM)?
    A. Ponazuril
    B. Ivermectin
    C. Sulfadiazine and pyrimethamine
12. What is a common sign of neonatal septicemia?
    A. Hyperexcitability
    B. Bone fractures
    C. Injected mucous membranes
13. How often should healthy foals suckle?
    A. Every 30 to 40 minutes
    B. Every 10 to 20 minutes
    C. Every 45 to 50 minutes
14. In general, how often should recumbent foals be repositioned?
    A. Every 4 hours
    B. Every 2 hours
    C. Every hour
15. What procedure is commonly performed to remove a dead fetus from the uterus?
    A. Fetotomy
    B. Cesarean delivery
    C. Oxytocin injection
16. Which of the following is *not* an option for use as a local anesthetic for perineal surgery in mares?
    A. Propofol
    B. Lidocaine
    C. XylazineH
17. What bone can rotate in a horse with laminitis?
    A. Sesamoid bone
    B. Carpal bones
    C. Distal phalanx
18. What is the term used to describe the horse with paralysis of the left arytenoid cartilage?
    A. Tying up
    B. Roarer
    C. Barker
19. What is the name of the surgical procedure that corrects dorsal displacement of the epiglottis?
    A. Tieback
    B. Staphylectomy
    C. Sacculectomy
20. Where along the trachea is a tracheotomy incision made?
    A. At the junction of the proximal and middle one third of the trachea
    B. At the junction of the distal and middle one third of the trachea
    C. Along the middle one third of the trachea

Answers: (1) B, (2) A, (3) C, (4) B, (5) B, (6) A, (7) A, (8) A, (9) C, (10) B, (11) C, (12) C, (13) A, (14) B, (15) A, (16) A, (17) C, (18) B, (19) B, (20) A. ∎

30

Food Animal Medicine and Surgery

TEACHING/LEARNING OBJECTIVES

1. List six ways to stimulate a newborn calf to breathe.
2. Explain why the neonatal calf must receive colostrum within the first 6 to 8 hours after birth.
3. Explain the potential sequelae of omphalophlebitis.
4. Explain how infections with *Actinobacillus lignieresii* and *Actinomyces bovis* are generally treated.
5. Name causes of pharyngeal trauma and abscessation in cattle.
6. Explain how metabolic acidosis develops in cattle that ingest excess carbohydrates.
7. Describe two methods of obtaining a sample of rumen fluid.
8. List causes of bloat and ways to treat them.
9. Describe common medical treatment of traumatic reticuloperitonitis in dairy cattle.
10. Compare abdominocentesis of monogastrics and large ruminants, and explain why the difference exists.
11. Explain causes of abomasal displacement and volvulus.
12. Define metaphylaxis and reasons for its use.
13. Describe the clinical course and treatment of winter dysentery.
14. Explain why pepsinogen levels increase in animals with ostertagiasis.
15. Explain why antibiotics are given to treat bovine viral diarrheal.
16. List ways to help prevent breakouts of bovine respiratory disease syndrome.
17. List methods currently used to treat septic arthritis in large ruminants.
18. Which digits bear the most weight in large ruminants?
19. List causes of laminitis in large ruminants and treatment methods.
20. Define the white line and describe causes of white line disease.
21. Describe ways to prevent sole ulcers in large ruminants.
22. Explain the reasons for applying wooden blocks to claws of large ruminants.
23. Explain how the spread of lymphosarcoma between animals can be prevented.
24. Explain where the organism *Anaplasma marginale* lives and the clinical signs that result from infection with this agent.
25. Compare contagious and environmental causes of mastitis and explain how the California Mastitis Test is performed.
26. Describe how to prepare the vulva and perineal area for examination in a cow experiencing dystocia.
27. What is the purpose of placing a Buchner suture?
28. What treatment is commonly performed for fibropapillomas of the penis and preputial prolapse in bulls?
29. Describe the necropsy findings that one might expect to find in ruminants with valvular endocarditis and pericarditis.
30. Describe dietary management techniques used to prevent urolithiasis in ruminants.
31. Compare the furious and dumb forms of rabies and explain how this infection is diagnosed.
32. List clinical signs and causes of polioencephalomalacia.
33. Explain the importance of diagnosing infection with *Moraxella bovis* as early as possible.
34. Describe the treatment of the most common tumor of cattle.
35. Explain the treatment for warts, ringworm, and rain scald.
36. Describe open and closed castration.
37. Explain why individual lambing pens are preferred over group pens.
38. List potential causes of enterotoxemia in goats and describe a treatment regimen.
39. Explain how stress can contribute to the development of respiratory disease in goats and copper toxicity in sheep.
40. Explain how tetanus and nutritional myodegeneration can be prevented.
41. Name the most common cause of urolith formation in small ruminants.

42. Describe the scrapie (large and small ruminants) and pseudorabies (swine) eradication programs that are now in place and the veterinary technician's role in enforcing the programs.
43. Describe the animal in which pregnancy toxemia typically occurs.
44. Name the organisms that cause pinkeye in sheep and goats.
45. What are clinical signs of contagious ecthyma in ewes, does, lambs, and kids?
46. List potential causes of rectal prolapse in sheep.
47. Name opportunistic pathogens of the gastrointestinal and respiratory systems and explain their role in clinical disease.
48. Name a gas anesthetic that should not be used with pigs susceptible to malignant hyperthermia.
49. List potential causes of tail biting in pigs and ways to prevent this behavior.
50. What is the relationship between the teat order and the pecking order in pigs?

KEY TERMS

Abaxial coronet
Abomasum
Agammaglobulinemic
Alopecia
Amniotic membrane
Anestrus
Anoxia
Anterior uveitis
Ataxia
Auriculopalpebral nerve
Balling gun
Blackleg
Blepharospasm
Blue ear disease
Bluebag mastitis
Brachygnathism
Buck
Buchner technique
California Mastitis Test (CMT)
Catarrhal colitis
Celiotomy
Cellulitis
Choke
Chorioallantoic membrane
Coffin joint
Conjunctivitis
Constrictor vestibuli muscle
Corium
Corpus cavernosum penis
Crepitus
Cull
Dead-end host

Dysphagia
Elastrator band
Emasculotome
Enterotoxin
Enucleation
Enzootic
Epiphora
Epistaxis
Epizootic
Epsilon toxin
Eructation
Evisceration
Supraorbital process
Ewe
Exophthalmos
Extirpation
Failure of passive transfer
Farrow
Fat liver syndrome
Fetotomy
Fimbriae
Flexor tendons
Foot rot
Founder
Gin chung
Gravel
Hard bag
Hardware disease
Heel bulbs
Hypopyon
Interdigital necrobacillosis
Interdigital ridge
Iodism
Keratectomy
Keratitis
Ketonemia
Ketonuria
Kid
Kohler milk culture
Kyphosis
Lacrimation
Lamb
Laminitis
Laparotomy
Left shift
Leukoencephalomyelitis
Limbus
Liptak test
Lumpy jaw
Macrophages
Mad Itch
Malignant edema
Malignant hyperthermia (MH)
Mastitis
Mastication
Medial canthus

Metaphylaxis
Milk fever
Mydriasis
Navicular bursa
Needle teeth
Negri bodies
Neonatal isoerythrolysis
Nervous ketosis
Omasum
Omphalophlebitis
Orf
Osteomyelitis
Ovine progressive pneumonia (OPP)
Oxytocin
Pale soft exudative pork (PSE)
Papillomatous digital dermatitis (hairy heel wart)
Paraphimosis
Parathyroid gland
Pastern
Perineal urethrostomy
Peyer patches
Phagocytosis
Phimosis
Physeal fracture
Pili
Pinocytosis
Pluriparas
Pollakiuria
Polymethylmethacrylate (PMMA) beads
Primary bloat
Prion protein
Prognathism
Pruritus

Pyuria
Rain scald
Redox potential
Reefing
Reticulum
Round foramen
Rumen transfaunation
Rumen trocharization
Rumenotomy
Rut
Secondary bloat
Seroconversion
Sole ulcer
Sore mouth
Stranguria
Streak canal
Subarachnoid space
Supernumerary teat
Syndesmochorial placentation
Tarsorrhaphy
Tenesmus
Thrill
Tunica albuginea
Urolithiasis
Vagus indigestion syndrome
Villous atrophy
Volatile fatty acid
Water belly
White line abscess
White muscle disease
Woody tongue
Zygomatic arch

Chapter Outline	Teaching Strategies
The role of the veterinary technician in food animal practice	For diseases described in this chapter, have the students begin to apply information learned in previous chapters. Ask them to choose antibiotic regimens for diseases, anesthetic regimens if surgery might be performed, and analgesic drugs. Have the students describe methods of restraint for various situations presented in the chapter.
Common diseases and conditions of cattle	
Care of the neonate and neonatal diseases	Review the differences in colostrum ingestion requirements in the kitten, puppy, calf, and foal. Discuss time requirements, how colostrum is transferred, and procedures to follow for failure of passive transfer. Demonstrate a method of measuring serum protein or IgG concentration.
Diseases of the digestive system	Review the anatomy and physiology of the digestive system of ruminants, including the process of fermentation. For each disease listed below, point out locations on illustrations.
Actinomycosis and actinobacillosis Pharyngeal trauma/abscessation	Explain how sodium iodide helps to control these infections.
Grain overload (carbohydrate engorgement, lactic acidosis)	Ask the students to research types of feed that are recommended for cattle. They can use the nutrition chapter in their textbook or any other sources, provided that they share the source. Have them explain what they will tell owners who ask what to feed their cattle. Show slides of normal and abnormal rumen fluid (gross and microscopic) that illustrate various colors, consistencies, and sedimentation characteristics.

CHAPTER 30 Food Animal Medicine and Surgery

Chapter Outline	Teaching Strategies
Rumen tympany (bloat)	Compare and contrast the causes and treatments of rumen tympany and gastric tympany and gastric dilatation volvulus in dogs.
Traumatic reticuloperitonitis (TRP, hardware disease)	On illustrations, have the students identify the centesis site for all four quadrants and describe anatomical landmarks. Show pictures of transudates and exudates and discuss their causes.
Abomasal displacement/volvus	On an illustration, indicate where the Liptak test is performed.
Diarrhea in the adult	Review the life cycle of *Ostertagia ostertagi* and compare type II and pre-type II ostertagiasis. Have the students determine ways in which the veterinary technician can be helpful in preventing, diagnosing and treating these various causes of chronic diarrhea.
Diseases of the respiratory system	
Bovine respiratory disease syndrome	Have the students discuss how preconditioning of calves before weaning and vaccination before transport may help to decrease the incidence of BRDS.
Diseases of the musculoskeletal system	
Regional analgesia and regional antibiotic perfusion techniques and polymethylmethacrylate (PPMA) implants	Use an illustration to point out anatomy of the limb that is pertinent for providing regional analgesia before claw amputation, corn removal, lameness exams, and foot rot.
Lameness	Show photos of animals with the following diseases. Give clues and ask students to name the disease.
Interdigital necrobacillosis (foot rot)	
Papillomatous digital dermatitis (PDD, hairy heel wart)	
Laminitis (founder)	
Interdigital hyperplasia (interdigital fibroma, corn)	
Sole (rusterholtz) ulcers	
White line disease	
Underrun heel and sole	
Claw amputation	
Wooden block application	
Blackleg and malignant edema	
Diseases of the hemolymphatic system	Compare clinical signs, prevention methods, and treatment of lymphosarcoma, anaplasmosis, and anthrax.
Lymphosarcoma	
Anaplasmosis	
Anthrax	Emphasize that this is a reportable disease.
Diseases of the reproductive system and mammary gland	
Mastitis	Review anatomy of the mammary gland. List the various ways of classifying mastitis along with the etiologic agents. Describe the ways that the disease is spread between animals and from the environment to the animal. Ask the students to research the drugs that are approved for administration to cows with mastitis along with withdrawal times. Have them determine the role of the veterinary technician in preventing, diagnosing, and treating this economically devastating disease.
Dystocia	Review the stages of labor. Compare stages of labor and causes of dystocia between calves, foals, kittens, and puppies.
Vaginal/uterine prolapse	Compare vaginal and uterine prolapse in terms of causes, recurrence potential, future use of the cow, timing of treatment, and treatment.
Retained placenta (retained fetal membranes)	Discuss theories regarding the causes of retained placentas.
Fibropapillomas of the penis	
Preputial prolapse	
Metabolic disorders	
Periparturient hypocalcemia (milk fever)	Compare milk fever with eclampsia in the bitch in terms of causes, time of onset relative to giving birth, clinical signs, and treatment of the dam and offspring. Review the function of the parathyroid gland in regulating calcium levels.
Ketosis (acetonemia)	List potential causes of ketosis in the cow and treatment options. Review the process of ketone formation.

PART FIVE SURGICAL AND MEDICAL NURSING

Chapter Outline	Teaching Strategies
Diseases of the cardiovascular system	Review the anatomy and physiology of the heart.
Vegetative or valvular endocarditis	Have the students explain how dependent edema and a left shift develop.
Pericarditis	
Diseases of the urinary system	
Urolithiasis	Have the students explain their role in helping to differentiate between colic and urethral obstruction in ruminants.
Contagious bovine pyelonephritis	Discuss urolithiasis and contagious bovine pyelonephritis in terms of gender predilection.
Diseases of the nervous system	Have the students discuss diagnostic procedures that would help differentiate the various neurologic diseases listed. Emphasize the importance of taking a thorough history as an aid to making a definitive diagnosis.
Rabies	Stress that this is a reportable disease.
Polioencephalomalacia (polio)	
Listeriosis	
Thromboembolic meningoencephalitis (teme)	
Obturator and sciatic nerve paresis and paralysis	Review the path of the obturator and sciatic nerves.
Diseases of the eye	Review the anatomy of the eye.
Infectious bovine keratoconjunctivitis (IBK, pinkeye)	
Ocular squamous cell carcinoma (oscc, cancer eye)	Point out landmarks that must be identified in order to perform the Peterson block.
Diseases of the skin	Have the students discuss the role of the immune system in the treatment of warts and ringworm. What steps should be taken if these diseases do not resolve spontaneously?
Cutaneous papillomas (warts)	
Dermatophytosis (ringworm)	
Dermatophilus (streptotrichosis, rain scald)	
Behavior	See Chapter 1.
Common surgical procedures performed on cattle	
Dehorning	Review the anatomical relationship between horns and frontal sinuses. Discuss potential sequelae if the sinuses are exposed as the result of a dehorning procedure. Point out the location of the cornual artery. Discuss reasons for dehorning cattle.
Castration	Compare the open and closed castration techniques with the use of an elastrator band. Discuss advantages and disadvantages of each method.
Laparotomy	Discuss intussusception, cecal volvulus, and abomasal displacement. On diagrams, point out the potential locations of these problems to help clarify the various incision sites.
Supernumerary teat removal	
Common diseases and conditions of small ruminants	
Care of the neonate	Compare the care of the neonatal large and small ruminant with hypoglycemia and hypothermia.
Diseases of the gastrointestinal system	
Johne disease	Discuss differences between Johne disease in large and small ruminants.
Enterotoxemia	Explain how an ELISA test works. Obtain a test kit for demonstration. Stress the importance of vaccinating goats.
Diseases of the respiratory system	
Pasteurella pneumonia	Compare the AGID and ELISA tests, including the cost of each.
Ovine progressive pneumonia (OPP)	
Diseases of the musculoskeletal system	
Foot rot	Emphasize that formalin is the last choice for treatment because it is a carcinogen and an environmental hazard.
Tetanus	Review the difference between a toxoid and antitoxin. Have the students discuss ways that the technician can help prevent tetanus before, during, and after dehornings, tail dockings, and castrations.

Copyright © 2006 by Elsevier, Inc. All rights reserved.

CHAPTER 30 Food Animal Medicine and Surgery

Chapter Outline	Teaching Strategies
White muscle disease	Review the requirements of a healthy diet for sheep and goats.
Diseases of the hemolymphatic system	Review the anatomy and physiology of the lymphatic system and the red blood cell.
Caseous lymphadenitis (CL)	Invite a food inspector to speak to your class or research the role of the food inspector. Discuss reasons for carcass condemnation and show photos of condemned carcasses.
Copper toxicity	Explain the role of the liver in the development of hemoglobinemia and the effects of hemoglobinuria on the kidneys.
Diseases of the reproductive system and mammary gland	
Pseudopregnancy	Have the students determine how to differentiate between real pregnancy and pseudopregnancy in small ruminants.
Mastitis	Review ways that small ruminants can contract mastitis. Compare the treatment with that of large ruminants.
Diseases of the urinary system	
Urolithiasis	Compare clinical signs of urolithiasis in the small and large ruminant. Review the shape of the urethra in small ruminants and point out locations where uroliths commonly form.
Diseases of the nervous system	
Caprine arthritis-encephalitis (CAE)	Discuss the phenomenon of seroconversion and how it affects the diagnosis of this disease.
Scrapie	Contact your state veterinarian to obtain information on the current scrapie eradication program and discuss the requirements of the program with the students. Emphasize that this is a reportable disease.
Pregnancy toxemia	Have the students explain how the veterinary technician can assist in differentiating pregnancy toxemia from other diseases on the differential list.
Diseases of the ophthalmic system	
Pinkeye	Compare pinkeye in the large and small ruminant.
Entropion	Discuss potential sequelae of untreated entropion in lambs.
Diseases of the integument	
Contagious ecthyma (sore mouth, orf)	Emphasize that this disease is zoonotic and that gloves must be worn when handling potentially infected animals.
Behavior	See Chapter 1.
Common surgical procedures performed on small ruminants	Point out the landmarks used to administer an epidural injection. Review the anatomy of the meninges and also point out needle placement for subarachnoid injection of anesthetic. Discuss reasons for dehorning kids. On a diagram, point out innervation of the rectum to demonstrate the effects of docking tails too short.
Common diseases and conditions of swine	Discuss concepts of all-in, all-out rearing.
Care of the neonate	Discuss reasons for giving iron dextran injections, docking tails, and removing needle teeth from piglets only a few days old.
Multisystemic diseases	
Erysipelas	Show photos of the diamond skin lesions and stress the importance of vaccination at weaning and every 6 months.
Pseudorabies (PRV, Aujeszky disease, mad itch)	Contact your state veterinarian to obtain information on the pseudorabies eradication program. Share this information with your students and discuss the role of the veterinary technician in helping to eliminate this disease.
Porcine reproductive and respiratory syndrome (PRRS)	Show photos that illustrate the classic cyanosis of various parts of the body.
Diseases of the gastrointestinal system	Review microscopic and gross anatomy of the intestinal tract.
Diarrhea in young pigs	Compare these diseases in terms of the age of onset, clinical signs, prevention, and treatment. Show histopathologic slides of each disease. Have the students determine ways that the veterinary technician may help to eliminate diseases on the differential list.
Diarrhea in the grower/finisher pig	Compare these diseases in terms of the age of onset, clinical signs, prevention, and treatment. Show histopathologic slides of each disease. Have the students determine ways that the veterinary technician may help to eliminate diseases on the differential list.

Copyright © 2006 by Elsevier, Inc. All rights reserved.

PART FIVE SURGICAL AND MEDICAL NURSING

Chapter Outline	Teaching Strategies
Diseases of the respiratory system	
Atrophic rhinitis	Explain the purpose of a specific pathogen-free program.
Swine influenza	Stress that swine influenza is zoonotic.
Mycoplasma pneumonia	According to the author of the chapter, most herds are affected by this organism to some degree. In light of this fact, have the students discuss the usefulness of vaccinating herds and treating herds with antibiotics in the drinking water.
Pleuropneumonia	Review the meaning of an animal being a carrier of a disease as opposed to having an active disease process. Explain how this might affect titer testing or vaccinating an animal for that disease.
Pasteurella pneumonia	Have the students discuss the fact that this bacterium is an opportunistic pathogen and the importance of knowing this fact as other respiratory infections are diagnosed.
Diseases of the musculoskeletal system	
Porcine stress syndrome	Have the students explain ways to prevent clinical signs of this disease in pigs being transported or undergoing surgery.
Diseases of the reproductive system	
Reproductive failure	Explain the benefit of exposing gilts to sows before breeding. Ask students to compare this method of immunization to using vaccines.
Diseases of the nervous system	
Salt poisoning	Review the process of osmosis as it relates to the development of cerebral edema. Discuss the ramifications of rehydrating the animal too quickly.
Behavior	Discuss the numerous ways and reasons why pigs display aggression.
Pot-bellied pigs	
Nutrition and husbandry	Have the students outline a diet regimen for the pot-bellied pig that is geared toward weight loss.

WORD GAME OR SCRABBLE

Provide the clues listed in the boxes. The answer fits onto the spaces provided. The circled letters must be unscrambled to form the answer to the bonus question. The bonus question can be asked first (just in case the answer to the other questions are too hard) and then the one letter provided might help a little.

EXAMPLE

Bonus question: Traumatic reticulopericarditis is commonly called _____ disease.

Fill in the blank letters. Clue:

A T R O P H I C R H I N I T I S — multifactorial disease in pigs caused by *B. bronchiseptica* and *P. multocida*
Q U I D D I N G — Definition: Dropping food out of animal's mouth
F U S O B A C T E R I U M N E C R O P H O R U M — Necrotic laryngitis is caused by this bacterium invading damaged mucosa
M. H A E M O L Y T I C A — Normally present in pigs' nasal flora but when in lungs it causes pneumonia
B R I S K E T — Prolonged exposure to high altitude can cause this disease in cattle
P N E U M O N I A — In cattle, most commonly caused by parainfluenza 3 and BRSV
W A R T — Also known as papilloma
H Y P O C A L C E M I A — Metabolic cause of parturient paresis

Alternatively, the words on the left can just be presented with the letters scrambled and the clue on the right will help the student unscramble them.

CRITICAL THINKING CHALLENGES

1. Present clinical signs of actual cases. Have the students ask questions that will help them determine

Copyright © 2006 by Elsevier, Inc. All rights reserved.

CHAPTER 30 Food Animal Medicine and Surgery

what diagnostic tests to perform. The students should describe how they would assist the veterinarian in performing the tests, including what equipment to gather and how to prepare the animal. Provide results of the tests. Ask the students to interpret the results and describe treatments. Play the role of the owner in each scenario and ask questions that a concerned owner would pose.

2. Contact a local rancher to obtain information about the average cost of raising beef or dairy cattle and the return per head. From a local food animal veterinarian, obtain information on the average cost to treat an animal (or whole herd) for different diseases (for example, enterotoxemia, caseous lymphadenitis, and PRRS) discussed in the chapter. This exercise stresses the economic impact on dairy and beef farmers of some animal diseases. Have the students present plans for prevention (or at least early detection) of diseases that the veterinary technician can implement in practice.

QUIZ

Respond to each statement below by placing one letter of the answer on each line. The letters in the boxes spell the answer to the Super Clue.

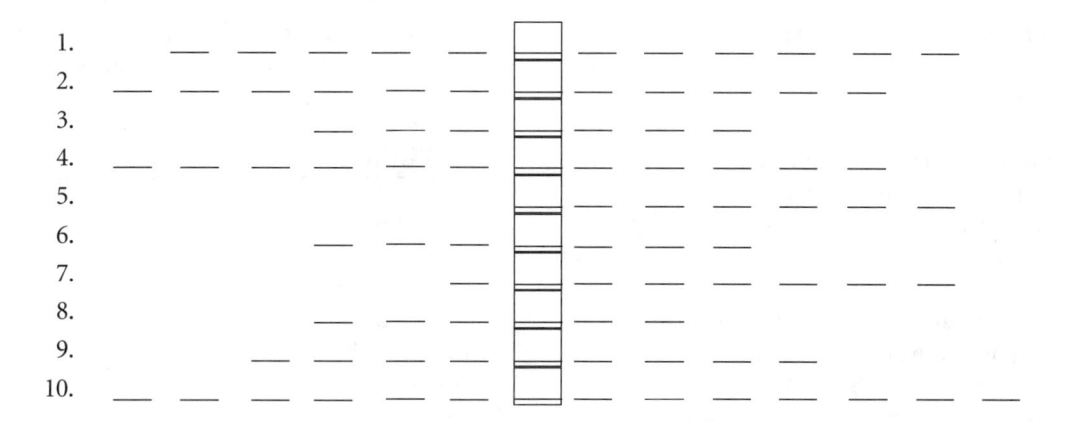

1. ___ ___ ___ ___ ___ | ___ ___ ___ ___ ___ ___
2. ___ ___ ___ ___ ___ | ___ ___ ___ ___ ___ ___
3. ___ ___ ___ ___ | ___ ___ ___
4. ___ ___ ___ ___ ___ ___ | ___ ___ ___ ___ ___
5. ___ ___ ___ ___ | ___ ___ ___
6. ___ ___ ___ | ___ ___ ___
7. ___ ___ | ___ ___ ___ ___ ___
8. ___ ___ ___ | ___ ___ ___
9. ___ ___ ___ ___ | ___ ___ ___ ___
10. ___ ___ ___ ___ ___ ___ | ___ ___ ___ ___ ___ ___

1. This is the inability to retract the penis.
2. This procedure is commonly employed by feedlots and involves treatment of cattle with long-acting antimicrobials upon arrival to the feedlot.
3. Pericarditis typically involves the formation of this type of fluid.
4. Baby pigs infected with this virus develop neurological signs, vomiting, and diarrhea while weaning and growing pigs develop a dry, nonproductive cough and flulike symptoms.
5. This is the most common cause of health problems and decreased life span in pet pigs.
6. *Anaplasma marginale* infection destroys red blood cells and causes this condition in cattle.
7. In healthy ruminants, most microbes should Gram stain this way.
8. This test helps to confirm the presence of left abomasal displacement.
9. Damage to this nerve may occur during dystocia or forced fetal extraction.
10. This is the process of obtaining ruminal contents and transferring it to another animal's rumen to help reestablish a population of normal flora.

Super Clue: This is the accumulation of fluid in the uterus that occurs during pseudopregnancy.

Answers: (1) paraphimosis, (2) metaphylaxis, (3) exudate, (4) pseudorabies, (5) obesity, (6) anemia, (7) negative, (8) Liptak, (9) obturator, (10) transfaunation, Super Clue: hydrometra. ∎

31

Nursing Concepts in Alternative Medicine

TEACHING/LEARNING OBJECTIVES

1. Explain the different objectives of shiatsu, trigger-point massage, sports massage, TTEAM, and Swedish massage.
2. What are the physiologic benefits of petrissage, effleurage, tapotement, friction, and vibration?
3. List signs of relaxation in a patient.
4. List signs that pressure is too great.
5. Name endangerment sites on animals.
6. List contraindications to massage therapy.
7. Explain how to strengthen the muscles around an animal's hips using a land treadmill.
8. List therapeutic benefits of ultrasound therapy.
9. Compare the advantages and disadvantages of continuous and pulsed modes of ultrasound therapy.
10. List the clinical uses of neuromuscular electrical stimulation (NMES).
11. Explain the differences between type I and type II muscle fibers.
12. Compare stimulatory, multifacilitory, and horizontal bioelectric therapy.
13. List the benefits of exercise for animals.
14. Explain to an owner how to make a cold pack at home.
15. List physiologic responses to cold therapy.
16. Briefly describe the theories of acupuncture.
17. Describe subluxation and the role of chiropractic therapy in managing this problem.
18. Explain why animals are better equipped to handle bacterial contamination of meats that humans.
19. Why should vegetables be lightly steamed and chopped or minced and grated before consumption?
20. List different forms in which herbs exist.
21. Compare Chinese herbal medicine and ayurvedic herbal medicine.
22. Compare the basic tenets of homeopathic and allopathic medicine.
23. Describe storage requirements of homeopathic remedies.
24. Define and explain constitutional and miasmic treatment practiced by homeopathic doctors.
25. Explain how pulsed electromagnetic field therapy works to help heal an osteoarthritic joint.
26. Compare the effects of using the North pole versus the South pole of a magnet for therapy.

KEY TERMS

Acupuncture
Aggravation
Allopathic medicine
Aquapuncture
Ayurvedic herbs
Continuity
Coupage
Cryotherapy
Depth
Duration
Echinacea
Effleurage
Electroacupuncture
Endangerment sites
Excursion
Flower essence therapy
Friction
Ginkgo
Ginseng
Holistic
Homeopathy
Implantation
Intention
Interneurons
Ischemic compression
Laser puncture
Low-level laser therapy (LLLT)
Ma huang
Massage
Materia medica
Meridian
Microcurrent therapy
Milk thistle
Moxibustion

CHAPTER 31 Nursing Concepts in Alternative Medicine

Myotherapy
Nebulization
Neuromuscular electrical stimulation (NMES)
Neutraceutical
Petrissage
Phonophoresis
Potency
Proving
Pulsed electromagnetic field therapy (PEMF)
Pulsed signal therapy (PST)
Repertorizing
Sequence
Shiatsu
Speed
Splinting
Sports massage
St. John's wort
Subluxation
Swedish massage
Tapotement
Tonification
Trigger-point massage
TTEAM
Type I muscle fibers
Type II muscle fibers
Ultrasound
Vibration

Chapter Outline	Teaching Strategies
Massage	Invite a massage therapist to demonstrate different types and techniques or obtain a video listed at the end of the chapter. Ask students to bring their pets to class and have them practice techniques.
Types of massage	
Techniques	
Contraindications	Discuss medical conditions from previous chapters that are contraindications to massage therapy.
Physical Therapy/ Rehabiliation	Have the students explain their role in each type of therapy. Ask them to research the costs of equipment required for some types of therapy.
Hydrotherapy	Review how to control resistance, buoyancy, and flexion/extension using hydrotherapy.
Land treadmill	Review the role of self-propulsion in walking on land and on a land treadmill.
Ultrasound	Discuss indications of ultrasound treatment.
Neuromuscular stimulation	Discuss the principles of fast- and slow-twitch muscle fibers. Review the anatomy of the muscle groups for which this therapy is commonly used.
Bioelectric stimulation	Compare neuromuscular and bioelectric stimulation therapies.
Passive range of motion	Review the anatomy of a commonly injured joint such as the stifle. Discuss the role of chondrocytes and synoviocytes in joint nutrition.
Exercises	
Cryo therapy- and heat therapy	
Contraindications	
Acupuncture	Have the students review the meridians of acupuncture. After viewing videos of acupuncture being performed on animals, the students can explain the placement of each needle.
Terminology and record keeping	
Acupuncture theories	
The Gate theory	
Endogenous Opioid theory	
Autonomic Nervous System theory	
Humoral theory	
Bioelectric theory	
Techniques	
Veterinary chiropractic	Invite a veterinarian certified in chiropractic medicine to discuss the use of this therapy with animals. Review the anatomy and physiology of the vertebral column and potential manifestations of subluxations.
History	
Alternative concepts in nutrition	
Home-prepared diets	Provide examples of home-prepared diets that are well balanced. Have the students explain what nutrients and micronutrients are in each component of the diet. Examine labels of commercial diets that could be rotated with these home-prepared diets to supplement missing requirements.

Copyright © 2006 by Elsevier, Inc. All rights reserved.

PART FIVE SURGICAL AND MEDICAL NURSING

Chapter Outline	Teaching Strategies
Nutraceuticals	Have the students visit a health food store and gather information on one or two nutraceuticals. Ask them to research the product and present their findings to the class to stimulate a discussion.
Herbal medicine	Stress the importance of understanding the effects of some of the commonly used herbs.
Herbs vs. drugs	Have the students make a chart listing commonly used herbs. The chart should include indications, contraindications, dosages, side effects, drug/herb interactions, and approximate costs. Students should be comfortable asking owners if they are currently giving their pets herbs or homeopathic treatments.
Western herbs	Compare western and Chinese herbal medicine.
Chinese herbal medicine	
Ayurvedic herbs	Ask the students to research the topics of ayurvedic, homeopathic, and Bach flower remedies and compare them with western medicine. Encourage the students to spend a day with a local veterinarian who performs one or more of these types of treatment. Ask the students to prepare a list of questions that they would like to ask of one of these practitioners and have the students take these questions with them to the clinics.

Veterinary homeopathy
  History and principles
  Practice	

Bach flower remedies	
Miscellaneous therapies	Review the physiologic and or psychologic effects of lasers, magnets, and aromatherapy.

Laser
    Precautions
  Magnets
  Aromatherapy	

CRITICAL THINKING CHALLENGES

1. Present case histories to the students and ask them to determine a therapy regimen for each animal. For each component of the regimen, the student should explain why they recommend it, what to do if the animal doesn't respond favorably or resists treatment, and how to have owners continue therapy at home.
2. Describe home-prepared diets and ask the students to determine what nutrients and/or micronutrients might be missing. Have them explain how to supplement the missing nutrients in another form of a home-prepared diet if the owner refuses to offer commercial diets.
3. Have the students contact a local veterinarian who practices alternative medicine and arrange to observe a session. The students can report their experiences to the class.

QUIZ

Respond to each statement below by placing one letter of the answer on each blank line. Place the answer to the Super Clue in the boxes from top to bottom.

1.
2.
3.
4.
5.
6.
7.
8.
9.

Copyright © 2006 by Elsevier, Inc. All rights reserved.

1. This condition describes a relationship between vertebrae that do not align perfectly.
2. This type of medicine is the most ancient known medicine and involves using plant materials to heal diseases.
3. This therapy, when applied to the skin, causes vasoconstriction, slowed nerve conduction, and decreased enzyme activity.
4. This form of therapy involves applying pressure with fingers on specific points in the body to increase circulation and stimulate the nervous system.
5. During this therapy, the therapist's hands never leave the patient's body and the speed of the therapy affects the outcome.
6. These objects have a North and South Pole, each of which is responsible for a different set of healing properties.
7. According to the theory of acupuncture, the life force or vital energy of the body circulates through these pathways.
8. This form of therapy involves kneading the skin to assist in removing metabolic waste and increasing circulation.
9. This form of therapy involves inserting needles into the skin in areas that represent meridians.

Super Clue: This system of medicine aims to balance the three Doshas found in all living organisms.

Answers: (1) subluxation, (2) herbal, (3) cryotherapy, (4) shiatsu, (5) vibration, (6) magnets, (7) meridian, (8) petrissage, (9) acupuncture, Super Clue: ayurvedic. ■

32

Veterinary Practice Management

TEACHING/LEARNING OBJECTIVES

1. Explain the role of primary, secondary, and tertiary care providers in veterinary medicine.
2. Explain how a facility design affects communication with animal owners, employee satisfaction, and patient care.
3. What area of a veterinary facility is mostly responsible for attracting new clients?
4. Name the four professional areas of activity within a hospital.
5. Describe the ideal reception area and examination rooms.
6. List ways in which nosocomial infections are transmitted and explain how they can be prevented.
7. Describe the requirements of a surgical area.
8. Describe the requirements of a necropsy area.
9. Explain why a surgery room should have only one entrance/exit.
10. Explain how the veterinary technician working in a large animal mobile unit must attempt to prevent the spread of infectious diseases.
11. Explain the effects of hospital cleanliness on a hospital's profitability.
12. Name the two most common methods by which new clients find a veterinarian.
13. Explain why one should never judge a client's ability to pay a bill by his or her appearance.
14. Explain why the client should pay all bills and discuss all issues with the veterinary staff before the pet is returned to them.
15. Discuss the benefits of client visits with their hospitalized pets.
16. Define direct cost and indirect cost and give an example of each one.
17. Define and provide examples of shopped fees.
18. Describe the usual controls for practice credit.
19. Explain how using fee slips in triplicate can help to control cash.
20. Explain the purpose of a petty cash fund and provide an example of its use.
21. List signs of poor business management.
22. Explain the role of the veterinary technician in minimizing malpractice complaints.
23. Explain why it is advantageous to promote programs instead of services.
24. What is the most common client complaint?
25. List animal care areas in which support staff should have in-depth knowledge.

KEY TERMS

Account receivables
Amortization
Consumer price index
Direct cost
Facility design
Gross income
Indirect cost
Macroshock hazards
Market segmentation
Mission statement
Net income
Nonshopped fees
Nosocomial infection
Pareto's Law
Petty cash
Primary care provider
Professional marketing
Secondary care provider
Shopped fees
Tertiary care provider

CHAPTER 32 Veterinary Practice Management

Chapter Outline	Teaching Strategies
Veterinary practice management areas	
Veterinary facilities	
Facility nomenclature	
Management of hospital areas	Obtain AAHA standards of excellence and have the class discuss them as they relate to patient care and communication with clients. Draw blueprints of various clinics/hospitals and have the students critique them. Have the students draw blueprints for an ideal clinic and ask their classmates to critique them. They can create a clinic name, describe the location, and write the mission statement.
Outside areas	
Outpatient area	
Inpatient area	
Surgical area	
Support area	
Traffic flow	
Large animal facilities	Have the students compare the duties of a veterinary technician in a small animal clinic and a large animal facility.
Large animal mobile units	
Large animal haul-in facilities	
Building maintenance	Have the students work together to determine ways to minimize outdoor and indoor building and ground maintenance.
General maintenance	Review the cost to purchase and repair equipment such as anesthetic machines, ultrasound machines, automatic processors, and autoclaves. Also, discuss the cost to the clinic, employees, patients, and clients if any of this equipment unexpectedly breaks down.
Managing equipment	
Maintenance	
Managing electrical	White out key words and phrases from Box 32-4 and make copies for the students. Ask them to fill in the blanks and explain each statement.
Equipment	
Veterinary healthcare team	Discuss the possible duties of each member of the veterinary team. Have the students divide the duties of the practice manager amongst the other staff to help understand the need for the position in larger practices. Invite members from the societies with specialty certification programs listed in Box 32-5 to speak to your class regarding the opportunities offered by these organizations.
Veterinary practice manager	
Ward staff	Discuss educational requirements and work experience of ideal candidates.
Receptionists	Discuss educational requirements and work experience of ideal candidates.
Personnel management	Emphasize that the veterinary technician may be called upon to perform all duties except those for which the veterinarian is specifically trained (for example, surgery, prescribing treatments, and making diagnoses).
Delegation principles	
Job descriptions	Provide sample job descriptions for various personnel in small animal, large animal, and mixed animal practices. Provide sample employee evaluation forms.
Hiring procedures	Have the students practice being the interviewer and interviewee in large and small animal practices using the questions in the chapter and any others that they deem fit. Students can actually treat this as a dress rehearsal for an actual interview. Have the students prepare questions that they would ask if they were actually being interviewed for a position. Students can constructively critique each other's verbal and nonverbal responses.
Role of veterinary technicians and veterinarians in management	
Patient management	
Inventory management	Use formulas in Box 32-7 to practice calculating turnover rates of items. Obtain sample inventory forms from computer programs to demonstrate the variety of methods of inventory maintenance. Review the relationship of inventory maintenance with building maintenance, OSHA requirements, and interpersonal communication. Discuss methods of assuring that the clinic does not run out of items.
Client management	
Value of the client	

Copyright © 2006 by Elsevier, Inc. All rights reserved.

PART SIX TOPICS IN PRACTICE MANAGEMENT

Chapter Outline	Teaching Strategies
Client selection of a veterinarian	Discuss the role of the veterinary technician in promoting a client's satisfaction with a clinic. Stress that most clients will spend more time communicating with support staff than with the veterinarian.
Evaluation of the client	
Client traffic flow management	
Office procedures	
Appointments	
Practice scheduling	Have the students attempt to make a schedule for an average practice (8 AM to 12 PM, 3 PM to 7 PM Monday through Friday and 9 AM to 1 PM Saturday). Remind students that full-time employees cannot work over 40 hours without earning overtime pay. All positions must be scheduled. Discuss the importance of cross-training and utilizing part-time employees.
Professional fees	Provide an example of a salary being prorated to a fee such as the cost of a spay or neutering procedure. Invite an accountant to speak to the students regarding salary and fee determination in veterinary medicine. Review the differences between shopped and nonshopped fees.
Collections and billings	Discuss the importance of printing out a written fee estimate before beginning treatment.
Cash control	
Business management	
Pet insurance	Obtain literature from pet insurance companies to share with the students. Determine how beneficial coverage might be for owners and the practice in various situations.
Client communication	
Client expectations	
Common complaints from clients	
The difficult client	
Professional marketing	
Practice marketing	
Internal marketing	The veterinary technician plays a key role in all aspects of practice marketing. Have the students discuss what they believe their role to be in terms of practice appearance, personal appearance, client reminders, handout material, and other communication methods mentioned in the chapter.
Client relationships	
Practice appearance	
Support staff utilization	
Full service care	
Client reminders	
Personal appearance	
Handout materials	
Sympathy and thank you communications	
Newsletter/e-mail	
Special services	
Sales point displays	
Animal care talks	
External marketing	Have the students collect samples of external marketing of local veterinary clinics/hospitals. Analyze these ads and discuss the role of the veterinary technician in their production and promotion.
Professional advertising	
Telephone yellow pages	
Internet web page	
Newspapers	
Radio and television	
Community activities	
Graduate technician self-marketing	Obtain the IAMS publication "How to Market Yourself—A Veterinary Technician Placement Program" and discuss methods that veterinary technicians can employ to help them increase their billable tasks. Review the importance of this goal for the entire veterinary staff. Encourage students to review information at www.NCVEI.org.

Copyright © 2006 by Elsevier, Inc. All rights reserved.

CHAPTER 32 Veterinary Practice Management

ACTIVITY

Describe the design of a couple of different clinics. Include some mistakes. For example, "The radiology room is as far away as possible from the surgery room and treatment area in order to avoid exposure of personnel to scatter radiation." "The surgery room must always have two entrances: one entrance for the prepped animal, surgeon, and surgical assistant and one entrance for all other personnel." "The recovery room must have a window so that postsurgical patients with an endotracheal tube in place can be observed periodically as the technician performs other duties." Ask the student to select the statements that are incorrect and choose from a list of reasons. This could also be set up as a true-or-false exercise.

CRITICAL THINKING CHALLENGES

1. Ask each student to contact a local veterinary clinic/hospital and request an interview with the owner or practice manager regarding the facility design. Ask if there is anything about the building's design that they would change if they could and why. Other questions might include:
   A. What would you like to change about the design of this facility and why?
   B. Are there trends in the field that dictate the need to change (reconstruction or reorganization)? Have the students also report their own impression of the facility's design to the class.
2. Invite veterinarians to speak to your class who have been successful and unsuccessful in starting up and running veterinary clinics/hospitals. Have students prepare questions in advance regarding starting up a veterinary facility.
3. Explain the increasing use of problem-based interview questions. Have the students practice asking and answering these questions while their classmates provide constructive critiques. Possible questions include:
   A. Tell us about a time when you had to assume a leadership role on a job.
   B. How did it come about and how did it turn out?
4. Disagreements between co-workers are unavoidable. Tell us about a time when you did not agree with a co-worker and how you resolved the conflict.

QUIZ

Respond to each statement below by placing one letter of the answer on each blank line. Place the answer to the Super Clue in the boxes from top to bottom.

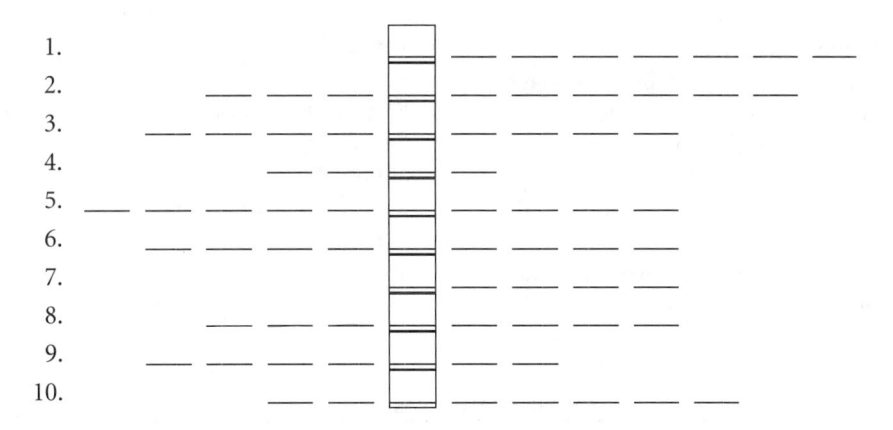

1. This procedure can help to stop the spread of disease throughout a herd or kennel and prevent it in the future.
2. These infections are acquired by patients while staying in the hospital.
3. This is the second-largest expense area of operating a veterinary practice.
4. This is always the best method of payment for services.
5. Doing this is important when communicating with a client because it gives the client an opportunity to clarify or confirm the technician's understanding.
6. The patient is often taken to this area after orthopedic surgery is performed to reduce fractures or place implants.
7. This type of cash is often used to purchase stamps and incidental supplies locally.
8. This type of facility offers overnight hospitalization.
9. This room should have only one entrance/exit.
10. These costs to operate a business are also known as overhead.

Super Clue: These fees do not have to be competitive with local clinics and are increased by the inflation rate on at least an annual basis.

Answers: (1) necropsy, (2) nosocomial, (3) inventory, (4) cash, (5) paraphrasing, (6) radiology, (7) petty, (8) hospital, (9) surgery, (10) indirect, Super Clue: nonshopped. ■

Copyright © 2006 by Elsevier, Inc. All rights reserved.

33

Medical Records

TEACHING/LEARNING OBJECTIVES

1. List as many reasons for keeping complete, detailed medical records as possible.
2. Explain how medical records can be used to support research.
3. Describe three types of physical patient records and name advantages and disadvantages of each.
4. Explain one major drawback of using the source-oriented medical record.
5. Discuss reasons why recording a patient's signalment is important.
6. Name the typical components of the patient's database in a veterinary hospital.
7. Define SOAP and explain its purpose.
8. Explain how a master problem list is a snapshot overview of a patient's medical history.
9. List reasons for asking owners to sign consent forms.
10. Give two reasons for keeping logs.
11. What are advantages of keeping both anesthetic forms and logs?
12. Define controlled substances and explain the meaning of the numbering sequence of Schedule I to Schedule V.
13. Explain how to correct entries in a medical record.
14. Define VMDB and explain its purpose.

KEY TERMS

American Animal Hospital Association (AAHA)
Comprehensive Drug Abuse and Control Act
Controlled substances
Database
Informed consent
Master problem list
Primary purpose for medical records
Problem-oriented medical record
Reportable diseases
Retrospective study
Secondary purpose for medical records
Signalment
SOAP
Source-oriented medical record
Veterinary Medical Database (VMDB)
Working problem list

Chapter Outline	Teaching Strategies
Functions of the medical record	Study already-completed medical forms from local hospitals or complete your own to point out examples of how the record supports primary and secondary purposes. Students can determine if the record is an example of a POMR or SOMR and can identify historical information, physical exam, database, master and working problem lists, and progress notes.

Primary purposes
  Supports excellent medical care
Secondary purposes
  Supports business and legal activities
  Supports research
	Contact the state veterinary school or obtain issues of *Veterinary Research* to learn about current research being conducted. Ask the students to determine the role of medical records for the researchers. Invite an investigator to speak to your class to explain the importance of recording accurate, legible, and thorough medical records and the impact of these records on his or her work and ability to get continued funding. This is an opportunity for the students to learn about opportunities in research settings for veterinary technicians.

CHAPTER 33 Medical Records

Chapter Outline	Teaching Strategies
Types of patient records	Explain the purpose of the AAHA. Obtain a copy of the AAHA's record keeping requirements for accreditation and discuss it with the class.
Letter-sized folders	
Card files	
Carbonized sheets (ambulatory large animal practices)	
Format of the patient record	See Functions of the Medical Record, above. Review commonly used abbreviations.
Source-oriented medical record	
Problem-oriented veterinary medical record	
Components of the POVMR	
Client and patient information	
History form	
Physical examination form	
Database	Emphasize that diagnoses and therapeutic plans can be determined based on information in the database.
Master problem list	Compare master problem list and working problem list and discuss the utility of each method.
Working problem list	
Progress notes	Review the individual components of a SOAP. Provide specific examples of information taken from SOAPs and ask the students to determine if it belongs under S, O, A, or P.
Ward treatment sheets and cage cards	
Pertinent forms	Point out that veterinary hospitals vary in the forms that they use depending on their specific needs.
Laboratory diagnostic summary and flow sheet	
Consultants	
Case summary and discharge Instructions	Discuss reasons for giving discharge instructions to owners. Emphasize the importance of reviewing it with the owner before the owner is reunited with his or her pet.
Consent and authorization forms	
Logs	
Radiology log	
Surgery log	
Anesthesia log	
Necropsy log	
Controlled substances log	Discuss DEA licenses, inspections, and storage and recording requirements for controlled substances.
Organization and filing	Compare the alphabetic and numeric filing systems and include advantages and disadvantages of each method.
File purging	
Lost records	
Ethical and legal issues	
Ownership of medical records	Review reasons for making copies of medical records and point out that these records are the property of the hospital.
Release of medical information	Present examples of medical release forms. Explain the legal implications of not requiring such forms to be signed by the owner.
Medical and legal requirements	Discuss methods of correcting entries and identifying the author of entries. Bring a copy of the state laws to class that govern how long records should be kept and restrictions on the release of medical information.
Veterinary medical database (VMDB)	
Computers	

Copyright © 2006 by Elsevier, Inc. All rights reserved.

ACTIVITY

Provide a few of the forms in the chapter already completed but with mistakes and ask the student to click on all of the mistakes that they can identify.

EXAMPLE

Essential information is missing such as

Owner's phone number
Scribbled out entries
Illegible words
Unsigned euthanasia authorization form
Abbreviated final diagnosis
SOAP report missing the "O," or letters in wrong order

CRITICAL THINKING CHALLENGES

1. Obtain blank medical record forms from several local veterinary hospitals. Ask the students to compare them focusing on potential advantages and disadvantages of each one. The students can work in pairs to create their own forms.
2. Contact the AVMA PLIT or your state's veterinary medical association. Request information on cases in which a veterinary hospitals were involved in lawsuits regarding data recording or record keeping. Discuss methods to prevent such errors.
3. Ask the students to work in pairs to review completed medical records and identify errors including omissions and inconsistencies.

QUIZ

Match each statement with the appropriate word/phrase at the right. There is only one correct answer for each statement.

1. This is essentially a list of final diagnoses rather than a list of symptoms. _____
2. In this filing system there are no duplicate files. _____
3. This schedule of controlled drug is the least addictive. _____
4. Entries in medical records should be made in this color of ink. _____
5. These document ongoing management of veterinary patients. _____
6. This consists of the age, breed, sex, and species of the veterinary patient. _____
7. Inventory records for controlled drugs must be kept in the medical record for how long? _____
8. These provide data for quick analysis and retrospective studies. _____
9. This association requires use of letter-sized folders and the POVMR approach to record keeping in order to receive accreditation from them. _____
10. Under this part of the SOAP, physiologic data are recorded. _____

A. Working problem list
B. Schedule V
C. American Animal Hospital Association
D. 1 year
E. Blue
F. Progress notes
G. Objective
H. Schedule I
I. Problem oriented
J. Subjective
K. Numeric
L. 8 years
M. Signalment
N. Alphabetic
O. 2 years
P. Assessment
Q. Master problem list
R. Logs

Answers: (1) Q, (2) K, (3) B, (4) S, (5) F, (6) M, (7) O, (8) R, (9) C, (10) P. ∎

34

Computer Applications in Veterinary Practice

TEACHING/LEARNING OBJECTIVES

1. Explain the difference between operating software and applications software.
2. List advantages of 32-bit programs.
3. Explain how Tablet PCs help the veterinary team, client, and patient.
4. Explain the advantage of having mirrored hard drives so that the cost is justified.
5. How and how often should computers be cleaned?
6. Explain how computerized billing tends to increase invoices and the number of professional staff in a practice and decrease burnout.
7. Explain how a paperless practice is protected in the event of a natural disaster or litigation.

KEY TERMS

Computer hardware
Operating software
Applications software
32-bit
Server
Tablet PCs
Microprocessor
Motherboard
Redundant (mirrored) hard drives
Surge protector
Data
Database
Travel sheet
Line item
Voice recognition software
Profit centers
Paperless

Chapter Outline

Computer hardware and software
Computer configurations
Maintenance tips

How to research, select, and purchase hardware and software

Typical uses of computers in veterinary practice
Data collection

Scheduling
Billing
Medical records
Client communications and mass mailings
Inventory management
Accounting and practice management
Implications for the future

Teaching Strategies

Discuss maintenance contracts, including their cost. Make copies of several types of maintenance contracts for the students to review.
Obtain copies of demo CDs from vendors and explore these with the class. Discuss advantages and disadvantages of each package. Have the students research costs of computerizing several different types of clinics.

Review ways that a database can be utilized to improve internal marketing, external marketing, and communications.

Chapter Outline	Teaching Strategies
Paperless vs. Less paper	Discuss the issue of data loss in the event of a natural disaster and the advantages of the paperless system.
Other applications for computer use in veterinary practice	Recommend that your students register with www.VetMedTeam.com and/or www.VSPN.org. Periodically during the semester have a student bring in information from the site on predetermined topics to discuss with the class.
The future is not far away	Reinforce the concept that while computerization may require an initial investment in time and money, the benefits to the animals, owners, and veterinary team outweigh these costs.

CRITICAL THINKING CHALLENGES

Ask the students to imagine that they work for the only veterinarian (a very busy one) in a small town. The clinic is not computerized. Have them prepare a presentation that will sell the veterinarian on the idea that computerizing the clinic would be a great advantage, despite its cost. Include specific examples of its benefits, how the system would be set up in the clinic, and approximately how much it would cost to purchase.

QUIZ

Circle T (true) or F (false) for each statement.

1. T F Unfortunately, no software program to date is able to address the issue of accounts receivables by identifying clients who have not been paying their bills.
2. T F Most veterinary software packages come with predetermined prices for products and services making the veterinarians' job much easier.
3. T F Operating software organizes and monitors peripheral devices such as printers, scanners, and disc drives.
4. T F The majority of scheduled appointments are generated from reminders.
5. T F The best way to clean inside the computer is with a diluted hypochlorite solution.
6. T F The use of a travel sheet is slowly becoming the most commonly used method to track services as they are rendered in the veterinary practice.
7. T F Hardware and software generally require replacement every 5 to 10 years.
8. T F Slots on computer cases must be covered tightly to prevent dust and hair from entering.
9. T F The mouse and modem are examples of hardware.
10. T F Windows 95/98/NT and 2000 are considered to be 32-bit programs.

Answers: (1) F, (2) F, (3) T, (4) T, (5) F, (6) F, (7) T, (8) F, (9) T, (10) T. ■

35

Zoonoses and Public Health

TEACHING/LEARNING OBJECTIVES

1. List individuals who are at risk of developing serious infection if bitten by an animal.
2. Describe situations in which animals are more likely to bite.
3. Describe the appropriate disposal of a carcass/materials that are suspected of being infected/contaminated with anthrax.
4. Clarify which animals may suffer peracute, acute, subacute, and chronic forms of anthrax and the clinical signs typically seen with each form.
5. Explain why necropsy should never be performed on animals suspected of having *B. anthracis* infection.
6. List reservoirs for *Chlamydia psittaci*.
7. Explain how psittacosis may be transmitted to humans.
8. Describe ways in which transmission of *Chlamydia psittaci* to humans can be prevented.
9. How do most people in the world contract brucellosis?
10. Describe clinical signs in humans infected with *B. melitensis* biovar *abortus* and *B. melitensis* biovar *melitensis*.
11. Describe the clinical course of campylobacteriosis in humans.
12. Explain how to collect blood for culture of *Bartonella henselae*.
13. Explain how cat-scratch disease is transmitted to humans and how it can be prevented in both cats and humans.
14. Describe individuals who are predisposed to infection with *C. canimorsus*.
15. Describe clinical signs of infection with *C. canimorsus* in dogs.
16. Compare clinical signs of *Erysipelothrix rhusiopathiae* infection in swine, turkeys, and humans.
17. If pasteurellosis is suspected in an animal, describe how to collect and store samples for diagnosis.
18. List the forms of plague in humans and describe the clinical course of each form.
19. Explain how plague is transmitted to humans.
20. Compare the clinical signs of the acute and chronic forms of Q fever in humans.
21. Where can the agents that cause rat-bite fever be found?
22. Name occupations with increased risk of exposure to *Salmonella* spp.
23. Explain how salmonellosis can be diagnosed.
24. What animals are commonly infected with tularemia and how do they become infected?
25. Describe clinical signs of the three forms of tularemia in humans.
26. What populations are at risk of developing clinical signs of cryptococcosis?
27. How is cryptococcosis diagnosed?
28. Explain how dermatophytoses are transmitted to humans and describe the lesions in both animals and people.
29. Explain how cryptosporidiosis can be transmitted in the small animal and large animal veterinary facility.
30. Discuss toxoplasmosis in sheep compared to other animals.
31. Explain how humans may become infected with *Toxoplasma gondii*.
32. Explain how cats may become infected with *Toxoplasma gondii*.
33. Explain how to handle an animal suspected of having monkeypox and include personal protective equipment required.
34. Describe the treatment for monkeypox.
35. List reservoirs of contagious ecthyma.
36. Explain how contagious ecthyma is transmitted to humans and how it is treated.
37. Describe how *Herpesvirus simiae* infection is transmitted.
38. Explain safety measures that must be taken by all personnel working with macaque primates.
39. Compare the clinical signs of lentogenic, velogenic, and mesogenic strains of the virus that causes Newcastle disease.
40. Explain measures that all veterinary personnel should take to prevent the spread of Newcastle disease.

41. Describe urban and sylvatic cycles of the rabies virus.
42. What clinical signs are expected to be seen in rabid dogs, cats, cattle, foxes, skunks, and raccoons?

KEY TERMS

Abattoir
Acute
Ampullitis
Bacillary peliosis
Bacillary angiomatosis
Biovar
Bite wound
Buboes
Carrier
Chronic
Coryza
Definitive host
Diamond skin disease
Endospore
Enzootic
Epizootic
Erysipeloid
Eschar
Exanthematous rash
Fastidious
Fowl cholera
Fulminant disease
Haverhill fever
Intermediate host
Kerion
Lymphadenopathy
Mechanical transmission
Neuralgia
Orchitis
Orf
Pathognomonic feature
Peracute
Pruritus
Rabbit fever
Reservoir
Reticuloendothelial structures
Saprophyte
Seminal vesiculitis
Snuffles
Spirillosis
Spondylitis
Streptobacillosis
Subacute
Tinea
Tinea barbae
Tinea capitis
Tinea corporis
Vector
Vesicles
Zoonosis

Chapter Outline	Teaching Strategies
	For each disease mentioned in Table 35-1, show the students photos of the organism from histologic preparations and of clinical manifestation in animals and people. Ask the students to describe what to do immediately if they suspect that an animal is infected with the disease or if they or any other staff member may have been exposed to it. Contact your state veterinarian for information regarding recognition and response to zoonotic diseases of livestock and poultry.
Animal-associated injuries: bite wounds	The veterinary staff can take specific measures to decrease the incidence of these injuries. Have the students discuss ways to accomplish this goal in the small and large animal practice. Students may need to review restraint techniques in Chapter 1. Ask them to discuss the role of communication in preventing these injuries. Point out which diseases are most likely to be seen in small, equine, food, and exotic animal practices.
Bacterial zoonoses	
Anthrax	Point out that although this disease is rarely diagnosed in the United States, it should still be considered a potential diagnosis if appropriate clinical signs are present.
Psittacosis (avian chlamydiosis)	Review the biphasic reproductive cycle of this bacterium. Emphasize effective methods of cage cleaning.
Brucellosis	Review the anatomy and physiology of the reproductive tract and how it is affected by this organism.
Campylobacteriosis	
Cat-scratch disease (*Bartonella henselae* infection)	Review current flea control methods.

CHAPTER 35 Zoonoses and Public Health

Chapter Outline	Teaching Strategies
Capnocytophaga infection	Review the treatment of all dog and cat bites.
Erysipelothrix infection	Emphasize the importance of sanitation in preventing this disease.
Pasteurellosis	Compare clinical presentations of this disease in various species of animals.
Plague	Review the clinical signs of *Yersinia pestis* infection in cats and dogs.
Q fever (coxiellosis)	Have students discuss their role in helping to prevent the transmission of this disease.
Rat-bite fevers: streptobacillosis and spirillosis	Compare clinical presentations of streptobacillosis and spirillosis.
Salmonellosis	Have the students describe how pet reptiles must be handled to decrease the possibility of contracting salmonellosis.
Tularemia	Explain how veterinary personnel might be exposed to this disease and how it can be prevented.
Mycotic zoonoses	
Systemic infections: cryptococcosis	Discuss veterinary staff who may be at risk of contracting cryptococcosis, clinical signs, and how to prevent it.
Superficial mycoses: dermatophytoses	Discuss common methods of diagnosing dermatophytosis.
Parasitic diseases	
Cryptosporidiosis	Point out that humans are reservoirs for this organism and review ways in which humans may be exposed to this agent.
Toxoplasmosis	Compare primary and congenital toxoplasmosis. Discuss precautions that all personnel (particularly pregnant employees) must take to prevent transmission of this disease.
Viral diseases	
Monkeypox	
Contagious ecthyma (orf)	
Herpesvirus simiae infection (B virus)	Review biosafety levels and their requirements. Discuss facilities in the United States in which a veterinary technician would need to be concerned about this disease.
Newcastle disease	Point out the economic impact of this disease on the poultry industry.
Rabies	Review the protocol of preexposure vaccination for veterinary personnel. Discuss steps to be taken when an owner or member of the veterinary team is bitten by a dog in the clinic. Include actions to take in the event that the dog is vaccinated against the rabies virus and unvaccinated.

Game: Tic-Tac-Toe

Q-fever question	Rabies question	Toxoplasmosis question
Cryptosporidium question	Newcastle question	Campylobacteriosis question
Brucellosis question	Cat-scratch disease question	Rat-bite fever question

This requires two players, or the class can be divided into two teams. You are the moderator who reads the questions. This can be played on an overhead projector. If they answer correctly, they gain possession of the box. If they answer incorrectly, the box remains open. The next time a player chooses that box a new question is asked on that topic.

CRITICAL THINKING CHALLENGES

1. Some zoonotic agents are capable of being (and recently have been) manufactured as biological weapons. Veterinary technicians and veterinarians can be the first to recognize or suspect infection of animals with these diseases and play a key role in

Copyright © 2006 by Elsevier, Inc. All rights reserved.

their prevention and diagnosis. In this regard the veterinary team plays a major role in public safety and education of owners. Either describe clinical signs or show photos of animals/humans with clinical manifestations of zoonotic diseases and have the students prepare a list of differential diagnoses. Have them describe the immediate treatment of the animal(s) and any persons who may be at risk of infection.

2. Ask the students to describe their response if a co-worker is severely bitten at work. Their discussion should include treatment of the co-worker as well as communication with owners regarding rabies and handling of the dog or cat.

QUIZ

Match each statement with the disease that it describes.

1. ___ Ingestion of rodent-contaminated food or water can cause this form of streptobacillosis.
2. ___ This food- and waterborne disease is the most common cause of diarrhea in the world.
3. ___ A Wood's lamp may help to diagnose this disease.
4. ___ The prevalence of this organism in livestock is related to the number of cats in pasture lands.
5. ___ Humans who work with infected animals can contract this disease by cleaning the cages or inhaling infective particles that have been aerosolized by sneezing and wing flapping by the bird.
6. ___ Endocarditis causes death in approximately 2% of humans infected with this organism.
7. ___ Many human cases of this disease occur in New Zealand and it is an occupational disease of sheep handlers, veterinarians, and abattoir workers.
8. ___ This disease may be acquired through bites from infected monkeys and aerosolization of the virus.
9. ___ In people, infection with this organism may cause cellulitis, which appears as a painful, raised, purplish lesion.
10. ___ This virus can be transmitted in the saliva of bats and is always fatal if contracted by humans.
11. ___ Fleas that ingest this organism will regurgitate it into bite wounds and die of starvation.
12. ___ This infection may manifest as bacillary peliosis or bacillary angiomatosis.
13. ___ This disease manifests as fowl cholera, coryza in rabbits, and atrophic rhinitis in pigs, rats, and calves.
14. ___ This disease may manifest in humans as reddish, pruritic papules that develop into fluid-filled vesicles or as a nonspecific upper respiratory problem.
15. ___ This disease is transmitted via the fecal-oral route and fecal carriage rates may exceed 90% in some reptiles such as iguanas, turtles, and snakes.
16. ___ This organism can be present in high numbers in pigeon or other bird droppings and exposure to highly infected aviaries or pigeon coops increases the risk of disease in humans.
17. ___ Veterinary personnel should keep a high index of suspicion for this disease in animals, especially rodents, that have a history of fever, conjunctivitis, respiratory signs, and nodular rash.
18. ___ Humans may become infected with this agent through dog and cat bites and scratches.
19. ___ This disease can be transmitted through aerosolization from infected birth fluids and ruminant placentae, wool, and hides and possibly through exposure to infected newborn or stillborn pets.
20. ___ This disease is transmitted via the fecal-oral route and the infective oocysts are resistant to many chemical disinfectants, including chlorination.
21. ___ Most veterinary personnel afflicted with this disease have acquired it from infected cats.

A. Monkeypox
B. Pasteurellosis
C. Tularemia
D. Cryptococcosis
E. Rabies
F. Q fever
G. Salmonellosis
H. Toxoplasmosis
I. *Herpesvirus simiae* infection
J. Anthrax
K. Cryptosporidiosis
L. Campylobacteriosis
M. Brucellosis
N. Haverhill fever
O. Psittacosis
P. Plague
Q. Erysipelothrix infection
R. Contagious ecthyma
S. Cat-scratch disease
T. *Microsporum canis*
U. *Capnocytophaga canimorsus*

Answers: (1) N, (2) L, (3) T, (4) H, (5) O, (6) M, (7) R, (8) I, (9) Q, (10) E, (11) P, (12) S, (13) B, (14) J, (15) G, (16) D, (17) A, (18) U, (19) F, (20) K, (21) C. ∎

36

Occupational Health and Safety

TEACHING/LEARNING OBJECTIVES

1. What is the role of the Occupational Safety and Health Administration (OSHA)?
2. Describe ways in which leadership can provide practice-specific safety training to ensure that all personnel are trained for their duties?
3. Explain how to store heavy supplies or equipment and chemicals.
4. Explain how to safely open an autoclave.
5. What is the function of a surge suppressor and what types of things may and may not be plugged into it?
6. Explain how to store flammable liquids and other materials.
7. Explain where portable heaters can and cannot be placed in a clinic?
8. Explain PASS.
9. Explain the Right to Know Law.
10. Define secondary container?
11. Explain how to dilute a chemical with water.
12. Describe how to clean up a chemical spill.
13. Explain how to dispose of light bulbs.
14. Describe personal protective equipment that should always be used when bathing or dipping a pet.
15. List means of becoming exposed to zoonotic agents.
16. Explain the concern of handling animals infected with parvovirus (a nonzoonotic agent) for an employee who has puppies or unvaccinated dogs at home and describe ways to prevent these problems.
17. Describe safety precautions that must be taken when performing dental procedures on animals.
18. What protective equipment must be worn when taking radiographs?
19. Explain how to dispose of radiographic processing chemicals.
20. Perform a leak check of an anesthetic machine.
21. List the potential dangers of long-term exposure to waste anesthetic gases.
22. Describe the procedure to follow if anesthetic is spilled.
23. List precautions that must be taken to reduce waste anesthetic gas when using a mask or tank for induction.
24. Describe storage conditions for compressed gases.
25. Describe safety precautions that must be taken when handling cytotoxic drugs.

KEY TERMS

Cold sterilization
Collimator
Cytotoxic drugs (CD)
Dosimetry badge
Ergonomic
Ground-fault circuit interruption (GFCI) type outlet
Hazardous Materials Plan
Hospital Safety Manual
Material Safety Data Sheet (MSDS)
Medical waste
National Institute of Occupational Safety and Health (NIOSH)
Occupational Safety and Health Act
Occupational Safety and Health Administration (OSHA)
OSHA Form 300A
Personal protective equipment (PPE)
Practice-specific safety training
Right to Know Law
Secondary container
Sharps container
Thyroid collar
Waste anesthetic gas (WAG)
Zoonotic disease

PART SIX TOPICS IN PRACTICE MANAGEMENT

Chapter Outline	Teaching Strategies
The objectives of a safety program	Have the students make a list of safety issues in the veterinary workplace before reading this chapter. As they study the chapter, ask them to add topics to the list. Emphasize that there are numerous safety concerns in the clinic/hospital and the student should be aware of these upon beginning a career in this field.
Your safety rights	Provide the students with the phone number, address, and e-mail address of OSHA.
Your safety responsibilities	Give the students a copy of the Occupational Safety and Health Act (the Act) and highlight major points. Discuss examples of situations that warrant disciplinary action or termination for willful violation of safety rules.
The leadership's rights	Review the procedure for inspection by an OSHA agent.
The leadership's responsibilities	Ask the students to imagine the ideal leadership to have on a job. Have them discuss the qualities of such leaders in the veterinary workplace.
General workplace hazards	Obtain copies of hospital safety manuals from local veterinary hospitals and discuss them as the chapter is studied.
Dressing appropriately	Review various dress codes and reasons for them. Emphasize that each clinic has its own dress code that must be respected.
Save your back!	Have the students practice lifting boxes or other inanimate items. Be sure that they bend their knees and keep their backs as straight as possible.
Clean up after yourself!	
Everything in its place	
Beware break time!	
Machinery and equipment	Review the concepts/functions of grounding, GFCE-type outlets, grounded plugs, and surge protectors.
Electrical	
Fire and evacuation	Review storage requirements of flammable liquids and other materials. Stress that one should always have at least two clear exits from the building. Review the information in Box 36-1. Emphasize that the alarm should be sounded and all employees should have left or be leaving the building before using the fire extinguisher.
Don't become a victim of violence	Discuss different types of alarm systems in veterinary hospitals and ways to contact police in the event of a robbery or other crime. Have the students review valuable items that are in the veterinary clinic and ways that they can be protected.
Hazardous chemicals—right to know	Obtain a copy of OSHA's Right to Know Law and discuss it with the class. Obtain copies of several Material Safety Data Sheets and review their contents with the students.
Special chemicals	Review special handling requirements for chemicals such as glutaraldehyde, formalin, and ethylene oxide. Bring the MSDS to class and discuss special requirements for these chemicals.
Medical and animal-related hazards	See Chapter 1 for restraint techniques.
Noise is noise	Review the rating system for hearing protective devices.
Bathing, dipping, and spraying areas	Bring a few medical dips and insecticide containing shampoos to class. Have the students read the labels specifically looking for instructions, safety information, ingredients, and any other information that pertains to employee and pet safety. Emphasize that students must become accustomed to reading this information and MSDS information before using products.
Zoonotic diseases	See Chapter 35 for a more extensive discussion of zoonotic diseases.
Viral infections	
Bacterial infections	
Fungal infections	
Internal parasites	
External parasites	
Protozoal infections	
Nonzoonotic diseases of concern	Review ways to decrease contamination of the rest of the clinic with nonzoonotic, contagious diseases such as parvovirus and agents in the feline upper respiratory disease complex.
A dirty mouth? Precautions for dentistry operations	See Chapter 28. Explain how aerosolized *P. multocida* can lead to cardiomyopathies in humans.

Copyright © 2006 by Elsevier, Inc. All rights reserved.

CHAPTER 36 Occupational Health and Safety

Chapter Outline	Teaching Strategies
Radiology	See Chapter 9. Review methods of checking gloves and aprons for holes. Discuss the importance of wearing and submitting dosimetry badges and review the process of periodic badge submission. Bring MSDS for radiographic processing chemicals to class for the students to read and discuss.
Anesthesia	See Chapter 19. Perform a leak-check of an anesthetic machine in class. Review the advantages and disadvantages of the three types of scavenging systems. Have the students describe extra precautions that they would take if inducing a patient with a mask or induction tank. Beginning with the moment that a patient is intubated to the few minutes after extubation, ask the students to list all precautions that they must take to minimize exposure to waste anesthetic gas.
Compressed gases	Review the reasons for keeping compressed gases in a veterinary clinic and discuss the types of injuries that can be caused by mishandling these cylinders.
Sharps and medical waste	Obtain a copy of your state's rules regarding disposal of hazardous medical waste and have the students compare them with the information in Table 36-1. Ask the students to practice the one-handed method of recapping a needle, both on the floor and on a tabletop.
Hazardous drugs and pharmacy operations	Obtain the manufacturer's information for several common cytotoxic drugs and have the students make lists of protective measures to take when handling them. Review the physiologic mechanism of some of these drugs.

CRITICAL THINKING CHALLENGES

1. Prepare a list of activities commonly performed by veterinary staff. Ask the students to list or describe protective equipment that should be worn when performing these tasks and any other concerns/precautions that should be taken. Have the students describe potential hazards to the employee if these precautions are not taken.
2. Have the students imagine that they are an OSHA representative performing an inspection of a veterinary clinic. Ask them to make a checklist of all areas of the hospital and describe what they would hope to find and what constitutes a violation.

QUIZ

Circle T (true) or F (false) for each statement.

1. T F Every employee is entitled to see private information about other employees if it is relevant to his or her safety at certain times of the year.
2. T F The leadership of a veterinary practice is responsible for providing safety training for all employees.
3. T F Chemicals should always be stored at or above eye level so that their labels are in clear view from across the clinic.
4. T F Food may be stored in the same refrigerator as vaccines, drugs, and laboratory samples as long as a separate shelf is clearly labeled for this purpose.
5. T F As long as equipment is turned off, overloaded or faulty electrical cords cannot overheat or short and start a fire.
6. T F When using a fire extinguisher, the correct sequence of events is to pull the pin, aim low (at the base of the fire), squeeze the handle, and sweep from side to side.
7. T F The Right to Know Law requires employees to wear all safety equipment that is prescribed by the manufacturer and the practice when using any product containing a hazardous chemical.
8. T F Chemical spills should be cleaned with a detergent soap and water and not a disinfecting soap.
9. T F Historically, glutaraldehyde has been used to preserve tissues in veterinary clinics.
10. T F Spray attachments for tubs should not be used to flush eyes because the streams of water from these devices may damage the corneas.
11. T F Although parvovirus is not a zoonosis, an employee in a veterinary clinic might infect his or her own pet with this virus after handling an infected pet at work.
12. T F *Pasteurella haemolytica* is one of the most common pathogens in the mouths of animals and can be aerosolized during dental operations.
13. T F The collimator allows one to control scatter radiation to some degree by restricting the primary beam.

Copyright © 2006 by Elsevier, Inc. All rights reserved.

14. T F The dosimetry badge worn when taking radiographs helps to collect scatter radiation.
15. T F A leak-check must be performed before every use of the anesthetic machine.
16. T F If anesthetic is spilled, it should be mopped up with detergent soap immediately.
17. T F Compressed gas cylinders that are empty can be stored in the clinic area as long as they are tagged as empty.
18. T F When disposing of a used needle and syringe, the needle should not be removed from the syringe.
19. T F Powder-free chemotherapy gloves should be worn when handling cytotoxic drugs.
20. T F For up to 24 hours after administering cytotoxic drugs to an animal, any laundry soiled with their bodily excretions is considered medical waste.

Answers: (1) F, (2) T, (3) F, (4) F, (5) F, (6) T, (7) T, (8) T, (9) F, (10) T, (11) T, (12) F, (13) T, (14) F, (15) T, (16) F, (17) F, (18) T, (19) T, (20) F. ∎

37

Euthanasia

TEACHING/LEARNING OBJECTIVES

1. Explain when is the appropriate time to begin to discuss the topic of euthanasia with an owner.
2. Describe some of the possible reflexes of animals when euthanasia solution is injected.
3. Describe various options for the location of euthanasia.
4. Name the dosage of sodium pentobarbital recommended for euthanasia.
5. List things that technicians do that indicate to the owners that their pet's body has been treated with dignity and respect.
6. Explain possible coping strategies for staff members who perform numerous euthanasias or for those who might be approaching burnout.

KEY TERMS

Euthanasia
Sodium pentobarbital
Burnout

Chapter Outline	Teaching Strategies
The decision	Review the nature of information that can be given to owners who are considering euthanasia for their pets. Some information is more appropriately imparted by the veterinarian; other Information is commonly shared by the veterinary technician, assistant, and receptionist. Have the students discuss this concept using several scenarios.
As the end draws near: the beginning of the end	Stress the importance of scheduling euthanasia procedures in advance during times of the day when business is expected to be slow. When this is not possible, it is still important to allow owners to spend time with their pet after the euthanasia is performed.
The stress of euthanasia	Review ways in which frequently performing euthanasia in a practice can lead to stress and ways to cope.
Euthanasia in the shelter and research facility	Compare reasons for euthanasia in the shelter, research setting, and clinic/hospital. Discuss ways in which technical staff in these settings might cope with the duties of performing euthanasia.
Euthanasia of large animals	Discuss methods of promoting safety for the owner and staff during the euthanasia of a large animal. Stress that this can be a very emotional event for the owner just as it for the owner of a small animal that is euthanized.

CRITICAL THINKING CHALLENGES

Provide several situations in which the owner of a beloved pet is considering euthanasia for a pet or has just had a pet euthanized. Situations might include the geriatric dog or cat in end stages of cancer, a retired racehorse with advanced osteoarthritis, a bird that appeared to be perfectly healthy yesterday, and a puppy with an advanced parvovirus infection. The owners should represent a variety of clients including the elderly person with no other relatives that the pet, the young couple without enough money to pay the bills, and the child who had the responsibility of caring for the bird. Have the students act out the roles of the owner, the veterinary technician, and the veterinary receptionist while you portray the veterinarian. Have the classmates critique

Copyright © 2006 by Elsevier, Inc. All rights reserved.

the act based on compassion, respect, and knowledge demonstrated.

QUIZ

Circle T (true) or F (false) for each statement.

1. T F The veterinary technician should help indecisive owners by providing information about the disease, treatments, prognosis, and costs.
2. T F Veterinary professionals can be extremely helpful to the owner considering euthanasia for a pet by communicating compassionately and respectfully.
3. T F Owners who have or are considering having their pet euthanized may feel guilt, helplessness, anger, and pain.
4. T F Many owners change veterinarians after the loss of a pet.
5. T F The term *euthanasia* should always be used when referring to intentionally ending a pet's life.
6. T F Being present for the euthanasia of a pet might help some clients begin to grieve and accept the death of their pet earlier.
7. T F It is recommended that owners pay for the euthanasia service after it is performed so that they can think clearly.
8. T F If owners wish to be present during euthanasia, a peripheral catheter should be placed in a back leg.
9. T F Frequently performing euthanasia is a possible cause of burnout in the veterinary profession.
10. T F The facial vein should be used for injection of euthanasia solution in large animals.

Answers: (1) F, (2) T, (3) T, (4) T, (5) F, (6) T, (7) F, (8) T, (9) T, (10) F. ■

38

Client Bereavement and the Human-Animal Bond

TEACHING/LEARNING OBJECTIVES

1. List needs that pets fulfill for elderly people.
2. Explain how urbanization has affected the position of pets in the family.
3. Define denial and give examples of client behavior that exemplify this emotion.
4. Define bargaining and give examples of client behavior that exemplify this emotion.
5. How should veterinary personnel respond to a client who feels angry with himself- or herself.
6. Explain ways that veterinary professionals can prevent professional grief from causing burnout.
7. List warning signs of depression in a client who has lost a pet and describe a way to help the client.

KEY TERMS

Anger
Anthropomorphism
Bargaining
Bereavement
Compassion
Denial
Depression
Empathy
Grief
Grief process
Guilt
Professional grief
Resolution
Venting

Chapter Outline	Teaching Strategies
The human-animal bond	Review physiologic and psychological benefits that some pet owners experience by having pets. Find clinical research that has been conducted to confirm the benefits and discuss results with the class.
The attachment between humans and animals	Begin a discussion that might allow student to empathize with people who have undergone pet loss. Ask them if they have ever known anyone who fits a description in Box 39-1. Have them describe the person's situation and express how they think the person felt at the time of the loss. Stress that empathy can be an important part of the veterinary technician's job.
Benefits of attachment	
Pet loss and veterinary medicine	Emphasize that veterinary personnel often become a part of the grieving owner's support system. Discuss ways that veterinary personnel can support these clients.
When the bond is broken	
Pet loss and the grief process	
The normal grief process	Explain that the grief process described by Dr. Kübler-Ross was originally developed to describe grief experienced by humans who are facing their own death or the death of a loved one. This fact should emphasize the increasingly elevated status that pets are assuming in our society today because many pet owners proceed through the same stages in response to the loss of a pet. Discuss the role of guilt during the bargaining and anger stages of grieving. Have the students locate books that deal with the grief process in children. If books are short the student can read them to the class and compare the style with the guidelines in Box 38-4.

Chapter Outline	Teaching Strategies
Denial and bargaining	
Anger	
Depression	
Resolution and acceptance	
Grief and the veterinary professional	Emphasize that, without realizing it, dealing with death and dying so frequently can negatively affect veterinary personnel. Have the students discuss ways to prevent and cope with these negative effects in the workplace.
Conclusion	

CRITICAL THINKING CHALLENGES

1. Have a student act out the role of a grieving owner in the denial stage of the grief process. The owner still has attachments to the pet listed in Box 38-1. Another student plays the role of the veterinary technician who must communicate according to the guidelines listed in Box 38-2. The rest of the class determines if the technician's language (verbal language or body language) is appropriate. Repeat this activity, working through all stages of the grief process.
2. Ask students to interview a friend or family member who has lost a pet. It doesn't matter how recently the loss occurred. During the interview the following questions should be posed:
   A. How did you lose your pet?
   B. What was the name of your pet?
   C. When did you lose your pet?
   D. Describe your relationship with your pet.
   E. How did you feel when you first heard that your pet had died or was dying?
   F. How did you react?
   G. How long was it before you got another pet?
3. Have the students identify as many stages of the grief process as they can.
4. Have each student contact a pet loss counselor and obtain information that can be brought to class to be shared. Ask them to highlight information that is not mentioned in the chapter or that may present a different approach to death and dying.
5. Invite a pet loss counselor to class to discuss the grief process as it is experienced by owners and veterinary professionals. Ask students to prepare questions in advance regarding the different types of counselors and their educational requirements, different types of therapy, and any other aspects of the profession.
6. Your office manager, miss E, used to be a congenial, easy-going, and fun person for whom to work. Recently, the clinic has become more busy, some of the original staff members have quit and it has been difficult to fill their places, and the crowding and noise at the clinic has increased. Gradually, miss E has become more withdrawn, has gained weight, and now always seems either very tired or very agitated. Assuming her symptoms are workplace-generated, what may be wrong with her? You and miss E are friends outside the workplace. Name one thing you can do to help her through this time in her life.

QUIZ

1. The acceptance stage of the grief process has also been called _____.
2. Clients experiencing the _____ stage of the grief process may have a change of appetite, withdraw from others, become irritable, and may have trouble sleeping.
3. The pet owner who starts to show you pictures from his recent vacation after being told that his pet cannot be saved after being hit by a car is experiencing the _____ stage of the grief process.
4. One way that a veterinary professional can help an angry client is to allow them to _____, or express their feelings.
5. The author _____ worked extensively with dying persons and their families in the 1960s and wrote the book *On Death and Dying*.
6. Veterinary professionals may be tempted to become defensive or respond in like manner when the client is experiencing the _____ stage of the grief process.
7. As a general rule, children under the age of _____ do not really understand that death is final.
8. The client who tries to negotiate with God for miracles upon hearing the news that his pet is dying is experiencing the _____ stage of the grief process.
9. One definition of _____ is: "ascribing human forms or attributes to a thing or being that is not human" (*Webster's American Dictionary, College Edition*).
10. The depression stage has also been called _____.

Answers: (1) resolution, (2) depression, (3) denial, (4) vent, (5) Dr. Elisabeth Kübler-Ross, (6) anger, (7) 8 years, (8) bargaining, (9) anthropomorphism, (10) grief. ■

Copyright © 2006 by Elsevier, Inc. All rights reserved.

39

Stress and Substance Abuse in Practice

TEACHING/LEARNING OBJECTIVES

1. Define stress and stressors and give an example of an external environmental and internal stressor that a veterinary technician might encounter in a clinic setting.
2. Define GAS and its three stages.
3. Explain the role of the adrenal glands in the fight-or-flight response to stress.
4. Explain the role of the pituitary gland in the fight-or-flight response to stress.
5. Describe the role of neurotransmitters in coping with stress.
6. List risk factors for substance abuse.
7. Explain the accepted protocol for intervening with a co-worker who is impaired.
8. List characteristics of the type A and type B personalities.
9. List examples of potential general environmental stressors, veterinary environmental stressors, personal stressors, client stressors, and career stressors.
10. Explain the benefits of appropriate nutrition, sleep, exercise, and mental recreation and their effects on stress resistance.
11. Describe how the phenomenon of burnout can relate to stress and substance abuse.

KEY TERMS

Adrenal glands
Autohypnosis
Autonomic nervous system
Dopamine
Endorphins
Epinephrine
General adaptation syndrome (GAS)
Impairment
Neurotransmitter
Norepinephrine
Pituitary gland
Polyphasic behavior
Rapid eye movement (REM)
Serotonin
Stress
Stress hardy
Stressors
Substance abuse
Substance dependence
Type A personality
Type B personality

Chapter Outline	Teaching Strategies
A definition of stress	
Good stress/bad stress	Discuss stressors commonly encountered in the veterinary clinic.
Choice	
Control	
Consequences	
Mental and physical effects of stress	
Fight or flight	Review the purpose of the fight-or-flight reaction of stress.
The pathway of stress	Review the anatomical and physiologic pathway of stress.
	Emphasize the activities that occur during each stage of the general adaptation syndrome (GAS).
Stress and the brain	Review changes in the brain that occur during times of stress.
Substance abuse and stress	Emphasize that abnormal neurotransmitter function plays a role in substance abuse development. Discuss risk factors that may contribute to substance abuse and addiction.

PART SIX TOPICS IN PRACTICE MANAGEMENT

Chapter Outline	Teaching Strategies
Abuse or dependence?	
Risk factors for substance abuse	
Recognizing and intervening	Review warning signs that substance abusers may exhibit in their personal and professional lives. Stress that impairment of a co-worker can place the whole clinic at risk of malpractice.
Stress and personality	
The stress-prone individual	Discuss characteristics of the person with the type A personality and explain that the personality is, to some degree, shaped by the environment.
The stress-hardy individual	Discuss characteristics of the person with the type B personality.
Identifying stressors	Review the stressors listed in the chapter and point out the importance of being able to recognize them in order to cope with them. Ask students if they can think of other stressors within these categories and/or additional examples of how to cope with those that are listed.
Life event stressors	
Environmental stressors	
Personal stressors	
Client stressor	
Career stressors	
Evaluation	
Coping with stress	
Stress resister habits	Emphasize the need for continual self-assessment of nutrition, sleep, exercise, and mental recreation habits. Students should review their own personal habits regarding these four aspects of their lifestyles.
Nutrition	
Sleep	
Exercise	
Mental recreation	
Mental health and awareness	Explain how to locate a mental health professional. Provide a list of questions that should be asked of any prospective counselor before seeking their services. Discuss the various types of professionals in this field.
Support	Discuss the importance of support from others and ways to foster various forms of support in the veterinary community.
Relaxation techniques	
Burnout, impairment, and treatment	Review potential physical manifestations of burnout and stress the importance of intervention.

ACTIVITY

1. Provide exercises to help students recognize indications of stress in oneself and others.
2. Develop descriptions of a technician's, veterinarian's or any co-worker's stressful situation and ask the student to identify all of the words/terms that apply.

EXAMPLE

A technician is in the seventh hour of an 8-hour shift. The phones have been ringing "off the hook" all night. You just got off of the phone with an angry client who is upset about the bill that she had to pay today for her pet's treatment. The technician scheduled to come in and relieve you calls in and says that he is sick (again) and will not be able to work that night. It's a very busy night and the veterinarian on duty says to you, "I hope you didn't have any plans for the evening. I need you to stay a few more hours." As you listen to the veterinarian, you can feel your heart rate increasing and your heart pounding in your chest and your stomach feels like it's in a knot. You are frustrated with this lack of responsibility shown by this co-worker. In fact, you respond to the veterinarian, " I can't depend on anyone around here. I'm the only dependable technician in this clinic and the most competent one here." After you take a few deep breaths and regain composure, your say to the veterinarian, "Of course I can stay." You'll make almost any sacrifice to receive approval from your boss.

A. Type A
B. Type B
C. Alarm phase of GAS
D. Adaptation phase of GAS
E. Exhaustion phase of GAS
F. Life event stressor

Copyright © 2006 by Elsevier, Inc. All rights reserved.

G. General environmental stressor
H. Veterinary environmental stressor
I. Environmental stressor
J. Personal stressor
K. Client stressor
L. Career stressor

Answer: A, C, H, K, L

PRACTICAL SITUATIONS

1. Fill out Table 37-3 to determine whether your personality is a strong Type A, a strong Type B, or somewhere in the middle. Then write three examples in which you exhibited characteristics consistent with your dominant personality type and (if possible) three in which you responded according to your nondominant personality type.
2. What causes you the most stress? Turn an 8½ by 11-inch sheet of paper sideways and divide it into four columns. Use the discussion of different types of stressors under "Identifying Stressors" in the chapter; in the first column, list one or two recent things you perceived as "very stressful" in each category: life event, environmental, personal, client or classmate, and career or school. In the second column, write down why you believe this caused you stress. In the third column, write down whether you were happy with the way you responded to each stressor. Now, using the "Coping With Stress" discussion in the chapter, write down in the fourth column some ways you could have modified your response or handled the situation differently so that, in the future, each stressor can become positive rather than negative, or may even be prevented.
3. Using the "Stress Resistor Habits" section in the chapter, record your own nutritional, sleep, exercise, and mental-recreation habits for 5 days. Are there areas in which you can improve or reduce your stress level? If so, list two changes you can make in each problem area to increase your resistance to stress.
4. Developing relaxation skills. As a class, perform one of the relaxation exercises listed in Tables 37-7 and 37-8. Afterward, have a class discussion of how the exercises made the class feel. Did the exercises increase their feeling of relaxation? Have everybody read the section entitled "Relaxation Techniques" in the chapter, which lists some other methods of relaxing. Discuss whether they use of these techniques and what other things they do relax.
5. Exploring personality-type recognition. Break the class in to small groups of two or three. Have each person write down secretly what his or her personality type was determined to be in the first written exercise and what he or she believes is the personality type of the other members of the group. Then have everyone reveal his or her response and discuss why he or she classified each person as they did. If there were discrepancies in answers, have them discuss why people may perceive a person differently than the quiz classifies him or her.

CRITICAL THINKING CHALLENGES

1. Present situations in the veterinary clinic that may begin as positive stress and turn into negative stress for the veterinary technician. For each one, ask the students to discuss choice, control, and consequences involved in the change from good to bad.
2. Invite a recovering substance abuser to your classroom. If possible, ask someone in the veterinary profession or at least in the medical profession. Ask him or her to complete the questionnaire in Table 39-2 and to share results with the students. Ask your guest to discuss their history and how they eventually got help.
3. Ask each student to describe, in writing, a previous or current stressor in his or her life and how they cope with it. They should reflect and determine if their coping behavior was appropriate. If not, how could they have better handled the situation? The students can turn these writings in anonymously if they like and you can read them to the class for discussion.
4. It is important to be able to recognize when someone else (co-worker, friend, relative, etc.) is experiencing overwhelming stress and to know how to respond. It is even possible that we contribute to that person's stress without realizing it. Ask the students to consider if they have ever been in such a situation and describe the events. This exercise can help us become more sensitive to the impact that we have on others with whom we work.
5. Invite a mental health professional to class to discuss the mental health profession and how to locate and choose a counselor. Ask the counselor to talk about stress and substance abuse in the veterinary profession.
6. Your office manager, Miss E., used to be a congenial, easy-going, and fun person for whom to work. Recently, the clinic has become busier, some of the original staff members have quit and it has been difficult to fill their places, and the crowding and noise at the clinic have increased. Gradually, Miss E. has become more withdrawn, has gained weight, and now always seems either very tired or very agitated. Assuming her symptoms are workplace-generated, what may be wrong with her? You and Miss E. are friends outside the workplace. Name one thing you can do to help her through this time in her life.

QUIZ

Place one letter of the response to each statement on each line. The boxes spell out the answer to the Super Clue.

1. __ __ __ __ __ __
2. __ __ __ __ __
3. __ __ __ __ __ __ __
4. __ __ __ __ __ __ __
5. __ __ __ __ __ __ __ __ __ __
6. __ __ __ __ __
7. __ __ __ __ __ __ __ __ __ __
8. __ __ __ __ __ __ __
9. __ __ __ __ __ __ __ __

1. If this person is elderly, angry, or grieving, he or she may be creating stress for the veterinary personnel.
2. This type of veterinary environmental stressor can be caused by telephones ringing, conversations in the background, and the seemingly constant barking of dogs.
3. Friends, spouses, and co-workers can often provide this to help cope with stress.
4. This nutrient is important in counteracting the impact of stress on the body.
5. According to the GAS theory, if a stressor continues to be threatening after the adaptation stage is reached, then this stage occurs.
6. An optimal amount of this is necessary to cope with stress every day; the type and duration needed are currently being researched.
7. This relaxation technique involves control of breathing as the word *relax* is repeated.
8. This is defined as psychological, sometimes physical, exhaustion caused by prolonged, uninterrupted exposure to a stressor or stressors.
9. This antidote to stress helps relieve tension and restores normal chemical balance.

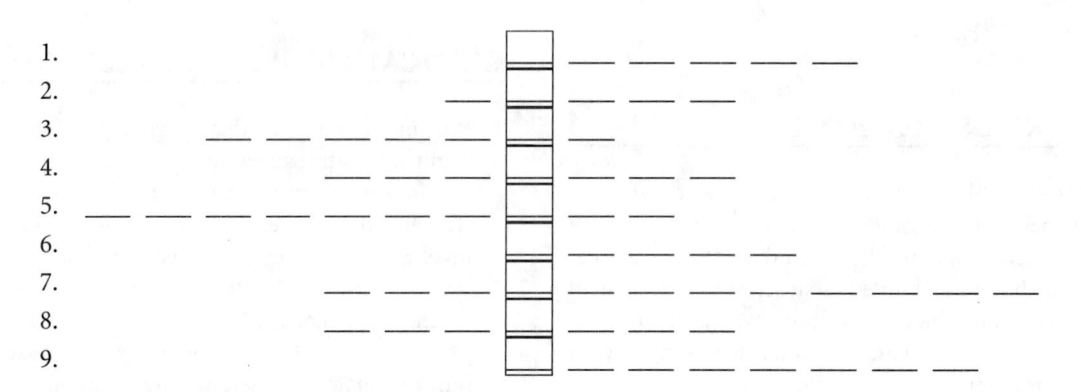

Super Clue: This hormone is released by the adrenal glands in response to stress.

Answers: (1) client, (2) noise, (3) support, (4) protein, (5) exhaustion, (6) sleep, (7) autohypnosis, (8) burnout, (9) exercise, Super Clue: cortisone. ∎

Test Bank

INTRODUCTION

AN INTRODUCTION TO THE PROFESSION OF VETERINARY TECHNOLOGY

1. The first veterinary technician-training program was established in the:
   A. 1920s
   B. 1940s
   C. 1960s
   D. 1980s
2. The acronym *NAVTA* stands for:
   A. National Association of Veterinary Technical Assistants
   B. National Association for Veterinary Technical Acclaim
   C. North American Veterinary Technician Association
   D. None of the above
3. A veterinary technician may choose a career path in:
   A. Private veterinary practice
   B. Zoos
   C. Aquariums
   D. Research facilities
   E. All of the above
4. A "specialty" or "referral" practice:
   A. Employs veterinarians who have completed special training in a particular aspect of veterinary medicine, such as dermatology, surgery, or internal medicine
   B. Specializes in the medical and surgical care of a particular species
   C. Refers patients to other practices as its exclusive function
   D. Requires all veterinary technicians who work there to have a referral from a veterinary specialist
5. Veterinary technicians have the opportunity to be recognized for a higher level of skill and interest in a particular area of veterinary technology. The first two academies in veterinary technology recognized by the NAVTA are in the areas of:
   A. Emergency/critical care and surgery
   B. Emergency/critical care and anesthesia
   C. Emergency/critical care and radiology
   D. Emergency/critical care and outpatient care
   E. None of the above
6. Presently, there is a shortage of veterinary technicians across the United States.
   A. True
   B. False
7. The greatest number of veterinary technicians is employed in which area?
   A. Industry/sales
   B. Mixed animal practice
   C. Feline practice
   D. Companion animal practice
8. Which organization accredits veterinary technical education programs?
   A. NAVTA
   B. AAVSB
   C. AVMA
   D. NEVTEA
9. The accreditation process for a veterinary technician education program includes
   A. Meeting curriculum, faculty, facility, and administration requirements
   B. Regular reporting to the accrediting agency
   C. On-site evaluations
   D. All of the above
10. Most states require veterinary technicians to obtain a given amount of continuing education in order to maintain licensure, registration, or certification:
    A. True
    B. False
11. Regarding the veterinary technician's job duties, which statement is most accurate?
    A. The veterinary technician is trained and works exclusively in animal care
    B. The veterinary technician's job duties may involve office management and use of the business' computer system in addition to his or her animal-care duties

C. The veterinary technician's job duties may involve client education and inventory control in addition to his or her animal-care duties
   D. B and C
12. In a private practice, the responsibilities of a veterinary technician may involve acting as receptionist
   A. True
   B. False
13. The veterinary technician can be a valuable support person for grieving or worried pet owners
   A. True
   B. False
14. Regarding difficult or angry clients, which statement is most accurate?
   A. These clients should be handled solely by the veterinarian in charge.
   B. Veterinary technicians do occasionally have to address these clients in the course of the workday.
   C. The veterinary technician must never deal with these clients due to the possibility of a lawsuit against the practice.
   D. Only the practice manager or veterinarian should deal with these clients because the veterinary technician is not trained to do so.
15. In the veterinary hospital pharmacy, it is illegal for the veterinary technician to:
   A. Acquire the proper license to purchase and dispense federally controlled substances
   B. Fill a prescription
   C. Stock the pharmacy
   D. Dispense medications to the client
16. Veterinary technicians are often skilled in which radiographic technique?
   A. Positioning the patient
   B. Setting the machine properly
   C. Taking exposures at the appropriate time
   D. All of the above
   E. None of the above (Because of possible exposure to harmful radiation, it is too dangerous for a veterinary technician to work around radiographic equipment.)
17. A radiograph is commonly referred to as:
   A. Chemotherapy
   B. An ultrasound image
   C. An MRI
   D. A "cat" scan
   E. An x-ray
18. It is legal for a veterinary technician to:
   A. Administer preoperative anesthetic agents
   B. Place an intravenous catheter
   C. Induce and maintain anesthesia
   D. Perform routine dental prophylaxis procedures
   E. All of the above
19. A veterinarian typically completes how many years of education at an accredited veterinary school?
   A. 2
   B. 3
   C. 4
   D. 5
   E. 6
20. What must a graduate of a foreign veterinary educational program do to become licensed to practice veterinary medicine in the United States?
   A. Pay a fee
   B. Pass a county examination
   C. Become certified by the Educational Commission of Foreign Veterinary Graduates
   D. Graduate from an accredited veterinary school
21. To achieve Veterinary Technician Specialist status, a veterinary technician must:
   A. Be a graduate of an accredited veterinary technology program and/or be legally licensed, certified, or registered to practice veterinary technology in her state
   B. Have successfully completed the educational, training, and experiential requirements established by the respective academy of specialists
   C. Have been reviewed and approved for specialist status by the academy
   D. All of the above
   E. None of the above (Veterinary technicians are not formally recognized as specialists.)
22. How many years of schooling does an accredited veterinary technology program provide?
   A. 2
   B. 3
   C. 4
   D. A or B
   E. A or B or C
23. A "veterinary technologist":
   A. Has the same credentials as a veterinary technician; the two terms are interchangeable
   B. Holds medical technologist and veterinary technician degrees
   C. Holds laboratory technologist and veterinary technician degrees
   D. Holds a Bachelor of Science degree in veterinary technology from a 4-year, accredited program
   E. Is qualified to perform laboratory tests that a veterinary technician is not qualified to perform
24. A veterinary technician has the letters "AS" to designate his or her degree, which stand for
   A. Animal Specialist
   B. Associate of Science
   C. Animal Science
   D. Animal Scientist
   E. Associate of Animal Science
25. A "veterinary technician" has the same qualifications as a "veterinary assistant."
   A. True
   B. False

26. The requirements for certification, licensure, or registration of veterinary technicians vary from state to state and may involve:
    A. Passing the Veterinary Technical National Examination (VTNE)
    B. Passing a state examination
    C. Passing both the VTNE and a state examination
    D. A or B or C, depending on the state one wishes to work in
    E. None of the above (Veterinary technicians take a county-based examination for licensure.)
27. American Association for Laboratory Animal Science–certified veterinary technicians care for the laboratory animals used in USDA-registered research and teaching facilities.
    A. True
    B. False
28. In general, it is widely accepted that veterinary technicians may:
    A. Prescribe medication
    B. Diagnose
    C. Prognose
    D. Perform surgery
    E. None of the above
29. In states where there are no laws to guide the professional actions of veterinary technicians, the interpretation and judgment of the _____ has the most impact on what a veterinary technician can and cannot do on the job.
    A. Veterinary technician himself
    B. Practice manager
    C. Local police force
    D. Supervising veterinarian
    E. Local judicial system
30. The laws that govern the practice of veterinary medicine and the legal roles of veterinary technicians are outlined in two documents known as:
    A. The practice act and the rules and regulations
    B. The laws of veterinary medicine and the laws of veterinary technology
    C. The rules governing the practice of veterinary medicine and the rules governing veterinary technicians
    D. None of the above
31. In a state that licenses veterinary technicians, a veterinary technician who receives a formal complaint of unethical conduct will be investigated by which agency?
    A. NAVTA
    B. State board of veterinary medicine
    C. AVTE
    D. State house and senate
    E. State board of veterinary technicians
32. A veterinary technician's license cannot be revoked once issued.
    A. True
    B. False
33. The first term below refers to laws that are written down, approved, and enforced by governmental bodies, and the second term refers to laws that have evolved over time based on established professional conduct, customs, and practices and are enforced by judges in a court of law.
    A. Legislative; common
    B. Legislative; ordinary
    C. Ordinary; legislative
    D. Ordinary; malpractice
    E. Criminal; civil
34. It is not possible for a veterinary technician to be sued as a result of her actions while working.
    A. True
    B. False
35. *Malpractice* or *professional negligence* by a veterinary practitioner is best defined by which of the following descriptions?
    A. Failure to follow the written laws of that state governing the practice of veterinary medicine
    B. Refusal to treat a particular patient
    C. Failure to provide a level of care equivalent to that provided by a reasonable practitioner of similar training under similar circumstances
    D. Failure to provide a reasonably safe environment for his employees and clients
36. The person most often held responsible for the injurious actions of a veterinary technician is the:
    A. Practice manager:
    B. Supervising veterinarian
    C. Veterinary technician himself
    D. Person who hired the veterinary technician
    E. Respondent superior
37. A veterinary technician's license is not permanent and must be periodically renewed according to the rules and regulations of the given state.
    A. True
    B. False
38. The ethics established by a society are called:
    A. Societal ethics
    B. Personal ethics
    C. Professional ethics
    D. Community ethics
    E. None of the above
39. A veterinary technician who feels it is wrong to place a pet up for adoption is being guided by her own set of principles regarding what is right and wrong. In this case, these principles would be known as:
    A. Animal ethics
    B. Societal ethics
    C. Community ethics
    D. Professional ethics
    E. Personal ethics
40. A *dosimeter* is:
    A. A special scale used to weigh very small animals
    B. A device used to monitor x-ray exposure

Copyright © 2006 by Elsevier, Inc. All rights reserved.

C. A machine that counts the pills used to fill prescriptions
D. A device that measures the dose of liquid medication to give an animal
E. None of the above

41. Concerning a profession's code of ethics, which statement is most accurate?
    A. It is established by members of the profession to help define and encourage conduct specific to that profession.
    B. It is established by members of the judicial system to define and encourage conduct appropriate to that profession.
    C. It provides guidelines by which people hire and train newly qualified professionals.
    D. Newly qualified professionals are not expected to adhere to it.

42. Which statement is part of the NAVTA Profession's Code of Ethics for veterinary technicians?
    A. Prevent and relieve the suffering of animals.
    B. Aid society and animals through providing excellent care and services for animals.
    C. Promote public health by assisting with the control of zoonotic diseases and informing the public about these diseases.
    D. Protect confidential information provided by clients.
    E. All of the above.

EXTRA CREDIT

43. Define *lavage*.
    A. To wash out or flush a wound, organ, or body cavity
    B. The physical rehabilitation of a muscle or group of muscles following orthopedic surgery
    C. A tool used to open the mouth for dental procedures
    D. Any massage technique that involves concomitant use of hot water
    E. A French poodle's bathtub

CHAPTER 1

RESTRAINT AND HANDLING OF ANIMALS

1. A good rule of thumb to follow when restraining animals for veterinary care is:
   A. Apply the maximum amount of restraint possible to ensure the safety of all involved.
   B. Apply the minimum effective amount of restraint that will keep the animal and personnel safe.
   C. Always apply the same amount of restraint: that which is usually tolerated by a member of the species being handled.
   D. Never use ropes when restraining animals.

2. The veterinarian and associated personnel are legally responsible for any injuries to the client while performing a veterinary procedure.
   A. True
   B. False

3. The _____, _____, and _____ will pin their ears back when upset or aggressive, while the _____ will prick its ears forward.
   A. Dog, cat, llama; horse
   B. Dog, horse, llama; cat
   C. Cat, dog, horse; llama
   D. Horse, llama, cat; dog

4. Concerning the punishment of a dog by hanging it or shaking it by the scruff of the neck, which statement is most accurate?
   A. This method of punishment is ineffective in dogs.
   B. This method of punishment should never be used because of the risk of injury to the dog.
   C. This method of punishment is particularly potent because it resembles the way a dominant dog will demonstrate its control over a submissive one.
   D. This method of punishment should be used frequently when trying to win the trust of a submissive dog that is terrified of humans.

5. An otherwise docile female animal is most likely to become aggressive toward her human handler when the handler:
   A. Feeds her in a new location
   B. Appears to be a threat to her suckling young
   C. Moves her to a new location
   D. Places a restraint device, such as a collar or halter, on her

6. Which type of aggression rarely poses a risk to veterinary hospital personnel during their workday?
   A. Pain-induced aggression
   B. Predatory aggression
   C. Territorial aggression
   D. Dominance aggression

7. The most commonly encountered type of attack in veterinary facilities is:
   A. Canine dominance-aggression biting
   B. Equine dominance-aggression biting
   C. Female rabbit territorial-aggression biting
   D. Canine fear biting

8. The most dangerous animal of all the species that veterinary personnel are asked to restrain is the:
   A. Dairy breed bull
   B. Adult, male Rottweiler
   C. Thoroughbred stallion
   D. Adult, female python

9. A duck hunter brings "Duke," his intact, adult, male, 100-lb Labrador retriever, in for a heartworm test. He has trained and worked closely with Duke since

Copyright © 2006 by Elsevier, Inc. All rights reserved.

the dog was 6 weeks old. You take the otherwise docile dog back to the treatment room, where he suddenly begins to growl, glare, and resist restraint. He will not allow you to place a muzzle. What action will most likely result in the most rapid, safe, and successful sample collection?
   A. Return Duke to his owner and tell him to bring the dog back in a few days to try again.
   B. Bring the hunter into the treatment room; Duke will probably calm down in the presence of his owner and trainer.
   C. Place Duke in a cage and try again in a couple of hours.
   D. Resort to whatever technique will restrain Duke, be it a cable snare, choke rope, or sedation. This dog must be taught a lesson to make future visits manageable.
10. Horses display aggression by:
    A. Biting
    B. Head butting
    C. Kicking
    D. A and C
11. A fight between two large pigs is usually handled by
    A. Lassoing each pig and pulling them apart
    B. Shooting each pig with a dart gun loaded with a sedative
    C. Placing a solid panel of plywood between them
    D. Making a very loud noise to scare the pigs so they separate
12. The best way to approach a horse is:
    A. Quickly and directly from the front
    B. Slowly and directly from the front
    C. Quickly and from the front and left side
    D. Slowly and from the front and left side
13. A handler is less likely to be seriously injured by a kick if she stands very close to (up against) a horse's hind quarters rather than 3 feet behind the horse.
    A. True
    B. False
14. You are standing alongside the withers of a stalled horse attempting to place a rope around its neck. The best action to take if the horse moves away from you is to:
    A. Yell "No!" and slap its neck quickly.
    B. Let it move away, leave the stall, then try again.
    C. Attempt to stay with the horse by moving along side and holding onto the mane.
    D. Kick the horse in the belly.
15. A foal is best restrained by:
    A. Placing one arm under the foal's neck and one hand grasping the base of the tail
    B. Placing both arms around the neck
    C. Placing a rope around its neck
    D. Picking it up off the ground
16. The position of a chain lead attached to a halter that will control most horses without being too severe is:
    A. Over the poll (behind the ears)
    B. Under the jaw
    C. Over the nose
    D. Under the upper lip against the gums
17. Concerning tying a horse, which statement is most accurate?
    A. Most of the time, it is necessary to tie a horse while performing a procedure.
    B. Tie a horse to an object at its shoulder level or higher.
    C. Tie the horse long; leave at least 3 feet of rope between the halter and the object to which it is tied.
    D. A tied horse that becomes frightened will tend to run forward into or over the object to which it is tied.
18. Under any circumstances, a handler should stand on the same side of the horse as the veterinarian working on the horse.
    A. True
    B. False
19. Which method is acceptable for the restraint of a haltered horse that will not stand still for a minor procedure or examination?
    A. Grabbing the skin of the neck just cranial to the shoulder and rolling it around the clenched fist
    B. Twisting the horse's ear
    C. Tying one leg up off the ground
    D. Casting the horse
20. When a lifted foreleg is used as a means of equine restraint, the person holding the leg should:
    A. Face the rear of the horse
    B. Face the front of the horse
    C. Place the hoof between his thighs just above the knees to free both hands
    D. None of the above; a lifted foreleg is not a safe means of restraining the horse
21. The first thing that should be done after leading a horse into the stocks is:
    A. Place hobbles on the rear legs
    B. Tie the horse's lead rope to the stocks with a slipknot
    C. Remove the horse's halter
    D. Close and latch the rear gate
22. Before performing an obstetric procedure, the clinician wraps a mare's tail up in gauze, ties a quick-release knot just below the fleshy portion, and runs off to answer her cellular phone. She calls to you to tie the tail up out of the way while she's gone. You should:
    A. Tie the free end of the gauze to the stocks with the tail pulled high above level of the horse's rump.

B. Tie the free end of the gauze to the stocks with the tail hanging low and just lateral to its normal position.
   C. Tie the free end of the gauze around the neck of the horse.
   D. Any of the above are acceptable methods of tying the tail.
23. Which statement regarding chemical restraint of the equine is true?
   A. A newly anesthetized colt should be slapped prior to beginning castration to ensure he won't be aroused by the initial incision.
   B. It is safe to stand close to a tranquilized horse that tends to kick when not sedated.
   C. Chemical restraint is used only as a last resort in the horse.
   D. Chemical restraint is used primarily to facilitate safe casting of the horse.
24. A cow in a narrow chute will avoid a human, so generally it is safe to move in and about chutes when driving cattle.
   A. True
   B. False
25. Which technique can be used to move cattle down an alleyway?
   A. "Tailing"
   B. Cattle prods
   C. Wiffle paddles
   D. All of the above
26. A _____ is often found at the end of a series of pens and alleyways and is the final capture and restraining device for cattle.
   A. Stocks
   B. Stall
   C. Corral
   D. Chute and head catch
27. Generally, the greatest danger to a handler working in close proximity to a tied cow's head is:
   A. Getting bitten
   B. Receiving a blow on the legs from the cow striking out with its foreleg
   C. Getting hit in the face when the animal throws its head
   D. Getting run over by the animal
28. A cow restrained by a halter tied to a fence becomes fidgety during an ear examination. The clinician asks you to "jack" her tail, i.e.,
   A. Grasp one third of the way down the tail and push it straight up and forward until it is vertical.
   B. Grasp one third of the way down the tail and give three quick jerks downward.
   C. Pinch the very tip of the fleshy part of the tail with a haemostatic forceps until she stands still.
   D. Wrap the tail in brown gauze and tie the free end to her halter.

29. Which species, when made very nervous or excited, is most prone to panicking and injuring itself as it attempts to escape an enclosure?
   A. Dog
   B. Horse
   C. Cat
   D. Cow
30. While horses generally kick straight to the rear, cattle usually kick forward and to the side with a hooking action.
   A. True
   B. False
31. The most prudent way to capture a mohair goat is:
   A. By roping it
   B. By grabbing its wool
   C. With a shepherd's hook
   D. By grabbing its tail
32. _____ are essential for the safety of veterinary personnel restraining pigs.
   A. Heavy leather gloves
   B. Durable work boots
   C. Hard plastic forearm covers
   D. Ear plugs
33. The first step to take when attempting to handle a large, aggressive dog is:
   A. Put on heavy leather gloves and grab the scruff of the neck.
   B. Place a muzzle.
   C. Catch the dog by the neck using a snare or a lead rope with a slip knot.
   D. Throw a towel over the dog's head.
34. Which species can usually be restrained for minor procedures by one handler setting it up on its rump?
   A. Goat
   B. Sheep
   C. Cat
   D. Rabbit
35. If a dog is too large for you to lift onto the examination table by yourself, you should:
   A. Leave him on the floor to be examined there.
   B. Get help so two of you can lift him.
   C. Try to get him to jump up onto the table.
   D. Either A or B.
36. You are restraining a Basenji dog for cephalic venipuncture. When the person performing the injection has placed the needle and is ready to inject the drug, he says to you, "Okay." He is most likely asking you to:
   A. Let go of the dog's foreleg.
   B. Lift the thumb that is occluding the vein.
   C. Talk softly to the dog.
   D. Gently push down on the dog to encourage him to lie down.

37. Which statement about muzzling dogs is true?
    A. Brachycephalic breeds should not be muzzled with gauze due to its potential interference with their breathing.
    B. Gauze roll bandage should not be used as a muzzling material because it can easily break.
    C. Some dogs' mouths can be restrained manually with the handler's hands.
    D. Although commercially made muzzles are available, they should not be used because they seldom fit properly.
38. Heavy tranquilization is the most foolproof method of keeping a snappy dog from biting and an agitated horse from kicking.
    A. True
    B. False
39. One of the most effective ways to capture and restrain an agitated cat is to:
    A. Gently grasp both front legs.
    B. Place one hand over its back and one hand under its belly.
    C. Grasp the scruff of the neck.
    D. Talk softly to the cat.
40. The feline's first line of defense is its teeth.
    A. True
    B. False
41. Above all else, the handling of exotic species must be performed:
    A. Rapidly and aggressively
    B. Gently and tentatively
    C. Slowly and carefully
    D. Efficiently and confidently
42. Which species is most likely to seek out a hiding place if it escapes its enclosure?
    A. Cat
    B. Dog
    C. Horse
    D. Bird
43. Which statement about bird capture and restraint is true?
    A. In raptors (birds of prey), the greatest source of injury to the handler is the beak.
    B. Always wear leather gloves when handling psittacines (parrots and parakeets).
    C. Pressure with the hand or fingers on the breast of a passerine (songbird) can cause suffocation.
    D. The psittacine bird's primary weapon is its claws.
44. Which statement concerning rabbit restraint is most accurate?
    A. A rabbit being carried with its hind legs unrestrained can kick out with enough force to permanently damage its spinal cord.
    B. Rabbits, like ferrets, should be hung by the scruff of the neck during restraint for subcutaneous injections.
    C. Although infrequently performed, carrying the patient by the ears is an effective way to subdue an aggressive rabbit.
    D. Rabbits prefer slick surfaces, so the stainless steel examining table is an ideal surface on which to place them.
45. Most dogs and cats don't need tranquilization when shipped on airlines, because they feel secure in their shipping containers if accustomed to them before the trip.
    A. True
    B. False
46. Describe four classic signs seen in a dog about to bite you because she is afraid of you.
47. What is the key to restraining a horse in lateral recumbency to keep it lying down?
48. Briefly describe, in five to six steps, how you would capture a dog that has escaped from the kennel and is running loose down the street.
49. What are the two most common errors made when positioning a dog for jugular venipuncture?
50. List the three most commonly accessed veins in the cat.
51. Other than preventing the spread of infectious disease from one patient to the next, why is it important for the handler to wash his hands well before handling a snake?

EXTRA CREDIT

52. A "twitch" is:
    A. The large piece of plywood used to restrain pigs
    B. The ring sometimes placed in the nasal septum of a bull
    C. A nerve-stimulating restraint device often applied to the upper lip of horses
    D. What happens to your left eyebrow just prior to taking an exam
53. *Buccal:*
    A. Is a term that refers to a metal fitting used to attach two straps of leather together
    B. Is a term that means "directed toward the cheek"
    C. Is a term applied to a horse that escapes from stocks frequently
    D. Was the name of Roy Rogers's famous mount

CHAPTER 2

HISTORY AND PHYSICAL EXAMINATION

1. Concerning the veterinary technician's role in the history-taking process of a patient, which statement is most accurate?
    A. Even the best veterinarian may be unable to solve the problems of a particular patient without an accurate and complete history.

B. The veterinary technician is usually not involved in any aspect of obtaining a patient's history.
C. If a good physical examination is performed, the patient's history is of little importance in establishing a diagnosis.
D. Questions asked should help lead the client toward a particular answer.
E. Questions asked follow an exact protocol regardless of the species or the problem being evaluated.

2. The signalment of the animal is the:
    A. Age
    B. Breed
    C. Sex
    D. Reproduction status
    E. All of the above

3. The client is usually most concerned with the "chief complaint," which is
    A. The animal's most severe clinical sign
    B. The reason the client brought the animal in for evaluation
    C. The animal's longest-standing problem
    D. A and C
    E. None of the above

4. The section of a patient's history that addresses the severity, duration, frequency, progression, trigger situations, time of day, and character of the problem is the:
    A. Environmental history
    B. Signalment
    C. History of the present illness
    D. Chief complaint
    E. Past medical history

5. Questions about the severity, duration, frequency, progression, trigger situations, time of day, and character of the problem should be asked about every new problem, in addition to the reason the client brought the animal in for evaluation.
    A. True
    B. False

6. It is *not* important to spend time asking detailed questions about a pet's environment, medications, or diet because this information is usually located elsewhere in its medical record.
    A. True
    B. False

7. A question about whether a dog is on heartworm preventive medication is part of the dog's:
    A. Environmental history
    B. History of the present illness
    C. Past medical history
    D. Medication history
    E. Dietary history

8. One of the goals of the history and physical examination is to allow the clinician to formulate a list of "differential diagnoses," which are:
    A. All of the diagnoses the patient has received in the past
    B. A list of possible diagnoses based on the history and clinical signs observed that the clinician will attempt to rule in or out using specific diagnostic tests
    C. All possible diagnoses for a given organ system
    D. None of the above

9. A complete "systems review" requires that the following be asked:
    A. One or two questions about the musculoskeletal system
    B. At least five questions about each abnormal body system
    C. One or two questions about each body system
    D. One or two questions about each abnormal body system
    E. None of the above

10. The systems review is part of a patient's medical history.
    A. True
    B. False

11. The _____ system is the most technically difficult and time consuming to examine completely; therefore, a complete examination of this system is usually reserved for the patient with known or suspected disease of this system.
    A. Urogenital
    B. Cardiovascular
    C. Nervous
    D. Respiratory
    E. Gastrointestinal

12. Once a new patient is placed in an examination room, the first aspect of its visit usually involves the veterinary technician or veterinarian:
    A. Drawing a blood sample to screen for metabolic abnormalities
    B. Obtaining a complete medical history and performing a physical examination
    C. Giving the necessary vaccinations
    D. Obtaining a fresh fecal sample to screen for parasites
    E. Informing the owner that payment at the time of service is required

13. Concerning a complete physical examination, which statement is most accurate?
    A. Each of the 10 body systems must be thoroughly examined.
    B. A complete physical examination always begins with a detailed neurologic examination.
    C. The physical examination must follow a strict protocol in the order of systems evaluated.
    D. Measurement of the vital signs is an important part of the complete physical examination.

14. Which body part or parameter is included in a complete integumentary examination?
    A. Tongue
    B. Anal tone

C. Eyes
   D. Ears
   E. Interdigital areas
15. During the physical examination, only observations that appear significant need be recorded.
    A. True
    B. False
16. If a scale is available, an animal should be weighed at every visit to the veterinarian.
    A. True
    B. False
17. Observation of the nose for nasal discharge often begins the examination of which body system?
    A. Special senses
    B. Digestive
    C. Respiratory
    D. General appearance
    E. Musculoskeletal
18. Difficulty breathing due to stenotic (constricted) nares is most commonly seen in which kinds of dogs?
    A. Brachycephalic
    B. Dolichocephalic
    C. Working
    D. Sporting
19. While examining an adult horse, you discover a respiratory rate of 10 breaths per minute.
    A. This is a normal respiratory rate.
    B. This is an elevated respiratory rate.
    C. This is a reduced respiratory rate.
    D. This is an impossible value for a horse, so realizing you made a mistake, you repeat your count.
20. The heart rates of small breed dogs are generally _____ than those of large breed dogs.
    A. Faster
    B. Slower
    C. The same as
    D. None of the above
21. The normal feline heart rate ranges from:
    A. 60 to 100 beats per minute
    B. 80 to 120 beats per minute
    C. 100 to 180 beats per minute
    D. 160 to 240 beats per minute
22. Regarding auscultation of lung sounds, which statement is most accurate?
    A. The lungs can be ausculted only behind the fourth rib, dorsal to the costochondral junction.
    B. The lung sounds of a normal cat are often heard only during inspiration.
    C. The lung sounds of a normal dog are often heard only during inspiration.
    D. Abnormal lung sounds are properly described as "pops" or "whines."
    E. The lack of normal respiratory sounds is not significant, because many healthy animals have no respiratory sounds.
23. A normal capillary refill time (CRT) is:
    A. 0 to 1 seconds
    B. 1 to 2 seconds
    C. 2 to 3 seconds
    D. 3 to 4 seconds
    E. 4 to 5 seconds
24. Mucous membranes are normally _____ in color and are often observed _____.
    A. Pink; interdigitally
    B. Almost white; interdigitally
    C. Pink; on the skin of the inner ear
    D. Pink; on the gingivae over the upper canine tooth
    E. Almost white; on the gingivae over the upper canine tooth
25. The only time a jugular pulse is considered a normal finding in a dog or cat is:
    A. In the standing animal
    B. In the sitting animal
    C. In an animal lying sternally
    D. Occasionally in a laterally recumbent animal
26. The oral cavity of a cat should *not* be examined when the cat is awake due to the risk of getting bitten.
    A. True
    B. False
27. In dogs and cats, the pulse rate is most often evaluated over the:
    A. Facial artery
    B. Femoral artery
    C. Lateral ear vein
    D. Ventral coccygeal artery
    E. Carotid artery
28. Abdominal palpation of a normal dog or cat will most likely reveal:
    A. The liver border approximately 5 to 10 cm beyond the last rib
    B. A very enlarged and firm bladder due to the animal's high stress level
    C. Two round structures approximately 8 cm in diameter in the cranioventral abdomen
    D. Primarily intestines slipping between the palpater's fingers
29. In the normal cat, the kidneys are readily palpated and should be approximately:
    A. 0 to 0.5 cm in length
    B. 0.5 to 1.5 cm in length
    C. 1.5 to 2.5 cm in length
    D. 2.5 to 3.5 cm in length
30. Which of the following terms or phrases correctly describes the location of a heart murmur?
    A. Mitral
    B. Caudal to the right elbow
    C. Ventral to the costochondral junction
    D. Left-sided

Copyright © 2006 by Elsevier, Inc. All rights reserved.

31. The term *grade* refers to the _____ of a heart murmur.
    A. Location
    B. Timing
    C. Duration
    D. Loudness
    E. Character
32. During digital rectal palpation of an intact male dog, the normal prostate gland can be palpated as:
    A. Firm, bilobed, and not painful
    B. Fluctuant, bilobed, and not painful
    C. Firm, bilobed, and painful
    D. Both A and B (The normal prostate gland is not painful and varies dramatically in size, shape, and firmness from dog to dog.)
33. The urinary bladder can usually be palpated in which part of the abdomen?
    A. Craniodorsal
    B. Cranioventral
    C. Caudodorsal
    D. Caudoventral
34. In a pregnant dog or cat, milk can be expressed from the mammary glands during the last:
    A. 1 to 2 months of gestation
    B. 4 weeks of gestation
    C. 1 to 2 weeks of gestation
    D. 1 to 2 days of gestation
35. Which of the following parameters are used to assess the brain during a nervous system examination?
    A. Cranial nerves and mental status
    B. Spinal reflexes and postural reactions
    C. Wheelbarrowing and hemistanding
    D. Hopping and conscious proprioception
36. A firm but gentle tap on an appropriate tendon and observation of the degree of contraction of the corresponding muscle is used in the measurement of:
    A. Spinal reflexes
    B. Postural reactions
    C. Painful stimuli
    D. Conscious proprioception
37. If the patellar tendon is tapped and no quadriceps muscle contraction occurs, a lesion is most likely present in the:
    A. Brain
    B. Spinal cord
    C. Cranial nerves
    D. Muscles of the foot
38. The normal response to a firm toe pinch is
    A. Some acknowledgment of pain, such as looking at the toe, pupillary dilation, or a growl
    B. Withdrawal of the leg
    C. Withdrawal of all four legs simultaneously
    D. A and B
39. A normal ocular examination generally includes:
    A. Yellow ocular discharge
    B. A white sclera
    C. A cloudy cornea
    D. The eyelids rolled inward
    E. Constriction of only one pupil when the light is shined in the corresponding eye or the opposite eye

The following four questions concern observations made or tests performed during a physical examination. Select the correct body system to which each observation or test corresponds:
   A. Eyes
   B. Gastrointestinal
   C. Respiratory
   D. Circulatory
   E. Genitourinary
   F. Neurologic
   G. Integumentary
   H. Musculoskeletal

40. Capillary refill time
41. Mammary gland palpation and expression of milk
42. Ability to swallow
43. Femoral or patellar reflex
44. Name the three pairs of peripheral lymph nodes palpable in the normal animal.
45. Name the two pairs of peripheral lymph nodes *not* generally palpable in the normal animal.
46. Briefly describe how you would perform a complete lung examination.
47. A heart murmur is heard over the right, cranioventral chest wall. Which heart valve is most likely diseased?
48. Name three functions present in an animal with normal cranial nerves.
49. How would you describe a heart murmur heard over the mitral valve that occurs throughout systole, gets louder throughout the duration of the murmur, and is of low-to-moderate intensity?

EXTRA CREDIT

50. A "comedo" is a:
    A. Blackhead
    B. Small tumor
    C. Cone-shaped footpad
    D. Stadium where dogs play football

CHAPTER 3

DIAGNOSTIC SAMPLING AND THERAPEUTIC TECHNIQUES

1. When you are performing venipuncture, always use the _____ needle possible for the vein chosen and direct the bevel _____.

A. Largest; upward
   B. Smallest; upward
   C. Largest; downward
   D. Smallest; downward
2. Why is the skin wiped with 70% isopropyl alcohol before venipuncture?
   A. It removes some superficial skin contaminants.
   B. It causes vasodilation.
   C. It improves visualization of the vein.
   D. All of the above.
3. You are drawing blood from a cat's medial saphenous vein using a 23-gauge needle on a 3-ml syringe. The blood begins to fill the syringe then stops flowing. One likely cause of this problem is:
   A. The syringe is too large.
   B. You have applied too much suction, causing the vein to collapse.
   C. The needle is too large.
   D. The needle is too small.
4. The easiest vein from which to draw 10 ml of blood from an 11-kg dog is the:
   A. Lateral saphenous vein
   B. Cephalic vein
   C. Jugular vein
   D. Marginal ear vein
5. When might the lateral saphenous vein be preferred to the cephalic vein for canine venipuncture?
   A. When an animal is especially sensitive to pain
   B. When a dog is very aggressive
   C. When a larger amount of blood is needed
   D. All of the above
6. How does arterial blood collection differ from venous blood collection?
   A. It is not necessary to occlude an artery to obtain a blood sample.
   B. Venous blood will rapidly fill a syringe in a pulsatile manner, while arterial blood must be aspirated using manual pressure on the plunger.
   C. For all venous blood samples, "heparinize" the syringe, collect the sample, expel air bubbles from the syringe, and promptly cap the needle with a rubber stopper.
   D. Veins are much more likely to form hematomas, so they require firm digital pressure for several minutes after phlebotomy.
7. Which urine-collection technique will produce a sample suitable for bacterial culture?
   A. Urinary catheterization
   B. Cystocentesis
   C. Manual bladder expression
   D. A and B
8. If attempting to manually express urine by bladder compression and moderate pressure does not induce urination:
   A. Exert firmer pressure until the pet urinates.
   B. Use an alternate method of emptying the bladder.
   C. Repeat the technique every hour until successful.
   D. Place the animal in alternate positions and repeat the technique until successful.
9. Which statement concerning the placement and maintenance of an indwelling urinary catheter is most accurate?
   A. Urinary catheters should be inspected for occlusion (blockage) and adequate urine production every 4 to 6 hours.
   B. Twice daily, gently cleanse the prepuce or vulva with a warm antimicrobial solution, rinse with water, and then dry.
   C. A normal, healthy patient will produce 1 to 2 ml urine/kg body weight/hr.
   D. All of the above.
10. A canine urinary catheter is advanced:
    A. Until resistance is met at the os penis
    B. Until resistance is met at the urethral flexure around the pelvis
    C. 1 cm past the point where urine initially flows
    D. 5 cm past the point where urine initially flows in dogs less than 20 kg and 10 cm past this point in dogs weighing 20 kg or more
11. Always prevent contact of the catheter with non-sterile items when placing urinary catheters.
    A. True
    B. False
12. Dogs usually require anesthesia or heavy sedation for urinary catheterization, while cats can be catheterized while fully awake.
    A. True
    B. False
13. To perform cystocentesis on a dog or cat, restrain the animal while it is:
    A. Standing
    B. In lateral recumbency
    C. In dorsal recumbency
    D. In the position preferred by the person collecting the urine
14. If blood flows into the syringe when cystocentesis is attempted:
    A. Continue filling the syringe with as much sample as can be collected.
    B. Reposition the needle without withdrawing it from the abdominal cavity and re-aspirate.
    C. Withdraw the needle immediately and try again with a clean syringe and needle.
    D. Withdraw the needle immediately and use an alternative method of urine collection.
15. Fecal samples intended for parasitology examination are usually placed in _____ and can be refrigerated for up to _____.
    A. Aluminum foil; 3 days
    B. Aluminum foil; 5 days
    C. A sealed, air-tight plastic bag; 3 days
    D. A paper towel; 5 days

For the next four questions, match the diagnostic procedure with its description.
- A. Transtracheal wash
- B. Thoracocentesis
- C. Abdominocentesis
- D. Gastrocentesis
- E. Peritoneal lavage

16. Drawing fluid from the abdominal cavity
17. Obtaining fluid samples from the lower respiratory tract (bronchi and lungs) for culture or cytology (microscopic examination of the cells present)
18. Drawing gas and fluid from a distended stomach in animals with gastric dilatation
19. Removing fluid or air from the pleural space
20. The viscosity (thickness) of a joint-fluid sample is determined by:
    - A. Stretching a fluid drop between the thumb and forefinger
    - B. Pouring 1 ml of sample onto a slide and recording how fast it spreads to the edges
    - C. Shaking the sample and recording how much foam develops
    - D. Recording the time it takes to expel 1 ml of sample through a 25-gauge needle out of a 6-ml syringe.
21. Preventing serious complications when obtaining any bone marrow aspirate requires:
    - A. Exact site selection
    - B. Precise needle length
    - C. Strict sterile and aseptic (noncontaminating) technique
    - D. Not obtaining more than 5 ml of bone marrow
22. How are bone marrow samples prepared for examination?
    - A. Centrifuge, pipette blood off of the sample, and submit the remaining bone marrow to a reference laboratory in a sterile tube.
    - B. Centrifuge and submit the entire sample in a sterile tube.
    - C. Place a drop of sample on a microscope slide, lie the slide flat, allow to air dry, stain, and submit.
    - D. Place a drop of sample on a slide, tilt the slide to separate blood from marrow, remove blood, make two "pull" slides of the remaining bone marrow sample, and submit.
23. For which technique is it acceptable to carefully redirect or move the needle without removing it from the body cavity? (Select all that apply.)
    - A. Cystocentesis
    - B. Fine needle aspiration
    - C. Bone marrow aspiration
    - D. Thoracocentesis
24. When you are performing a transtracheal wash, it is important to remove at least 90% of the fluid infused to prevent "drowning" of the animal.
    - A. True
    - B. False
25. For which technique is it only necessary to wipe the area with alcohol before performing the procedure? (Select all that apply.)
    - A. Bone marrow aspiration
    - B. Fine needle aspiration
    - C. Arthrocentesis
    - D. Intravenous catheter placement
26. A(n) _____ catheter is used to infuse small volumes of fluid into a vein and is usually in place for only a few minutes.
    - A. Butterfly
    - B. Over-the-needle
    - C. Through-the-needle
    - D. Guide-wire
27. Why is an intravenous catheter flushed with heparinized saline after placement?
    - A. To ensure proper placement in the vein
    - B. To help prevent blood from clotting in the catheter
    - C. To help prevent phlebitis (vein inflammation)
    - D. A and B
28. What must be absolutely avoided when placing a long through-the-needle catheter into a jugular vein?
    - A. Aspiration of blood back through the catheter once it is placed
    - B. Repositioning the animal's head once the catheter is placed
    - C. Backing the catheter out through the introducer needle during placement
    - D. Securing the catheter to the neck after placement
29. Medications and fluids, with the exception of small boluses of heparinized saline, are never administered via an arterial catheter.
    - A. True
    - B. False
30. If pain, redness, swelling, and discharge are noted at an intravenous catheter site:
    - A. Rewrap the catheter more loosely.
    - B. Tell the veterinarian, remove the catheter and save it in a sterile location for possible bacterial culture, and place a new one in a different vein.
    - C. Flush the catheter with heparinized saline, place antibiotic ointment over the site of entry into the skin, and rewrap with clean gauze and tape.
    - D. Remove the catheter, rescrub the limb, and place a smaller-diameter catheter more proximally in the same vein.
31. In addition to during placement, when is an intravenous catheter flushed with heparinized saline?
    - A. Before administering intravenous medications
    - B. After administering intravenous medications
    - C. Every 4 to 6 hours in a catheter not receiving a continuous infusion of fluids
    - D. All of the above

Copyright © 2006 by Elsevier, Inc. All rights reserved.

32. Vocalization and signs of discomfort by a patient receiving medications intravenously are:
    A. Normal, as most intravenous medications are slightly irritating
    B. Abnormal, and injection should be immediately stopped if they occur
    C. Abnormal and may indicate leakage of the drug out of the vein
    D. B and C
33. Concerning subcutaneous administration of fluids and medications, which statement is most accurate?
    A. Aspiration to check for needle placement into a vein is not necessary before administering agents subcutaneously.
    B. The ideal location for subcutaneous administration in dogs and cats is between the shoulder blades.
    C. If multiple vaccinations or medications are to be administered, space injection sites several centimeters apart.
    D. All of the above.
34. To avoid penetrating the sciatic nerve during intramuscular injection into the hind leg of a dog, cat, or goat, place the needle:
    A. Proximal to the femur into the gluteal muscles and direct it caudally
    B. Just caudal to the midshaft of the femur bone and direct it craniall.
    C. Just caudal to the midshaft of the femur bone and direct it caudally
    D. Into the lateral semimembranosus or semitendinosus muscles and direct it caudally

For the next three questions, match the method of administration with the situation for which it may be used.
    A. Intradermal
    B. Intranasal
    C. Intratracheal
    D. Intraosseous
35. Fluid administration in a tiny kitten
36. Administration of some vaccines
37. Administration of emergency cardiopulmonary resuscitative drugs
38. To place an intraosseous catheter into the femur, the _____ is shaved and aseptically prepared.
    A. Hip region
    B. Lateral midfemur region
    C. Medial midfemur region
    D. Lateral stifle region
39. What helps prevent the introduction of skin bacteria into the bone during intraosseous-catheter placement?
    A. A careful surgical clip and scrub of the area to be penetrated
    B. A stab incision made through the skin with a scalpel before catheter penetration
    C. Avoiding the use of a bone that has been penetrated multiple times in an attempt to place the catheter
    D. A and B
40. If you must administer an ophthalmic solution and ointment to the same patient, always administer the ointment first then wait 3 minutes before applying the solution.
    A. True
    B. False
41. Always wear gloves when administering medication
    A. Into the eyes
    B. Into the ears
    C. That will be absorbed into the skin (transdermally)
    D. A and B
42. How might you administer an antiseizure drug to a convulsing animal in which you are unable to access a vein?
    A. Intrarectally
    B. Intranasally
    C. Intraperitoneally
    D. A and B
43. Oral medications are best administered to cats by:
    A. Hiding the pill in a bit of canned food
    B. Pulverizing the pill and mixing it with a bit of canned food
    C. Placing the pill at the back of the cat's pharynx and holding the mouth closed until the patient swallows
    D. A or B
44. If you aspirate food from a gastrostomy tube before feeding, you should:
    A. Consult the veterinarian.
    B. Administer 5 ml of water before and after feeding.
    C. Withdraw as much of the previous meal as possible from the stomach before feeding.
    D. Feed as scheduled, as this is a normal and expected finding.
45. In a feline, how is a nasogastric tube best secured?
    A. Glue the tube to the skin just lateral to the nostril.
    B. Tape the tube to shaved skin just lateral to the nostril, on the bridge of the nose, and onto the forehead.
    C. Glue or suture the tube to the skin just lateral to the nostril, on the bridge of the nose, and on the forehead.
    D. None of the above; a feline nasogastric tube is not secured, because it is only used for one-time administration.
46. Which statement concerning pharyngostomy (PG) versus esophagostomy (EG) tubes is most accurate?
    A. Red rubber feeding tubes or silicone tubes are used for pgs, while only silicone tubes are used for EGs.

B. PGs and EGs are secured in the same manner.
C. General anesthesia (rendering the animal unconscious) is only required for placement of EGs.
D. A commercially made applicator may be necessary to perform a PG in a very large dog.

47. From where is blood routinely collected in cattle?
   A. Jugular vein
   B. Ventral coccygeal vein
   C. Facial vein
   D. A and B

48. What site is commonly used to collect blood from pigs?
   A. Left anterior vena cava
   B. Right anterior vena cava
   C. Left or right anterior vena cava
   D. Ventral coccygeal vein

49. The transverse facial artery should *not* be used for arterial sample collection in the conscious horse because of the painful nature of a needle stick at this site.
   A. True
   B. False

50. Ideally, the _____ portion of a voided urine sample is collected.
   A. Initial
   B. Midstream
   C. Final
   D. A and B

51. How is urine collected from a cow? (Select all that apply.)
   A. Stimulate her to void urine by stroking the perineal area.
   B. Stimulate her to void urine by opening and closing the vulvar lips.
   C. Stimulate her to void urine by obstructing her nose and lips until she struggles.
   D. Place a urinary catheter.
   E. Perform cystocentesis.

52. You are attempting to obtain urine from a mare by catheterization. You repeatedly insert the catheter the recommended 10 cm into the vaginal canal but are not entering the urethra. What may be the problem?
   A. You are sliding the catheter over the transverse fold, which overlies the urethral orifice.
   B. You need to direct the catheter along the dorsal vaginal vault to enter the urethra.
   C. You did not properly lubricate the catheter.
   D. You are entering the cervix, which lies caudal to the urethral orifice.

53. In the private-practice setting, bovine rumen fluid is commonly collected by:
   A. Rumen trocharization
   B. Abdominocentesis
   C. Orogastric intubation
   D. Esophagostomy tube

54. In addition to an 18-gauge, 3.75-cm needle, what can be used to perform abdominocentesis in large animals?
   A. Teat cannula
   B. Spinal needle
   C. Stainless steel bitch urinary catheter
   D. All of the above

55. If fluid does not flow from the needle during large-animal abdominocentesis:
   A. Attach a syringe and apply negative pressure.
   B. Insert another needle several centimeters away from the initial one.
   C. Try another area.
   D. All of the above.

56. What structure must the technician take care to avoid during equine thoracocentesis?
   A. The mediastinum, found just ventral to the costochondral junction of the right sixth and seventh ribs
   B. The caudal vena cava, found at the dorsal aspect of the thoracic cavity
   C. The lateral thoracic vein, coursing subcutaneously over the ventral thorax
   D. A and C

57. For which procedure is it necessary to anesthetize the area by injecting 1 to 2 ml of 2% lidocaine before sampling?
   A. Cystocentesis
   B. Transtracheal wash
   C. Placement of an intravenous catheter in a feline cephalic vein
   D. Obtaining blood from an equine carotid artery

58. Proper placement of a needle or catheter into a vein is best confirmed by:
   A. Feeling it "pop" through the vein's wall
   B. A mild pain reaction by the patient
   C. Visualizing the needle going into the vein
   D. Blood flowing into the syringe hub or out of the catheter

59. How is intraarterial injection avoided when administering medications into the jugular vein in large animals?
   A. By using the right jugular vein only
   B. By using the proximal one third of the neck only
   C. By placing the needle first without the syringe attached and observing the nature of the blood emerging
   D. All of the above

60. Intravenous catheters are routinely placed in the _____ vein in hogs.
   A. Jugular
   B. Auricular
   C. Orbital
   D. Brachiocephalic

61. Concerning intramuscular injections, which statement is most accurate?
    A. It is critical to aspirate before injecting medication intramuscularly to ensure the needle is not in a vein.
    B. When administering medications into the semimembranosus/semitendinosus muscles of horses, inject the leg that is on the same side that you are standing.
    C. Intramuscular injections are best made into the dorsal gluteal muscles in bovines.
    D. In large animals, the area to be injected can be struck several times before needle insertion to cause vasodilation, which enhances medication absorption.
62. "Little Bo," the clinic's resident sheep, is due for her intramuscular tetanus vaccination. Where can you administer this to her?
    A. Semimembranosus/semitendinosus muscles
    B. Neck muscles
    C. Triceps muscles
    D. All of the above
63. When administering intramuscular injections to pigs, it is important to use a needle at least _____ long to avoid an intrafat injection.
    A. 1.25 cm
    B. 2.50 cm
    C. 3.75 cm
    D. 7.50 cm
64. To prevent pharyngeal or esophageal trauma when using a balling gun to administer tablets:
    A. Place it as deeply into the mouth as possible, until resistance is met.
    B. Forcefully eject the tablet.
    C. Elevate the patient's muzzle during administration.
    D. Place the tip gently over the base of the tongue, not too deeply in the mouth.
65. Rehydration of vomiting baby pigs is usually accomplished with _____ fluids.
    A. Oral
    B. Subcutaneous
    C. Intravenous
    D. Intraperitoneal
66. What precaution will help avoid aspiration pneumonia (due to gastric or rumen fluid entering the lungs) when performing nasogastric or orogastric intubation?
    A. Using a tube of sufficiently small diameter to fit in the ventral nasal meatus
    B. Kinking the tube during removal
    C. Raising the animal's head before and during removal
    D. Removing the entire tube in a single, slow sweep
67. Concerning the administration of oral medications to horses, which statement is most accurate?
    A. Liquid or paste medications can often be administered with a syringe, whose tip is placed into the interdental space at the side of the mouth and contents emptied onto the base of the tongue.
    B. After medicating a horse orally with a syringe, allow it to drink water immediately to help wash the medication down before the animal spits it out.
    C. Tablets are usually administered to horses, as to ruminants, with a balling gun.
    D. All of the above.
68. When aseptically preparing and infusing medication into mammary glands, clean the _____ side of the udder first and infuse the _____ side first.
    A. Far; near
    B. Far; far
    C. Near; far
    D. Near; near
69. A transtracheal wash is performed and the veterinarian leaves the trachea and skin unsutured. How can the veterinary technician best manage the site?
    A. Do not clean or bandage it.
    B. Leave it unbandaged and clean the skin surface every 4 to 6 hours for the first 3 days.
    C. Leave it unbandaged and flush inside the skin wound with a dilute antiseptic solution every 12 hours for the first 3 days.
    D. Cover the area with antibiotic-coated sterile gauze and a bandage for 24 hours.
70. Due to anatomic obstacles, _____ males are *not* routinely catheterized to obtain urine.
    A. Equine
    B. Ovine and caprine
    C. Canine
    D. Feline
71. The "three-syringe technique" is used to:
    A. Obtain blood samples from very long catheters
    B. Obtain a urine sample from a urinary catheter
    C. Administer an irritating substance intramuscularly
    D. Perform thoracocentesis
72. The marginal ear vein may be used to obtain blood samples for all of the following procedures except to:
    A. Sample for the erythroparasite *Babesia* spp.
    B. Sample for the erythroparasite *Hemobartonella* spp.
    C. Measure blood glucose
    D. Perform a CBC and serum chemistry panel
73. The veterinarian hands you a patient and asks you to place an intravenous (IV) catheter, start IV saline at maintenance rate, administer intramuscular antibiotics, offer feed and water, and draw blood for a complete blood count and chemistry panel. She then walks away. What procedure is best performed first and why?

74. Briefly describe the technique used to obtain a sample of canine vaginal cells for microscopic examination; include patient positioning, procedure, and sample preparation for microscopic examination.
75. Briefly describe the technique used to administer a warm-water enema to a dog.
76. What are the borders of the intramuscular-injection region on the neck of a horse or cow?
77. What are the techniques and precautions used during the preparation for and administration of intramammary infusions designed to prevent?

EXTRA CREDIT

78. *Flashback* is the term most often applied to:
    A. Urine entering a urinary catheter during catheter placement
    B. Blood entering a needle hub or catheter during intravenous procedures
    C. Fluid flowing out of a nasogastric tube spontaneously
    D. A veterinary technician's memory of a procedure learned in school that is recalled while at her first job
79. The term *clean stick* is applied to:
    A. An intramuscular injection in which no blood is aspirated before medication administration
    B. An intramuscular injection in a food animal that does not reduce the value of the carcass
    C. A vessel being punctured only once during an intravenous procedure
    D. A tree branch before you and your dog play fetch with it

CHAPTER 4

WOUND HEALING, WOUND MANAGEMENT, AND BANDAGING

1. How soon after injury is wound healing initiated?
    A. Immediately
    B. 30 minutes
    C. 2 to 4 hours
    D. 6 to 8 hours
    E. 10 to 12 hours
2. Upon injury, a significant increase in wound strength begins to occur after:
    A. 12 to 24 hours
    B. 1 to 2 days
    C. 3 to 5 days
    D. 7 to 10 days
    E. 10 to 15 days
3. Granulation tissue, the red tissue underlying a scab, is made up of:
    A. New capillaries
    B. Fibroblasts
    C. Fibrous tissue
    D. A, B, and C
    E. None of the above
4. The formation of new epithelium on the wound surface generally occurs after _____ in a sutured wound and _____ in a nonsutured wound.
    A. 0 to 12 hours; 3 to 5 days
    B. 0 to 12 hours; 7 to 10 days
    C. 24 to 48 hours; 3 to 5 days
    D. 24 to 48 hours; 7 to 10 days
    E. 24 to 48 hours; 14 to 16 days
5. If the skin surrounding a wound is very tight and under tension, _____ will be limited.
    A. Wound contraction
    B. Epithelialization
    C. Fibroblast migration
    D. Granulation tissue formation
    E. None of the above
6. Once a full-thickness layer of skin has formed at the edges of a wound, the process that acts to further reduce the size of the wound is:
    A. Macrophage activity
    B. Wound contraction
    C. Scab formation
    D. Scar formation
7. Which statement concerning wound healing is most accurate?
    A. The final phase of wound healing is wound contraction, which may occur for several years.
    B. During the final phase of wound healing, wound strength increases to its maximal level due to remodeling of collagen fibers in the scar.
    C. A scar, made up of collagen fibers, is actually stronger than the normal tissue surrounding it.
    D. The final phase of wound healing is known as the *maturation phase* and is always completed by 60 days after the initial injury.
8. A laceration in a healthy, robust animal will heal at the same rate as one in a sick, old, or debilitated animal.
    A. True
    B. False
9. Which of the following is most likely to interfere with the normal healing of a surgical wound?
    A. Use of a sharp blade for incision
    B. Exact alignment of the incision margins during skin closure
    C. No movement of the skin margins after closure
    D. Adequate blood supply to the incision
    E. Bacterial contamination and infection of the incision
10. Always apply an antibiotic ointment when preparing a laceration for surgical repair.
    A. True
    B. False
11. After the skin around a laceration has been prepared for surgical repair by clipping the hair and

performing a surgical scrub of the area, the veterinary technician should then:
- A. Lavage the wound using a forceful jet of a sterile balanced electrolyte solution.
- B. Lavage the wound using a forceful jet of a sterile balanced electrolyte solution with added antiseptic solution.
- C. Lavage the wound gently by pouring a sterile balanced electrolyte solution over the wound.
- D. Lavage the wound gently by pouring a sterile balanced electrolyte solution with added antiseptic solution over the wound.

12. Which factor is important to consider when making a decision about how to treat a wound?
- A. Time since the injury
- B. Degree of wound contamination
- C. Animal's physical status
- D. Location of the wound
- E. All of the above

13. For heavily contaminated wounds treated more than 12 hours after injury, immediate surgical closure is crucial to achieving adequate healing.
- A. True
- B. False

14. Allowing a wound to heal completely without surgical closure is known as:
- A. First intention healing
- B. Second intention healing
- C. Third intention healing
- D. Healing by contraction and epithelialization
- E. B and D

15. Which statement about bandages is true?
- A. The tertiary bandage layer contacts the wound surface (if a wound is present) and may be adherent or nonadherent and occlusive or semiocclusive.
- B. A dry-dry bandage has as its primary layer an adherent material soaked in saline.
- C. An occlusive primary layer allows air to penetrate the wound.
- D. If a wound is exudative, a semiocclusive primary layer is indicated.

16. When applying a bandage or cast to the distal limb, the entire foot should always be covered to protect it from abrasion.
- A. True
- B. False

17. Apart from obvious complications, an outpatient wearing a cast should generally be rechecked at least:
- A. Every other day
- B. Weekly
- C. Every 2 weeks
- D. Every 3 days

18. A large Rottweiler comes in with a fractured tibia at 6 PM. Surgical repair is scheduled for 9 AM the following morning. The most appropriate way to manage the fractured leg overnight is to:
- A. Apply a Robert-Jones bandage.
- B. Apply an Ehmer sling.
- C. Apply a Velpeau sling.
- D. Apply hobbles to the hind legs.

19. After performing an ovariohysterectomy (spay) on a 6-month-old Great Dane, the veterinarian asks you to apply an abdominal compression bandage. It is 12 noon. You plan to remove this bandage:
- A. At 2 PM, after your lunch break
- B. After 6 PM
- C. First thing tomorrow morning
- D. When the owner picks the dog up tomorrow

20. The biggest advantage to using an Ehmer sling rather than a 90-90 flexion sling to immobilize the canine or feline hind limb after reduction of craniodorsal coxofemoral luxation (replacing a dislocated hip) is:
- A. The Ehmer sling uses less material and so can be applied more rapidly.
- B. Only the Ehmer sling internally rotates and adducts the hip joint.
- C. The Ehmer sling completely raises the foot off the ground, while the 90-90 flexion sling allows weight bearing on the foot during walking.
- D. The Ehmer sling does not rotate or adduct the hip joint, thus placing the joint in an ideal position for healing.

21. When discharging a patient wearing a cast, client education is essential and should include instructing the client to:
- A. Check the animal's toes daily for warmth, discoloration, and swelling.
- B. Check the cast daily for a foul odor.
- C. Observe for areas of skin chafing from the cast.
- D. Keep the cast covered with a plastic bag or other waterproof material when the animal is outside.
- E. All of the above

22. A foul odor emanating from any part of a cast indicates:
- A. Severe infection
- B. Tissue damage
- C. The cast has become wet
- D. The animal has been licking the cast

23. Primary surgical closure is indicated in the treatment of an abrasion.
- A. True
- B. False

24. Blistering at the site of a burn indicates a:
- A. First-degree burn
- B. Second-degree burn
- C. Third-degree burn
- D. Fourth-degree burn

25. The best way to bandage a full-thickness, severe burn is with:
    A. A sterile, wet-to-dry primary bandage layer
    B. Antibiotic ointment under a sterile wet-to-dry primary bandage layer
    C. A sterile, dry-to-dry primary bandage layer
    D. A sterile, occlusive primary bandage layer with a heavily padded secondary layer
26. An injury in which skin and varying amounts of ligaments, tendons, muscle, and bone are torn off a limb is commonly known as a:
    A. Dragging injury
    B. Descarifying injury
    C. Degloving injury
    D. Necrotic injury
27. Which statement about decubital ulcers is most accurate?
    A. Active, well-muscled, healthy animals are at the greatest risk for the formation of decubital ulcers.
    B. Decubital ulcers are generally very easy to treat.
    C. Once a decubital ulcer develops, it is best treated with a tight, occlusive bandage, and the animal should be kept immobile and recumbent to allow the ulcer to heal.
    D. Decubital ulcers form over bony prominences.
28. Basic wound care in large animals is significantly different than that in small animals.
    A. True
    B. False
29. It is often necessary to treat wounds on large animals in the field. If clippers were unavailable, what would be the best way to remove the hair surrounding a laceration?
    A. Lather the wound edges with an antiseptic scrub and shave the hair with a razor or scalpel blade.
    B. Trim the hair as closely as possible with scissors.
    C. Use a chemical depilatory product to remove the hair.
    D. If clippers are unavailable, the hair surrounding a laceration can remain, as long as the area is scrubbed well with an antiseptic cleanser.
30. Wounds on the limbs of large animals should always be bandaged.
    A. True
    B. False
31. *Proud flesh* is:
    A. The term applied to the tissue in a severe laceration less than 6 hours old.
    B. The necrotic tissue trimmed from the edges of a severe, full-thickness burn
    C. The bright red tissue seen in a decubital ulcer
    D. Excessive granulation tissue than can form on the limbs of horses during wound healing
32. The layers of an equine lower-limb bandage placed over a nonsutured wound are applied in the following order:
    A. Topical medication, nonadhering dressing, rolled conforming gauze, elastic wrap, padded layer, brown gauze
    B. Topical medication, rolled conforming gauze, nonadhering dressing, brown gauze, padded layer, elastic wrap
    C. Topical medication, nonadhering dressing, rolled conforming gauze, padded layer, brown gauze, elastic wrap
    D. Topical medication, padded layer, nonadhering dressing, rolled conforming gauze, brown gauze, elastic wrap
33. How does an equine lower-limb support bandage differ from a lower-limb wound bandage?
    A. The two bandages are identical.
    B. The support bandage is more heavily padded.
    C. In the support bandage, the wound dressing, inner conforming gauze layer, and wide elastic tape around the top and bottom are not used.
    D. The final layer is applied more tightly in a support bandage.
34. Why must the thick bandage placed under a large-animal limb splint extend well above and below the ends of the splint?
    A. To adequately support the limb
    B. To prevent pressure sores
    C. To prevent wood shavings from getting under the splint
    D. None of the above
35. How often should a splint be reset in a foal?
    A. Daily
    B. Every other day
    C. Once weekly
    D. Twice weekly
36. The biggest complication that occurs when meticulous technique is not followed in the casting limbs of large animals is:
    A. Cast sliding down the limb
    B. Repeat fracture
    C. Pressure necrosis (tissue death)
    D. Hoof-wall deformities
37. How is a broom handle used in the application of an equine limb cast?
    A. A broom handle? A broom handle is not used in the application of an equine limb cast.
    B. A broom handle, threaded through a loop of wire attached to the hoof wall, is used to apply traction to the limb to keep it straight during cast application.
    C. A broom handle is incorporated into the cast to increase the cast's strength.

D. A broom handle, because it is made of wood, is a good instrument to use to mix the plaster used to create the cast.
38. Heavy padding should never be placed under a cast.
   A. True
   B. False
39. It is important to avoid wrinkling the stockinet and fiberglass when applying a cast due to the risk of pressure sores forming at the sites of wrinkles.
   A. True
   B. False
40. When casting an equine limb, after the initial layer of casting material is applied, external traction of the limb is often removed and an assistant is asked to support the leg at the metacarpal or metatarsal bone. What is the best way for the assistant to hold the limb?
   A. Firmly, using the fingertips of both hands
   B. Gently, using the fingertips of both hands
   C. Gently, with the limb resting on the palms of both hands
   D. Firmly, with both hands wrapped all the way around the casted limb
41. When applying casting materials around the limb, overlap successive layers by:
   A. 0 to ¼ roll width
   B. ¼ to ½ roll width
   C. ⅓ to ½ roll width
   D. ½ to ¾ roll width
42. The exercise program for an equine patient with a limb cast is best described as:
   A. Hand-walking several times daily
   B. Light exercise
   C. Moderate exercise
   D. Stall confinement only
43. When removing an equine limb cast, the cuts in the cast should be made longitudinally along the:
   A. Dorsal and palmar or plantar surfaces
   B. Medial and lateral surfaces
   C. Dorsal surface only
   D. Palmar or plantar surface only
44. How is a wooden block often used when casting a cow with one fractured digit (claw)?
   A. The block is placed under the unaffected claw.
   B. The block is placed under the affected claw.
   C. The block is placed between the claws.
   D. None of the above are correct; wooden blocks are not used when treating bovine limb fractures.
45. In addition to casts, what type of external skeletal fixation is often used in cattle with fractured lower hind limbs?
   A. Robert-Jones bandage
   B. Velpeau sling
   C. Modified Thomas splint
   D. Meissner splint
46. Name three reasons why it is important *not* to disrupt a healthy granulation tissue bed in a wound. In other words, name three functions of granulation tissue.
47. List, in order, the six steps taken in the application of any bandage. Assume that no wound is present. Include "splint application" as one of the steps.
48. Unfortunately, two common causes of patient burns often occur in the animal hospital. What are they?
49. How is a wooden, wedge-shaped block often used in the application of an equine limb cast? Why is it used?
50. When casting a bovine lower limb, what special technique is used to reduce pressure-sore formation at the dewclaws?

EXTRA CREDIT

51. Which of the following delays all phases of wound healing?
   A. Acetaminophen
   B. Caffeine
   C. Corticosteroids
   D. A rough rugby game
52. "Dead space" is:
   A. Necrotic, or dead, tissue in a wound
   B. A large gap between the cut tissue edges of a wound
   C. Space remaining in tissues as a result of failure of proper closure that allows the accumulation of blood or serum
   D. A boarding kennel after all of the dogs go home at the end of a busy holiday weekend

CHAPTER 5

BASIC NECROPSY PROCEDURES

1. Pathogenesis is:
   A. An alteration or abnormality in a tissue
   B. The sequence of events that lead to or underlie a disease
   C. A tissue alteration or abnormality that is invisible to the naked eye
   D. The science and study of disease
2. An owner's permission must be granted prior to performing a necropsy on his pet.
   A. True
   B. False
3. If a necropsy must be delayed, the carcass should be:
   A. Kept at room temperature
   B. Refrigerated
   C. Frozen
   D. Refrigerated or frozen

Copyright © 2006 by Elsevier, Inc. All rights reserved.

4. The carcass of a small animal awaiting necropsy should be stored:
   A. Uncovered with identification (ID) tags attached to the animal
   B. Wrapped in a clean towel with ID tags attached to the towel
   C. In a thin plastic bag with ID tags attached to both the animal and bag
   D. In a paper bag with ID tags attached to both the animal and bag

5. Why must a necropsy be performed as soon as possible after death?
   A. Decomposition occurs rapidly and can render tissues unfit for analysis.
   B. The procedure should be performed before rigor mortis sets in.
   C. Airborne bacteria immediately begin to grow and multiply on the body surface, thus contaminating it and invalidating all findings.
   D. All of the above.

6. The terms *focal, multifocal,* and *diffuse* are used to describe the _____ of multiple lesions.
   A. Location
   B. Shape
   C. Distribution
   D. Consistency

7. The most widely used general-purpose fixative for tissue preservation is:
   A. 10% formalin
   B. 50% formalin
   C. 10% buffered formalin
   D. Bouin fixative

8. Your practice has a special knife and other tools dedicated for necropsies. The most important reason for this is:
   A. To assure the knife is sharp and the forceps in perfect working order.
   B. So those performing necropsies always know where they are located.
   C. To avoid the spread of pathogens.
   D. Instruments used for necropsy are made especially for this purpose and are generally very expensive.

9. The best way to find out how to individually package and send various tissue and fluid samples to a diagnostic laboratory is to:
   A. Call and ask someone at the laboratory or look in a reference provided by them.
   B. Ask the veterinarian performing the necropsy.
   C. Memorize the methods of sample preparation and handling.
   D. Consult a veterinary-pathology textbook.

10. Small, thin, flat sections of tissue are generally:
    A. Placed in a container of fixative
    B. Placed on a pieces of cardboard, to which the tissues will adhere, and the tissue-cardboard pairs placed in fixative
    C. Placed in a container, provided by the diagnostic laboratory, specially designed to keep the tissue flat; the container is then placed in fixative
    D. Placed in an ice-cube tray filled with water and then frozen

11. Rinse all tissue specimens prior to placing in preservative.
    A. True
    B. False

12. When a patient dies or is euthanized, it is critical to record the exact time of death in the animal's record and provide it to the person performing the necropsy.
    A. True
    B. False

13. After the examination of external structures, the adult, nonruminant mammal is placed in _____ recumbency and dissection begins with _____.
    A. Dorsal; the mouth
    B. Left lateral; the eyes
    C. Right lateral; a midline incision extending from the mandibular symphysis to the axilla
    D. Sternal; the vertebral column and spine

14. The preferred fixative for whole brains, bones, and intact spinal cords is:
    A. 10% formalin
    B. 50% buffered formalin
    C. 10% buffered formalin
    D. Bouin fixative

15. Place the three necropsy procedures in the correct order that they should be performed.
    A. Examine joints; open body cavities; review preliminary findings with the clinician.
    B. Review preliminary findings with the clinician; open body cavities; examine joints.
    C. Open body cavities; examine joints; review preliminary findings with the clinician.
    D. Review preliminary findings with the clinician; examine joints; open body cavities.

16. Proper attire for performing the dissection of a large animal whose suspected cause of death is a bacterial species that can infect by being inhaled includes:
    A. Gloves and mask
    B. Apron and boots
    C. Gloves, boots, and mask
    D. A and B

17. Which internal structures should be weighed and measured?
    A. All organs in the three major body cavities: peritoneal, pleural, and pericardial
    B. The heart and all organs found to be abnormal in size or shape
    C. The liver, kidneys, and heart
    D. All of the above plus the eyes, brain, and testes

18. The head is best removed using a _____ approach.
    A. Dorsal
    B. Ventral
    C. Right lateral
    D. Left lateral
19. Choose the one way the equine necropsy differs from that of the small mammal and ruminant.
    A. The equine diaphragm is always weighed and measured.
    B. The chambers and vessels of the equine heart are examined in reverse order from those of the small mammal and ruminant heart.
    C. The equine reproductive and urinary tracts are examined prior to the abdominal and thoracic organs.
    D. All equine limb joints should be opened.
20. Concerning fetal dissection, which statement is most accurate?
    A. The fetus is placed in left lateral recumbency.
    B. The fetus is weighed and then measured from crown to rump, which is the distance from the tip of the nose to the tip of the tail.
    C. The body cavities are carefully opened so that the organs may be sampled in the body with sterile tools and an aseptic (noncontaminating) technique.
    D. Due to its small size, the brain is never collected.
21. Birds suspected of having infectious or zoonotic diseases should be submitted to a diagnostic laboratory for necropsy.
    A. True
    B. False
22. What special precautions must be taken when performing necropsies on birds?
    A. Wear a mask, protective clothing, and gloves.
    B. Perform the necropsy in a ventilation hood that draws airborne contaminants up into it and away from the prosector.
    C. Wet the carcass by immersing it in warm, soapy water or disinfectant.
    D. A and C
23. Concerning the necropsy of birds, which statement is most accurate?
    A. For very small birds (e.g., hummingbirds), the entire carcass can be fixed after the body cavities are opened.
    B. Small birds are examined exactly as are small mammals.
    C. Place birds in sternal recumbency for necropsy.
    D. Place birds in right lateral recumbency for necropsy.
24. You are assisting in the necropsy of a mouse, and the prosector asks you to inflate the lungs. What substance is placed in the lungs to inflate them?
    A. Room air
    B. 100% oxygen
    C. 100% carbon dioxide
    D. Formalin
25. Tissues placed in formalin are usually completely preserved within:
    A. 0 to 12 hours
    B. 24 to 48 hours
    C. 3 to 4 days
    D. 7 days
26. Which statement concerning a small-animal cosmetic necropsy is most accurate?
    A. A cosmetic necropsy is equal in value to a complete necropsy in determining the cause of death.
    B. A cosmetic necropsy can be performed when the disease processes are limited to the eyes or central nervous system.
    C. A cosmetic necropsy is completed by stuffing the body cavities with paper towels and suturing the ventral abdominal incision.
    D. All of the above
27. When submitting an animal for necropsy, extensive and detailed information concerning what three aspects of the case should be included on the form (not including the animal's, veterinarian's, and owner's names)?
28. If rabies is suspected, what part of the carcass must be submitted to an appropriate laboratory to confirm the diagnosis?
29. How are multiple, small tissue specimens from different parts of the body best packaged for preservation and labeled?
30. How should a ruminant be positioned for necropsy? Why?
31. During the necropsy of a very small mammal or bird (e.g., mouse or small hummingbird), what special technique is applied to the collection, preservation, and submission of the spinal cord?

EXTRA CREDIT

32. The calvaria is:
    A. The room in an animal hospital reserved for necropsies
    B. The saw designed specifically to cut bones
    C. The skull cap
    D. The equine-mounted army regiment

CHAPTER 6

CLINICAL PATHOLOGY

1. The veterinary technician need not concern himself or herself with the routine care and maintenance of in-house laboratory equipment because a

manufacturer-provided technician usually performs this service.
A. True
B. False

2. Which test is included in a complete blood count (CBC)?
A. Packed cell volume (PCV)
B. Red blood cell (RBC) count
C. Hemoglobin determination
D. A and B
E. All of the above

3. Which part of a CBC must be performed manually by trained personnel?
A. White blood cell (WBC) differential
B. RBC indices
C. Blood-film evaluation
D. Platelet count

4. The preferred anticoagulant for a sample on which a CBC will be performed is _____ and is available in a Vacutainer tube with a _____ top.
A. Ethylenediamine tetraacetic acid (EDTA); red
B. EDTA; purple
C. Heparin; purple
D. Heparin; green
E. None of the above

5. The type of anticoagulant present in a red-top Vacutainer tube is:
A. EDTA
B. Heparin
C. Citrate
D. Plasminogen
E. None of the above (There is no anticoagulant in a red-topped tube.)

6. Concerning proper care of the light microscope, which statement is most accurate?
A. The microscope is never covered so as to prevent damage to the eyepiece glass.
B. The 10×, 40×, and 100× objectives are all occasionally used with immersion oil to increase resolution of the image.
C. Immersion oil should be wiped off of an objective lens immediately after use.
D. The objective lenses may be cleaned with tissue paper, a paper towel, or lens paper.

7. A handheld refractometer is used to determine:
A. RBC indices
B. Urine specific gravity
C. Plasma protein concentration
D. B and C
E. All of the above

8. In hematologic testing, the size of the collection tube used is *not* important as long as an adequate amount of blood is drawn for the test being run.
A. True
B. False

9. Always include _____ when submitting a blood sample to a reference laboratory for a CBC.
A. Unstained blood films
B. Blood films stained with a modified Wright's stain
C. At least 1 ml of the patient's serum
D. Blood films stained with new methylene blue

10. The PCV is:
A. Another term for a WBC count
B. The percentage of total blood volume accounted for by RBCs
C. Another term for a RBC count
D. The total number of RBCs in a sample after it has been centrifuged

11. What sample does a veterinary technician performing a CBC in the animal hospital most often use to determine the plasma protein?
A. The plasma obtained from a heparin tube after centrifugation
B. The plasma obtained from a citrate tube after centrifugation
C. Whole blood in an EDTA tube
D. The plasma at the top of the microhematocrit tube after centrifugation

12. You are counting WBCs manually using the Unopette manual platelet count system. Your final count is far below the normal range for that species. What is the fastest and easiest way to double-check the accuracy of your count?
A. Count the WBCs in the other chamber of the hemacytometer.
B. Send the sample to a reference laboratory for verification.
C. Repeat the test using a fresh blood sample.
D. Have another veterinary technician perform the entire test using the same blood sample.

13. Concerning the buffy coat, which statement is most accurate?
A. The buffy coat is a white band of concentrated WBCs.
B. The buffy coat should be increased in diameter if the WBC count is greatly reduced.
C. The buffy coat is found at the interface of the plasma and air in a centrifuged microhematocrit tube.
D. The buffy coat is used to roughly estimate dramatic increases or decreases in the hematocrit.

14. How are the RBCs of birds and reptiles different from those of mammals?
A. Birds and reptiles have nucleated mature RBCs, while the mature RBCs of mammals are not nucleated.
B. Birds and reptiles have no RBCs.
C. The RBCs of birds and reptiles have the same function as mammalian WBCs.
D. Avian and reptilian RBCs have blue-staining granules, while mammalian RBCs are agranular.

15. Which of the following can be estimated by multiplying the number present in ten 100× (oil immersion) fields by 15,000?
    A. Lymphocytes
    B. RBCs
    C. Eosinophils
    D. Platelets
16. When evaluating a blood film, first scan the smear on low power (10×).
    A. True
    B. False

For the next five questions, match the term with its description.
    A. Metarubricyte
    B. Acanthocyte
    C. Rouleaux
    D. Polychromasia
    E. Spherocyte
    F. Reticulocyte

17. An RBC that appears smaller than a normal RBC and has no central pallor (pale area)
18. A nucleated RBC
19. An RBC with a membrane abnormality that causes it to develop multiple, irregularly spaced, club-shaped projections on the cell surface
20. A variation in the color of a patient's RBCs
21. An RBC that contains bluish-colored dots or strands when stained with new methylene blue
22. On a blood film, groupings of RBCs resembling stacked coins are normal in:
    A. Dogs and cats
    B. Cats and cattle
    C. Horses and cats
    D. Cattle and horses
23. You are reading a canine blood film and notice that many of the neutrophils contain small bluish-gray cytoplasmic inclusions, cytoplasmic vacuolation, and a light-blue cytoplasm. What action do you take?
    A. You find out which feline patient's blood film this actually is; these are attributes of normal feline neutrophils that are never seen in canine neutrophils.
    B. You report the neutrophils as "toxic."
    C. You discard the stain you used and replace it with fresh stain.
    D. You take no action because these are attributes of normal canine neutrophils.

For the next seven questions, match the WBC with its description.
    A. Monocyte
    B. Lymphocyte
    C. Neutrophil
    D. Eosinophil
    E. Basophil

24. This is a small to medium-sized cell with a thin rim of light- to dark-blue cytoplasm and a round, often eccentric nucleus.
25. This WBC has dark-blue granules.
26. This cell has a gray-blue, often grainy cytoplasm and a variably shaped nucleus.
27. This WBC has a segmented nucleus, colorless to pale-blue cytoplasm, and distinct reddish-orange granules in the cytoplasm.
28. This WBC has a deeply staining, clumped, segmented nucleus (3 to 5 lobes) with relatively clear cytoplasm or a very faint, almost indiscernible, dusting of tiny granules.
29. This cell is often confused with a band neutrophil.
30. In cattle, this kind of cell is often large and bizarre-looking.
31. A patient's total WBC count is 10,000 cells/µl. In your 100-cell WBC differential, you counted 50 neutrophils. What is the absolute number of neutrophils present per microliter of blood?
    A. 500
    B. 2500
    C. 5000
    D. 50,000
32. While good blood-sampling technique is important in obtaining accurate hematology results, which test will be totally invalidated if tissue injury occurs during venipuncture?
    A. Coagulation assay
    B. Plasma protein determination
    C. Buffy coat analysis
    D. Basket-cell count
33. A fresh urine sample is best analyzed:
    A. Immediately
    B. Within 3 hours
    C. Within 5 hours
    D. After refrigeration for 2 hours
34. Which statement about chemical reagent strip analysis of urine is true?
    A. The test should only be performed on the supernatant of centrifuged urine.
    B. The urine must be at room temperature if accurate results are to be obtained.
    C. Even significantly discolored urine will not affect the results.
    D. The manner in which the strips are stored is not critical to the test outcome.
35. A feline urine sample with a specific gravity of 1.010 is relatively concentrated.
    A. True
    B. False
36. A positive blood test on a urine chemical reagent strip indicates the presence of:
    A. Myoglobin
    B. Hemoglobin

C. RBCs
D. Any of the above

37. The epithelial cells that may be present in urine sediment, in decreasing order of size (largest to smallest), are:
    A. Squamous, transitional, renal tubular
    B. Transitional, squamous, renal tubular
    C. Renal tubular, transitional, squamous
    D. Squamous, renal tubular, transitional

38. Which statement about casts and crystals in urine sediment is true?
    A. They must be classified according to type and recorded.
    B. They can be ignored as insignificant findings and need not be recorded.
    C. They may indicate the presence of disease.
    D. A and C

39. The biggest advantage to staining urine sediment before examination is:
    A. The stain improves the detection of RBCs.
    B. The stain improves the detection of WBCs.
    C. The stain improves the detection of bacteria.
    D. The stain improves the detection of viruses.

40. In liquid reagent-based chemistry analyzers, a solution that contains a known concentration of specific substances is called a:
    A. Reagent
    B. Primary sample
    C. Standard
    D. Concentrate

41. An in-house chemistry analyzer appears to be giving incorrect results. The sample quality is known to be good and the machine is maintained exactly according to the manufacturer's directions. What is the best first step you should take to handle this problem?
    A. Call the technical support division of the manufacturer.
    B. Turn the machine off for 5 days then try analyzing the samples again.
    C. Analyze a control product and compare the results obtained with the expected values provided by the manufacturer.
    D. Discard all reagents (wet) or test cards (dry) and purchase new ones.

42. Postprandial (after-eating) serum-sample analysis is often complicated by:
    A. Lipemia
    B. Hemolysis
    C. Leukocytosis
    D. Hyperbilirubinemia

43. The best Vacutainer tube to use for serum analysis in an emergency situation is one with a
    A. Purple top
    B. Green top
    C. Red top
    D. Blue top

44. How must a blood sample in a clot tube be handled to ensure accurate blood chemistry results?
    A. The serum should be left on the clot and the entire tube refrigerated immediately after centrifugation.
    B. The serum should be left on the clot and the entire tube refrigerated within 2 hours of centrifugation.
    C. The serum should be separated from the clot immediately after centrifugation.
    D. The serum should be separated from the clot within 2 hours of centrifugation.

45. Slides prepared for cytologic analysis from a bodily fluid, tissue impression, or fine needle aspiration of a mass should always be stained before submission to a reference laboratory.
    A. True
    B. False

46. Describe, in four steps, how a PCV is obtained from an anticoagulated blood sample that is in a Vacutainer tube.

47. What three physical properties of urine are evaluated and recorded prior to chemical testing and microscopic examination?

48. Briefly describe the preparation of a urine sample for unstained sediment evaluation.

49. List four common causes of inaccurate results from in-house blood chemistry analyzers.

50. Define *anisocytosis*.

EXTRA CREDIT

51. Kohler illumination is:
    A. A microscope light source that consists of a halogen bulb
    B. Another term for darkfield illumination
    C. A method of illumination, by adjustment of the substage condenser, for obtaining the best image detail
    D. The light reflected off of a cow's nose

52. Azurophilic is:
    A. A term describing the affinity of glucose for its substrate on a urinalysis reagent test strip
    B. Appearing blue
    C. Appearing red
    D. A term describing a technician who loves dogs with bright blue eyes

CHAPTER 7

PARASITOLOGY

1. Which statement concerning animal parasites is most accurate?
    A. *Cestode* means wormlike.
    B. Parasitism is most severe in animals younger than 1 year of age.

C. All animal parasites are capable of infesting or infecting a broad range of animal species.
D. The nematodes have complex life cycles involving the use of an intermediate host or transport host.

2. Most important gastrointestinal parasites are diagnosed by examination of the:
   A. Feces
   B. Vomit
   C. Blood
   D. Urine

3. An owner asks you how her 5-week-old puppy could have roundworms at such a young age. You tell her the puppy could have been infected by the:
   A. Transplacental (prenatal) route
   B. Transmammary route
   C. Transcutaneous route
   D. A and/or B

4. In general, control of _____ is difficult because the eggs are highly resistant to environmental insult and remain viable in spite of weather extremes.
   A. *Toxocara, Parascaris, Ascaris,* and *Toxascaris* spp.
   B. *Haemonchus* spp.
   C. *Trichuris vulpis*
   D. A and C

5. Which pair of nematodes primarily infests the host by burrowing through the skin?
   A. Whipworms and hookworms
   B. Roundworms and intestinal threadworms
   C. Roundworms and hookworms
   D. Intestinal threadworms and hookworms

6. The common name for trematodes is:
   A. Whipworms
   B. Flukes
   C. Tapeworms
   D. Pinworms

7. *Strongyloides stercoralis* is unique because it is one of the only common intestinal nematodes of dogs and cats that is passed in the feces in a larval form *not* encased in an egg.
   A. True
   B. False

8. _____, _____, and _____ pass their eggs in dog feces and are commonly diagnosed by fecal-flotation techniques.
   A. Tapeworms; heartworms; hookworms
   B. *Dirofilaria* spp.; *Dipetalonema* spp.; *Dipylidium* spp.
   C. Ascarids; hookworms; whipworms
   D. Intestinal threadworms; coccidia; *Giardia* spp.

9. "Marty" is an adult, indoor-only Siamese cat who experiences recurrent tapeworm infections. After his most recent treatment for this infection, about what did you counsel his owner to prevent another infection with this parasite?
   A. Litter-box sanitation
   B. Flea control
   C. Diet
   D. Preventing the cat from interacting with the family's pet parrot

10. *Dipylidium caninum* in small animals is diagnosed primarily by:
    A. Finding the proglottids around the host's anal region or on his hocks (tarsi)
    B. Fecal sedimentation
    C. Direct fecal smear
    D. Fecal flotation

For the next four questions, match the parasite with its characteristics.
   A. *Dirofilaria immitis*
   B. *Dipetalonema reconditum*
   C. A and B
   D. None of the above

11. Nonpathogenic filarial nematode of dogs
12. The adults inhabit the right ventricle and pulmonary arteries of infested dogs and cats.
13. The mosquito transfers the parasite from an infected to a noninfected host.
14. Diagnosed by microfilarial detection and characterization techniques such as fresh blood/saline preparations or the filtration-concentration test.

15. Which coccidial species is considered nonpathogenic in dogs and cats?
    A. *Isospora* spp.
    B. *Toxoplasma gondii*
    C. *Cryptosporidium* spp.
    D. *Sarcocystis* spp.

16. Which patient is least likely to be shedding *Toxoplasma gondii* organisms?
    A. A 4-month-old kitten that wandered up to the owner's front door as a stray at the age of 3 months
    B. A sick, 5-year-old cat recently adopted from the local animal shelter, whose history is unknown
    C. A 10-year-old cat that has not been outside in over 8 years; the owner has no other pets
    D. A 1-year-old barn cat who hunts mice to supplement her diet of dry cat food

17. Which equine parasite has larval stages that migrate through the cranial mesenteric artery and its branches?
    A. *Strongyloides westerii*
    B. *Strongylus equinus*
    C. *Strongylus vulgaris*
    D. *Anoplocephala magna*

18. The most important gastrointestinal parasites of cattle and sheep in the United States are the _____, which are diagnosed by seeing _____ in the feces.
    A. Trematodes; leaf-shaped larvae
    B. Cestodes; blood
    C. Strongyle nematodes; strongyle-type eggs
    D. Trematodes; strongyle-type eggs

19. Sulfonamide antibiotics are indicated in the treatment of:
    A. Tapeworms
    B. Coccidia
    C. Large and small strongyles
    D. Intestinal threadworms
20. The tapeworms studied in this chapter are generally considered nonpathogenic to the infected animal and are usually not even treated in horses and cattle.
    A. True
    B. False
21. Of the common domestic animal species, only _____ are infected by pinworms.
    A. Sheep
    B. Goats
    C. Cattle
    D. Horses
22. The biggest advantage to housing cattle and sheep away from wet, swampy pastures lies in:
    A. Reducing exposure to snail populations, whose members act as the intermediate hosts for *Fasciola hepatica*
    B. Reducing the opportunity for *Trichomonas foetus* to complete its water-dependent life cycle
    C. Improved control of *Eimeria* spp.
    D. Reducing exposure to the earthworm, the intermediate host for *Moniezia* spp.
23. A strongyle-type egg found in swine feces can be identified as:
    A. A stomach or a large-intestinal worm
    B. A lungworm
    C. A kidney worm
    D. B or C
24. A pig without access to earthworms cannot be infected by:
    A. *Hyostrongylus rubidus*
    B. *Metastrongylus* spp.
    C. *Stephanurus dentatus*
    D. B and C
25. Fleas are *not* host specific and will attack many animals as well as humans.
    A. True
    B. False
26. Which insecticide is considered the most toxic, especially to puppies and kittens younger than 6 months of age?
    A. Pyrethrins
    B. Lufenuron
    C. Fipronyl
    D. Organophosphates
27. Which flea-control agent is safe for judicious use in nursing animals?
    A. Lufenuron
    B. Fipronyl
    C. Imidacloprid
    D. Pyrethrins
28. In general, flea collars alone effectively control flea populations on pets.
    A. True
    B. False
29. The larvae of equine botflies, whose eggs can be seen attached to the hair of the horse, inhabit the horse's:
    A. Small intestine
    B. Cecum
    C. Stomach
    D. Rectum
30. Which parasite has a larval form that lives in the subcutaneous tissue and eventually emerges from a hole in the skin?
    A. *Cuterebra* spp.
    B. *Wohlfahrtia* spp.
    C. *Hypoderma* spp.
    D. All of the above
31. For which species must treatment be applied at a specific time of year?
    A. Cattle grubs
    B. Lice
    C. Sheep nose bots
    D. Canine whipworms

For the next three questions, match the mite with the species and locations it infests.

A. *Notoedres cati*
B. *Chorioptes* spp.
C. *Otodectes* spp.
D. *Cheyletiella* spp.
E. *Demodex* spp.

32. Lives in the ears of dogs, cats, and other related animals
33. Lives in hair follicles of dogs, cats, cattle, sheep, humans, and horses
34. Lives on the body of cattle, sheep, goats, and rabbits
35. Mites are diagnosed by the morphologic appearance of the adults, which most often requires.
    A. Thorough skin scrapings
    B. Close examination of the skin and hair with the unaided eye
    C. The adhesive-tape test
    D. That cut hair samples be sent to a parasitologist for species identification.
36. The larvae of blowflies and screwworm flies are known collectively as:
    A. Bots
    B. Maggots
    C. Grubs
    D. Cercariae
37. In the United States, no species of tick inhabits the ears of the common domestic animals.
    A. True
    B. False

38. For which parasite is a direct fecal-saline smear the best diagnostic test?
    A. *Trichomonas* spp.
    B. *Toxocara* spp.
    C. *Toxoplasma gondii*
    D. *Amblyomma* spp.
39. One advantage of the zinc sulfate centrifugal flotation (ZnSO$_4$) technique over the other flotation techniques is:
    A. The simplicity of performing the ZnSO$_4$ technique
    B. The reduced cost of supplies required for the ZnSO$_4$ technique
    C. The ZnSO$_4$ technique does not destroy fragile cysts and larvae that are often destroyed by other flotation methods
    D. A and B
40. The number of eggs or larvae found in the feces and the severity of parasitism are directly related; that is, more eggs equals more severe disease.
    A. True
    B. False
41. What technique is used to quantify the number of parasitic eggs and larvae per gram of feces?
    A. Willis technique
    B. Stoll dilution or Stoll centrifugation technique
    C. Baermann funnel technique
    D. Formalin-ethyl acetate sedimentation technique
42. The two most effective techniques for detecting blood microfilarial infections are:
    A. The direct blood smear and the saline-blood preparation
    B. The saline-blood preparation and the microhematocrit technique
    C. The Knott and filter techniques
    D. The direct blood smear and the Knott technique
43. If neither the motile trophozoites nor the cysts of *Giardia* are seen on a direct fecal-saline smear, and giardiasis is suspected, which test should you next perform on the feces?
    A. ZnSO$_4$ centrifugal flotation
    B. Maceration technique
    C. Stoll Dilution technique
    D. Direct fecal smear made with distilled water rather than saline
44. Which parasite can infest humans who eat raw or insufficiently cooked infected meat?
    A. *Trichinella spiralis*
    B. Toxoplasma gondii
    C. Taenia spp. (tapeworms)
    D. All of the above
45. Concerning canine heartworm disease, which statement is most accurate?
    A. An "occult" heartworm infection is one in which there are no obvious clinical signs.
    B. From the time of the initial infection, it can take up to 60 days for serologic tests, which detect adult heartworms, to show a positive result.
    C. Because heartworm disease is easily prevented by daily or monthly preventive medications, it is generally considered more prudent to prevent the disease than to treat it.
    D. Treatment necessitates the use of a microfilaricide followed by an agent effective for the adult heartworms.
46. What is the common and full scientific name of the most frequently encountered parasite in pigs?
47. For each of the four stages of the flea life cycle, name and describe the stage, where organisms in that stage live or are usually located, and what, if anything, they feed on.
48. Describe the premise on which fecal-egg flotation techniques are based. In other words, how do they work?
49. Why are fecal-flotation techniques unsuitable for trematode eggs (with the exception of *Troglotrema* and *Paragonimus* spp.)?
50. How is it possible for an animal to be severely parasitized yet the diagnostic test for that parasite, properly performed, is negative?

EXTRA CREDIT

51. A *schizont* is:
    A. Part of the life cycle of *Isospora* spp.
    B. Part of the life cycle of the cestode parasites
    C. Part of the life cycle of the trematode parasites
    D. A newborn German-breed puppy
52. "Warbles" are
    A. Flies that lay their eggs in feces
    B. Flies that lay their eggs in a row just above the claws of cattle
    C. Seen as lumps on the backs of infested cattle
    D. The sounds a hungry cat makes when it wants to be fed

CHAPTER 8

CLINICAL MICROBIOLOGY

1. Which stain is most useful for differentiating the bacterial species present on a sample smear?
    A. Wright's stain
    B. New methylene blue
    C. Gram stain
    D. Giemsa stains

For the next four questions, match the diagnostic test with its description.
    A. Bacterial isolation by culture with subsequent identification schemes

B. Nucleic acid (DNA or RNA)–amplification system using polymerase chain reaction (PCR)
   C. Demonstration of specific microbial antigens
   D. Demonstration of a specific immunologic response using serum antibody levels or skin tests
2. The most frequently used method in bacteriology to demonstrate the presence of microbial species and identify them specifically
3. In this diagnostic method, the presence of only one contaminating microorganism can result in false positive results:
4. The newest method of bacterial identification
5. Allows the differentiation of closely related organisms based on the presence of a unique genetic sequence
6. To obtain accurate and useful results, your biggest concern when collecting a sample for culture is:
   A. To obtain at least 5 ml of exudate, body fluid, or tissue
   B. The brand of culture swab used
   C. The speed with which the sample is collected
   D. Avoidance of contamination from adjacent tissues or excretions
7. How should you submit 5 ml of urine, collected by cystocentesis, to a professional laboratory for aerobic bacterial culture?
   A. Saturate a sterile swab with the urine and submit it in the appropriate transfer media.
   B. Remove the needle, express the air from the syringe, cap the tip of the syringe, and submit the entire syringe.
   C. Transfer the urine to a sterile blood-collection tube (without anticoagulant) and submit the tube.
   D. B or C
8. During collection and transport to a reference laboratory, handling a specimen as if it contains anaerobes will *not* jeopardize the viability of aerobic bacteria.
   A. True
   B. False
9. The Coggin test for equine infectious anemia is based on:
   A. Serum antibody detection
   B. Serum antigen detection
   C. Isolation by bacterial culture
   D. Virus isolation
10. Concerning the pathogens that cause infectious diseases, which statement is most accurate?
    A. Bacterial isolation and identification by culture is critical because it is impossible to narrow down the list of possible infecting agents by any other method.
    B. All bacterial species are essentially alike, eliminating the need for special selective transport or culture media.
    C. Knowing the species and organ system affected allows the laboratory technician to narrow down the list of possible pathogens in a sample.
    D. If specimens will not be processed until the next day, samples should be kept at room temperature.
11. Although bacterial culture and antimicrobial sensitivity testing are important in diagnosing and selecting treatments for infections, _____ is the most important laboratory procedure used for microbiologic diagnosis.
    A. Direct microscopic examination (of exudates, impression smears from body tissues, or infected body fluids)
    B. The immunohistochemical assay
    C. Establishing the presence of a microbial toxin
    D. The nucleic acid–amplification assay (PCR)
12. For which type of organism must the laboratory be contacted prior to submitting the sample for culture so they will be ready to begin processing it as soon as it arrives?
    A. Coliforms (includes fermentative gram-negative enteric bacilli such as *Escherichia coli*)
    B. Fungi
    C. Viruses
    D. Antibodies
13. Obligate anaerobic bacteria:
    A. Require a special culture container from which all oxygen has been removed
    B. Grow poorly in the presence of oxygen
    C. Cannot grow at all in the presence of oxygen
    D. A and C
14. Allow inoculated primary-isolation media to incubate for _____ for most bacterial species before a final "no growth" report is issued.
    A. 24 hours
    B. 48 hours
    C. 72 hours
    D. 5 days
15. When gram-stained, fungi (yeast) appear gram positive, or _____ in color.
    A. Dark blue or purple
    B. Green
    C. Yellow
    D. Pink or red
16. On stained smears, bacteria are best identified using the:
    A. 4× objective
    B. 10× objective
    C. 40× (high-dry) objective
    D. 100× (oil-immersion) objective
17. The four-quadrant streaking method of solid-media inoculation of plates is specifically designed to:
    A. Detect motile bacteria
    B. Detect gram-negative species
    C. Detect gram-positive species

D. Dilute the specimen in such a way that isolated colonies develop, each representing a single bacterial cell
18. When incubating inoculated media, plates are placed _____ and screw tops are _____.
   A. Upside down; kept loose
   B. Right-side up; kept loose
   C. Upside down; screwed on tightly
   D. Right-side up; screwed on tightly
19. Concerning the preliminary evaluation of primary cultures, which statement is most accurate?
   A. Species identification of bacterial growth that results from environmental contamination or indigenous flora is essential.
   B. Most bacterial infections are caused by three or more agents.
   C. In general, if there is scant growth of three or more bacterial species, the result probably reflects normal flora.
   D. Usually, large, rough, granular, irregular, spreading, or heavily pigmented colonies, especially in small numbers, are significant and should be selected for further identification.
20. Lack of color or a color change surrounding colonies on the normally red blood-agar plates is caused by:
   A. MacConkey isolates
   B. A change in pH
   C. Hemolysis
   D. Gram-negative bacteria
21. When recording the relative abundance of growth of each type of colony, grown first in broth subculture and then on primary-isolation plates, using the 1+ to 4+ scale, a "1+" means:
   A. The colony type is only present in the initial streak lines with which the specimen was inoculated.
   B. The colony was isolated from broth subculture, but no growth is present on the primary plate.
   C. One colony of that type is present on the plate.
   D. A or B.
22. Once significant colonies have been selected on primary growth media, the next step is to perform a(n):
   A. Gram stain
   B. Slide catalase test
   C. Oxidase test
   D. Glucose fermentation test
23. Which of the following bacterial groups is usually considered a potential pathogen?
   A. *Micrococcus* spp.
   B. Nonhemolytic *Streptococcus* spp.
   C. Beta-hemolytic *Streptococcus* spp.
   D. Alpha-hemolytic *Streptococcus* spp.
24. Concerning the low-volume microbiologic laboratory seen in private veterinary practice, which statement is most accurate?
   A. Presumptive (not definitive) bacterial identification is usually sufficient.
   B. Commercial identification kits are an accurate, cost-effective alternative to conventional media.
   C. Commercial identification kits allow the identification of most bacterial groups within 4 to 24 hours after isolation.
   D. All of the above.
25. Concerning the shape of bacteria, "cocci" are round and "rods" are narrow and elongated.
   A. True
   B. False
26. When culturing _____, special inoculation techniques should be used to quantify bacterial colony counts.
   A. Urine
   B. Blood
   C. Nasal exudate
   D. Feces

For the next 10 questions, match the bacterial group with its significant characteristics.
   A. Spirochetes
   B. *Campylobacter* spp.
   C. *Streptococcus* spp.
   D. *Pseudomonas* spp.
   E. *Staphylococcus* spp.
   F. *Pasteurella* spp.
   G. *Mycobacterium* spp.
   H. *Clostridium* spp.
   I. Enterobacteriaceae family
   J. Actinomycetaceae family

27. Gram-positive cocci that occur in grapelike clusters; they are usually divided into catalase-positive and catalase-negative groups.
28. Branching, filamentous, gram-positive rods; grow best when cultured anaerobically, are seen in pyogranulomatous lesions, and include *Nocardia* spp. and *Dermatophilus congolensis*.
29. Small, gram-negative rods; oxidase negative, usually grow on MacConkey agar, and normally inhabit intestinal tract so are frequent contaminants; species include *Escherichia coli* and *Salmonella* spp.
30. Spiral-shaped, motile organisms; very difficult to grow in most laboratories; diagnosis is usually by serology (blood testing) or direct examination of the organisms in urine (dogs) or colonic mucosa (pigs); *Leptospira* spp., *Borrelia burgdorferi*, and *Brachyspira hyodysenteriae* are members of this group.
31. Small, gram-negative, oxidase-positive coccobacilli; exhibit a typical weak glucose-fermentation reaction in a TSI tube; tend to be nonreactive in commercial identification kits; are usually associated with respiratory infections or feline abscesses.

32. Curved, gram-negative rods; recognized by dark-field or phase-contrast microscopy by their darting motility; should be sent to a reference laboratory for isolation; cause abortion, infertility, or a zoonotic enteritis.
33. Gram-positive cocci occurring singly, in pairs, or in short chains; hemolysis on blood agar is important for clinical interpretation.
34. Acid-fast, small, short (occasionally pleomorphic) rods; stain poorly with Gram stain; rarely isolated because special media and procedures are required; more frequently seen in the liver, intestines, or feces of birds; cause tuberculosis in some animals and in humans.
35. Common soil and water bacteria; opportunistic pathogens of wounds and otitis; the most common pathogen produces water-soluble, yellow-green pigments that diffuse into the media; a distinctive odor aids recognition; should be routinely tested for susceptibility.
36. Large, gram-positive, spore-forming, anaerobic rods; cause diseases such as tetanus, botulism, and canine or feline enteritis (diarrhea).
37. Antimicrobial susceptibility testing is performed because some microorganisms are resistant to a given antibiotic.
    A. True
    B. False
38. Which of the following groups most frequently requires routine antimicrobial susceptibility testing?
    A. Slow-growing bacteria
    B. Anaerobic bacteria
    C. Gram-negative bacteria
    D. Gram-positive bacteria (other than *Staphylococcus* spp.)
39. The "MIC" obtained by the broth dilution susceptibility test in reference laboratories is defined as:
    A. The species of bacteria whose inhibition requires the least amount of a given antibiotic
    B. The size of the largest-diameter zone of inhibition
    C. The size of the smallest-diameter zone of inhibition
    D. The lowest concentration of antimicrobial that macroscopically inhibits growth of the organism.
40. Which statement concerning antimicrobial susceptibility testing using the agar diffusion test is most accurate?
    A. Always use a pure culture of bacteria for inoculation.
    B. MacConkey agar is the most practical media to inoculate.
    C. The antimicrobial disks are best made in-house using therapeutic drug solutions.
    D. It is important to be aware of frequent false-resistant results when testing cephalosporin activity.
41. When measuring zones of inhibition around antibiotic-impregnated disks, which statement is most accurate?
    A. Large colonies growing within a clear zone of inhibition should be ignored.
    B. Swarming growth into clearly outlined zones of inhibition should be ignored.
    C. The zone diameter is measured starting at the edge of the disk and does not include the disk diameter.
    D. The end-point of growth surrounding the zone of inhibition should include the faint growth of colonies detected only with difficulty.
42. The zones of inhibition, once measured, are recorded on the final report:
    A. In millimeters
    B. In centimeters
    C. Using one of three terms derived from a standard table that translate the diameter of each zone of inhibition into the isolate's resistance level to the antibiotic
    D. Using the terms *zone* or *no zone*
43. Disease caused by dermatophytes is also known as:
    A. Ringworm
    B. Enteritis
    C. Systemic mycosis
    D. A yeast infection
44. Dermatophyte test media (DTM) cultures should be recorded as "negative" only if no growth or color change has occurred in approximately:
    A. 24 hours
    B. 5 days
    C. 10 days
    D. 15 days
45. Which colonies grown on DTM are most likely pathogenic?
    A. Darkly colored brown or black colonies
    B. A media color change to red that preceded or occurred simultaneous to the growth of white-to-tan colonies
    C. A media color change to red that occurred after the growth of white-to-tan colonies
    D. White-to-tan colonies with no media color change
46. The three most important systemic fungal infections are serious zoonoses (infect humans) and are best identified by:
    A. Culture in a reference laboratory
    B. In-house culture in an approved biohazard safety hood
    C. In-house direct microscopic examination of the agents in the tissue, or yeast, phase
    D. In-house observation of their ectothrix on hairs or delicate hyphae in skin scales
47. On microscopic examination of exudate from otitis externa (external ear infection), you observe many

oval, bottle-shaped, monopolar-budding organisms. You record your findings as:
   A. *Malassezia* spp., or yeast
   B. *Sporothrix* spp.
   C. *Nocardia* spp.
   D. Coccidiomycosis
48. In general, the most frequently used method for diagnosis of viral disease is:
   A. Direct examination of infected animal cells for viral-inclusion particles
   B. Viral antigen detection
   C. Electron microscopy
   D. Isolation by culture
49. Test kits frequently used in private practice that use a color change to diagnose diseases such as canine parvovirus, feline leukemia, and influenza are all examples of:
   A. Enzyme-linked immunosorbent assays (ELISA)
   B. Immunoperoxidase method assays
   C. Hemagglutination assays
   D. None of the above
50. Testing that detects the concentration of antibody, and therefore an animal's immune response to a certain infecting agent (usually a virus), is often referred to as:
   A. Viral isolation
   B. Histology
   C. Mycology
   D. Serology
51. The veterinarian tells you that "acute" and "convalescent" blood samples will be needed for submission to a reference laboratory for serum antibody levels. You proceed to take the first sample today and schedule an appointment for _____ from now for the second blood draw.
   A. 24 hours
   B. 3 days
   C. 7 days
   D. 14 days
52. What practice must be observed when submitting acute- and convalescent-phase blood samples?
   A. Only use brand new needles, syringes, and tubes.
   B. Freeze the first serum sample until the second is obtained then submit both samples together.
   C. Ship the samples to the laboratory on ice to prevent thawing of the frozen serum.
   D. All of the above
53. Which immunologic disorder can be diagnosed in a low-volume, in-house laboratory?
   A. Autoimmune disorder
   B. Gammopathy
   C. Failure of passive transfer
   D. A and C
54. Nosocomial infections in veterinary hospitals probably occur at a similar frequency as those in human hospitals; that is, _____ of hospitalized patients acquire these infections.
   A. Less than 1%
   B. 1% to 2%
   C. 3% to 5%
   D. 7% to 10%
55. Nosocomial infections are most frequently seen in:
   A. Large, referral-type practices
   B. Small, private practices
   C. Exotic-animal hospitals
   D. Small-animal hospitals
56. The most important vehicles for the spread of nosocomial agents are:
   A. Food bowls
   B. Towels and bedding
   C. The hands of hospital personnel
   D. Cage surfaces
57. Most patients with nosocomial infections are
   A. Geriatric
   B. Severely debilitated
   C. Undergoing treatment with antibiotics
   D. Neonatal
58. A blood transfusion from an animal infected with a blood-borne pathogen can be a source of a nosocomial infection.
   A. True
   B. False
59. To reduce the incidence of nosocomial infections, veterinary hospitals should only use disinfectants that:
   A. Contain at least 0.1% sodium hypochlorite (bleach)
   B. Are registered by the Environmental Protection Agency
   C. Are labeled as part of a three-step cleaning system
   D. Are not diluted prior to use
60. A minimal immunization requirement for veterinary-hospital personnel includes:
   A. Rabies vaccine
   B. Tetanus toxoid
   C. Hepatitis B
   D. A and B
61. The most practical decontamination procedure for much of the glassware, instruments, and equipment used in a small microbiologic laboratory is:
   A. Chemical sterilization
   B. Irradiation
   C. Incineration
   D. Steam autoclaving
62. A properly labeled culture-specimen container includes what four pieces of information?
63. How is sample collection for asymptomatic carriers of ringworm different from that of animals showing clear lesions?
64. What is "failure of passive transfer"?

Copyright © 2006 by Elsevier, Inc. All rights reserved.

EXTRA CREDIT

65. In bacteriology, the term *normal flora* is best defined as:
    A. Nonpathogenic bacteria
    B. The microorganisms indigenous to a given organ system or body surface
    C. The microorganisms indigenous to the gastrointestinal tract
    D. The bacteria growing on plants in and around animal hospitals
66. The term *titer* refers to:
    A. The concentration of antibiotic required to inhibit the growth of a bacterial species
    B. The serum antibody level
    C. The concentration of immunoglobulin in a sample of colostrum
    D. What you have to do to your dog's collar when he keeps slipping out of it and escaping

CHAPTER 9

DIAGNOSTIC IMAGING

1. All hard copies of radiographs, computed tomography (CT) scans, ultrasound images, and magnetic resonance imaging (MRI) studies are:
    A. The owner's property
    B. The hospital's property
    C. Part of the patient's record
    D. B and C
2. For a radiograph to be considered admissible as evidence in a court of law, at least the _____ must be permanently imprinted onto it prior to developing.
    A. Patient name or identification number, owner name, hospital name, and date of the examination
    B. Lead markers indicating the extremity examined (right or left) or the side on which the animal is lying (right or left)
    C. Time of exposure in a series of timed examinations
    D. Brand of film used
3. The term *radiographic technique* generally refers to:
    A. The patient's position during exposure
    B. The machine's exposure settings (e.g., kVP, mAs) during a given examination
    C. The methods used to restrain the animal during exposure
    D. Type of film screen used
4. X-rays cannot penetrate:
    A. Bone
    B. The interior walls of most animal hospitals
    C. Lead
    D. B and C
5. Concerning the filaments in the x-ray tube that produce electrons, which statement is most accurate?
    A. The small filament may melt more rapidly than the large filament if an excess load is placed on it.
    B. The large filament is used to obtain images of higher quality.
    C. The small filament provides a larger focal spot (target region) for electrons at the anode than the large filament.
    D. Use of the small filament is generally restricted to the higher mAs settings used in grid radiography of thicker body parts.
6. Why are rotating-anode x-ray machines more powerful than stationary-cathode x-ray machines?
    A. The former allow greater dissipation of heat.
    B. The former allow the use of a smaller focal spot with higher tube currents.
    C. The former allow the use of shorter exposure times.
    D. All of the above.
7. Always place the thinnest part of the area you are radiographing toward the cathode side of the x-ray tube.
    A. True
    B. False
8. The primary source of radiation exposure to the technician during radiography is scattered radiation, which can best be defined as:
    A. Radiation produced when no collimator is used
    B. Lower-energy x-ray photons that have undergone a change in direction after interacting with structures in the patient's body
    C. High-energy x-ray photons from the primary x-ray beam
    D. Lower-energy x-ray photons produced when radiographing thick body parts
9. The acronym kVP stands for _____ and controls the _____ of x-ray photons produced.
    A. Kilovolts produced; speed
    B. Kilovolts produced; number
    C. Kilovolt peak; number
    D. Kilovolt peak; speed
10. For safety reasons, portable x-ray units should never be handheld:
    A. True
    B. False
11. You have just taken a thoracic radiograph at 50 kVP and 100 mA at 1/10 second. The pet's breathing caused his chest to move during the exposure, resulting in a blurry image. On the retake, how can you correct for this motion to create a clear image of the same density?
    A. Reduce the time to 1/20 second.
    B. Reduce the MA to 50.

C. Increase the kVP to 60.
   D. Reduce the time to 1/20 second and increase the mA to 200.
12. You have radiographed a fractured femur in a large dog. The resulting image is too gray; that is, you can see many shades of gray and a lot of detail in the muscle layers, but the bone is also too gray, and bony fragments are difficult to see. How can you best correct your settings to create a clearer image of the fractured bone?
   A. Increase the mAs.
   B. Decrease the mAs.
   C. Increase the kVP.
   D. Decrease the kVP.
13. Which statement is most accurate concerning the effects of a change in focus-film distance (FFD) when taking radiographs?
   A. The mAs setting must be changed according to a standard mathematical formula.
   B. In general, reduce the mAs by 1 unit for every FFD increase of 1 cm.
   C. The kVP and mAs need not be changed when the FFD is changed.
   D. The FFD is usually changed from one exposure to another throughout the day according to the body part examined.
14. How does one obtain the correct machine settings when taking a radiograph?
   A. The technician must memorize the settings.
   B. A veterinary-radiology textbook will have a chart of correct settings.
   C. Settings are obtained from a "technique chart" created, by trial and error, specifically for the machine one is using.
   D. A or B
15. Concerning the use of film holders (cassettes) in veterinary radiography, which statement is most accurate?
   A. A "nonscreen" cassette is made of nonrigid cardboard or plastic.
   B. The most commonly used cassettes in companion-animal practice are rigid and contain an image-intensifying screen.
   C. Screened cassettes are relatively inexpensive and are generally used three to five times, then discarded.
   D. A and B
16. Care of image-intensifying screens involves:
   A. Cleaning them with a special solution or 70% isopropyl alcohol at least once monthly or whenever screen artifacts are seen on a radiograph
   B. Washing once monthly with a mild detergent and rinsing well with distilled water
   C. Removing them from the cassette every 6 months for cleaning by the manufacturer
   D. A and C

17. In general, image-intensifying screens are fragile and are easily ruined by placing film in them when they are damp or by splashing darkroom chemicals onto them.
   A. True
   B. False
18. Only one type of radiographic film is available; it is suitable for all screen types and nonscreen uses.
   A. True
   B. False
19. The purpose of a grid is to:
   A. Allow only the primary x-ray beam to pass through and prevent scattered radiation from reaching the film.
   B. Increase the resolution of thicker body parts.
   C. Provide lines on the developed x-ray that are a known distance apart, thus allowing the accurate measurement of body structures.
   D. A and B
20. Most mistakes made in veterinary radiography are related to:
   A. Improper grid use
   B. Improper machine settings
   C. Improper processing techniques
   D. Animal movement during exposure
21. Which statement concerning hand processing versus automatic-film processing of radiographs is most accurate?
   A. Automatic processors are generally slower than hand-processing techniques.
   B. Both techniques require the use of fresh solutions and a well-ventilated darkroom.
   C. Automatic processors require much less maintenance than manual-processing tanks.
   D. Some newer automatic processors remove the need for a totally lightproof darkroom.
22. X-ray film should be handled carefully and held only by the corners both when loading cassettes and after exposure during processing.
   A. True
   B. False
23. X-ray film recycling and special units attached to fixer tanks allow the recovery of _____, a valuable and reusable substance.
   A. Halide
   B. Calcium tungstate
   C. Silver
   D. Mercury

For the next four questions, match the image characteristic with its description.
   A. Radiographic detail
   B. Radiographic contrast
   C. Radiographic density
   D. All of the above
24. This must be optimized to produce an image of diagnostic quality.

Copyright © 2006 by Elsevier, Inc. All rights reserved.

25. This refers to the number of shades of gray in an image and is most affected by the kilovoltage used during exposure.
26. This is most affected by movement or placing the body part to be radiographed too far from the film.
27. This term refers to how black a film is overall, that is, whether the film is overexposed, underexposed, or ideally exposed.
28. After exposing and developing an x-ray, you find the film totally white. What is the most likely cause of this problem?
    A. The film is unexposed.
    B. The film is underexposed.
    C. The film is overexposed.
    D. The grid was upside down.
29. In a practice using automatic x-ray processing equipment, the veterinary technician is expected to
    A. Calibrate the roller speed monthly.
    B. Keep the processor clean and add fresh developer and fixer solutions as needed.
    C. Provide a service overhaul on a regular basis, usually once every 3 months.
    D. All of the above.
30. What is necessary to prevent "fogging," or partial exposure, of x-ray film in the darkroom?
    A. Absolutely no light leakage into the room
    B. A lock on the door to prevent entrance during film processing
    C. A safelight of correct wattage and filter type for the film used
    D. All of the above
31. Your small-animal technique chart says "use Potter-Bucky grid" for abdominal measurements of greater than 10 cm. What does this mean?
    A. Place the cassette on top of the table for measurements of less than or equal to 10 cm and in the tray underneath the table for those greater than 10 cm.
    B. Remove the film from the cassette for measurements of greater than 10 cm.
    C. Place the cassette in the tray underneath the table for measurements of less than or equal to 10 cm.
    D. Place the cassette on top of the table for measurements of greater than 10 cm.
32. Which diagnostic imaging method is best suited to the production of a continuous, moving image?
    A. Magnetic resonance imaging (MRI)
    B. Fluoroscopy
    C. Computed tomography (CT)
    D. Nuclear medicine
33. A film badge that measures the amount of radiation to which veterinary personnel are exposed is best worn:
    A. Inside the lead apron at the waist
    B. Outside the lead apron at the waist
    C. Outside the lead apron on the collar at the level of the thyroid gland
    D. Outside the lead apron on a string around the neck so it hangs at heart level
34. Which type of contrast media can be used for any type of contrast examination including oral, urogenital, intravenous, intraarterial, intrathecal, and in the respiratory tract?
    A. Radiolucent gases such as air
    B. Insoluble, nonionic, radiopaque media such as iohexol
    C. Insoluble, inert, radiopaque media such as barium sulfate
    D. Soluble, ionic, radiopaque media such as iothalamate
35. The risk of life-threatening reactions necessitates the placement of intravenous catheters and constant patient monitoring when using radiographic contrast agents:
    A. Orally
    B. Intravascularly or intrathecally
    C. Rectally
    D. In the bladder
36. Roentgens, rads, and rems are:
    A. Terms used to measure the depth of penetration of an ultrasound beam
    B. Types of contrast agents used in veterinary radiography
    C. Units of measurement used in diagnostic radiography
    D. Terms used to measure radiation exposure
37. A technique in which a radiographic contrast agent is administered orally and a series of abdominal films taken immediately and at 15-, 30-, and 60-minute intervals until the contrast reaches the beginning of the large intestine is known as a(n):
    A. Lower gastrointestinal study
    B. Upper gastrointestinal study
    C. Esophageal study
    D. Barium enema
38. Radiographic evaluation of the kidneys using contrast media intravenously is known as:
    A. An intravenous pyelogram or IVP
    B. A renogram
    C. A Renografin
    D. An intravenous renogram
39. Which contrast agent should never be injected into the urinary bladder?
    A. Barium sulfate
    B. Diatrizoate
    C. Iohexol
    D. Iothalamate
40. Myelography is used to evaluate the:
    A. Muscles
    B. Spinal cord
    C. Nerves in the limbs
    D. Brain

41. Survey films are:
    A. Radiographs taken when contrast media is used
    B. Printed ultrasound images
    C. Radiographs taken without the use of contrast media
    D. Fluoroscopic images
42. Concerning positioning animals for radiography, which statement is true?
    A. A basic set of diagnostic films includes right lateral, left lateral, and dorsoventral images.
    B. The primary beam should always be centered on the lesion itself if the lesion's location is known.
    C. Use the smallest x-ray film that will adequately allow visualization of the lesion or suspected area of disease.
    D. Regardless of whether dorsoventral or ventrodorsal positioning will cause a debilitated or injured animal undue stress, at least one of these views must be obtained.
43. In addition to providing proper positioning and immobilization, the most important reason to use restraint devices such as sandbags, wooden blocks, and cassette holders is to reduce radiation exposure to personnel taking the radiograph.
    A. True
    B. False
44. Which statement comparing x-rays to ultrasound waves is most accurate?
    A. X-rays are most similar to audible sound and ultrasound waves to visible light.
    B. X-rays are dangerous to the unprotected user and ultrasound waves are harmless.
    C. A radiograph is black and white with shades of gray and an ultrasound image is generally projected in the actual color of the tissues examined.
    D. Generally, ultrasound penetrates tissues more deeply than x-rays and so allows visualization of deeper or thicker structures.
45. Ultrasound produces a more detailed image of bone than radiography.
    A. True
    B. False
46. Two transducers are available for ultrasound imaging in the small-animal practice in which you work 5 MHz and 7.5 MHz. Which of these will be used to examine the abdomen of an adult Chihuahua that weighs 5 kg?
    A. 5 MHz
    B. 7.5 MHz
47. An "echogenic" ultrasound image is _____ the surrounding structures.
    A. Relatively brighter than
    B. Relatively darker than
    C. More focused than
    D. Less focused than
48. In diagnostic ultrasound imaging, an area of darkness that occurs deep to very dense material, such as bone, is known as:
    A. Acoustic enhancement
    B. Refraction or "edge" artifact
    C. Shadowing
    D. "Mirror-image" artifact
49. For which structures is diagnostic ultrasound suitable?
    A. Abdominal organs
    B. Tendons
    C. Eyeballs
    D. All of the above
50. Teleradiology has enhanced the field of veterinary imaging by:
    A. Reducing the exposure of personnel to harmful radiation
    B. Allowing imaging data to be stored permanently
    C. Allowing the practitioner to send digital and analog data to veterinary specialists across phone and cable lines for a faster delivery
    D. Reducing the strength of the magnetic field required to produce high quality mri images
51. The advantage of digital radiograph is:
    A. Parameters of brightness and contrast can be adjusted after the image is obtained so that exposure techniques do not have to be as precise.
    B. Parts of an image can be magnified to enhance the interpretation of exotic imaging.
    C. Films, screens, and processing are not required.
    D. All of the above.

For the next four questions, match the diagnostic modality with its description.
    A. Magnetic resonance imaging (MRI)
    B. Nuclear medicine
    C. Computed tomography (CT)
    D. A and C
52. This modality is used to treat hyperthyroidism and thyroid tumors and is used diagnostically in "bone scanning."
53. The use of a powerful magnet in this diagnostic modality precludes the use of metal objects on or near the patient or personnel during imaging.
54. The most common veterinary use of this modality is in brain and spinal cord imaging.
55. The presence of radioactivity in patients treated with this modality requires the veterinary technician caring for these patients to insist on comprehensive instruction in radiation principles and safety.
56. Describe what is happening inside the x-ray tube during the first and second step of the switch in a two-step exposure system.
57. How often should the developer and fixer solutions used to hand-process radiographs be changed?

58. Name five important protection practices essential for reducing x-ray exposure to safe levels.
59. Why is hair removal and the application of a generous amount of ultrasound gel an important part of patient preparation for an ultrasound examination?

EXTRA CREDIT

60. Why is the "A" in the term *mAs* always capitalized?
    A. It is capitalized by convention.
    B. Capitalized this way, the term is not mistaken for a typo or misspelled word ("mAs").
    C. In the metric system, the second letter of an abbreviation is always capitalized.
    D. Because the "A" refers to Andre M. Ampere, the physicist credited with the discovery of electric currents.
61. Screen craze is:
    A. A white speckle-patterned artifact, seen best in the black area of an x-ray, caused by worn-out intensifying screens
    B. A linear artifact produced when the x-ray film placed into a screened cassette is accidentally folded or creased
    C. A spattered-droplet-patterned artifact seen when developer is accidentally splashed onto undeveloped film
    D. A mental condition seen in veterinary technicians who take a lot of radiographs

CHAPTER 10

VETERINARY ONCOLOGY

1. Cancer chemotherapy can often be performed easily in private veterinary practices, whereas radiation therapy requires referral to an institution with the appropriate equipment and facilities.
    A. True
    B. False
2. *Cancer* is best defined as:
    A. Systemic symptoms indirectly associated with the presence of a tumor
    B. A disease only treatable with chemotherapy or radiation therapy
    C. An uncontrolled growth of cells on or within the body
    D. B and C
3. Concerning tumor classification as benign versus malignant, which statement is true?
    A. Benign tumors are called *benign* because they do not cause significant problems.
    B. Generally, only malignant tumors exhibit uncontrolled growth.
    C. Generally, only malignant tumors are capable of local tissue destruction.
    D. Generally, only benign tumors are capable of metastasis.
4. Which statement about the behavior of and prognosis for certain cancer types is true?
    A. The incidence and behavior of a cancer type in dogs is generally equivalent to that type in cats.
    B. More than 100 histologic types of cancer exist, and each may require special treatment and carry a different prognosis.
    C. High-grade tumors are less aggressive and slower growing than low-grade tumors.
    D. The suffix *carcinoma* or *sarcoma* indicates a benign tumor.
5. _____ and _____ have been indicated in the transformation of healthy cells into cancer cells.
    A. Inherited genetic defects; hormones
    B. Viruses; diet
    C. Trauma; immune-system dysfunction
    D. All of the above
6. The best approach to a canine or feline patient with a suspected tumor is to:
    A. Advise the owner to "just watch it."
    B. Have the owner carefully record the pet's appetite, urination, defecation, and activity levels daily for 3 months; then have them come in for a recheck appointment.
    C. Immediately obtain a complete history from the owner and physical examination of and minimum database for the patient.
    D. Surgically remove the tumor as soon as it becomes large enough to be palpated (felt).
7. Geriatric patients diagnosed with cancer are best *not* treated too aggressively due to the possibility of severe side effects with treatment and the poorer prognosis in older patients.
    A. True
    B. False
8. The best site from which to obtain blood samples on suspected or confirmed cancer patients is the:
    A. Lateral saphenous vein
    B. Cephalic vein
    C. Jugular vein
    D. Bone marrow
9. Which views should you take if asked to radiograph the chest of a newly diagnosed or suspected cancer patient?
    A. Right lateral and left lateral
    B. Dorsoventral and ventrodorsal
    C. Right lateral, dorsoventral, and ventrodorsal
    D. Right lateral, left lateral, and ventrodorsal (or dorsoventral)

10. Concerning the use of cytology in the diagnosis of cancer, which statement is true?
    A. Cytology is the study of individual cell morphology for the purpose of obtaining a clinical diagnosis.
    B. Incorrect sample collection and preparation can lead to inaccurate results.
    C. Cytologic analysis is not always necessary because some tumors can be diagnosed on the basis of their gross (visible to the naked eye) appearance.
    D. A and B
11. In addition to writing the animal's name and patient identification number on the frosted edge of a slide for cytologic evaluation, always write the _____ on the slide, and always label using _____.
    A. Specific location from which the sample was obtained; a lead pencil
    B. Specific location from which the sample was obtained; indelible (permanent) ink
    C. Owner's last name; a lead pencil
    D. Owner's last name; indelible ink
12. A definitive (absolutely accurate) diagnosis of the cancer type is generally obtained by:
    A. Abdominal ultrasound
    B. Cytologic evaluation of the mass
    C. Radiologic evaluation
    D. Histopathologic evaluation of the mass
13. _____ is the microscopic examination of cells smeared on a slide, whereas _____ is the microscopic examination of whole-tissue samples.
    A. A fine needle aspiration; a biopsy
    B. Cytology; histopathology
    C. An impression smear; cytology
    D. A biopsy; an impression smear
14. Impression smears of core needle biopsies are best made by:
    A. Placing the entire sample in formalin overnight, removing a small piece the next morning, and gently "dabbing" the piece several times on a clean glass slide
    B. Rolling the sample across a clean glass slide before placing it in formalin
    C. Macerating (mincing) a small piece of the sample, placing it on a clean glass slide, and smearing the preparation with a second clean slide
    D. A referral laboratory due to the complicated nature of the procedure
15. For proper fixation, biopsy specimens should be no thicker than _____, and the fixative-to-tissue ratio should be at least _____.
    A. 1 mm; 11
    B. 1 cm; 101
    C. 5 cm; 11
    D. 10 cm; 101
16. When preparing for the surgical resection of a cancerous tumor, it is especially important to:
    A. Shave and clip the skin.
    B. Perform an additional surgical scrub.
    C. Clip an extra-wide area around the surgical site.
    D. Schedule the surgery for late in the day.
17. Chemotherapy is:
    A. The treatment of cancer with chemical agents
    B. The treatment of cancer with radiation
    C. The term applied to any form of cancer treatment
    D. The treatment of cancer with cryosurgery
18. The basic mechanism responsible for many of the toxicities often associated with chemotherapy, such as nausea, vomiting, diarrhea, and hair loss are due to:
    A. The teratogenicity of these modalities
    B. Cytotoxicity to cells with a high turnover rate
    C. The severe stress placed on the patient's body by the treatment
    D. The mutagenicity of these treatment modalities
19. It is the nadir of leukopenia (lowest white blood cell count) that most often determines the highest dose of a cancer drug that a patient will tolerate.
    A. True
    B. False
20. Some side effects associated with radiotherapy can develop months to years after treatment and usually involve permanent changes such as necrosis or fibrosis of normal tissues.
    A. True
    B. False
21. A feline patient recently treated with radiotherapy for squamous cell carcinoma on her ears is cleaning and rubbing her ears with her paws. The best thing to do until the veterinarian can be consulted is:
    A. Apply an Elizabethan collar.
    B. Clean the treated areas of the ears appropriately.
    C. Administer analgesics as needed.
    D. All of the above
22. In pet cancer management, euthanasia should only be recommended after all available methods of treatment have failed.
    A. True
    B. False
23. The spreading of cancer cells from a primary tumor to a secondary location is called:
    A. Paraneoplastic syndrome
    B. Carcinogenesis
    C. Extravasation
    D. Metastasis
24. A chondrosarcoma is:
    A. A sarcoma originating from cartilage that is benign
    B. A sarcoma originating from cartilage that is malignant
    C. A sarcoma originating from epithelial tissue that is benign

D. A sarcoma originating from a bone that is malignant
25. Which statement is true?
    A. The personnel administering and restraining the animal being treated with chemotherapy drugs must wear appropriate gloves, gowns, and face shields.
    B. The use of Luer-lock syringes can increase the chance of inadvertent cutaneous exposure during drug infusion.
    C. Chemotherapy drugs reach their highest levels in excreted urine and feces approximately 5 days after administration.
    D. Surgical masks must be worn while reconstituting of chemotherapeutic agents.
26. List five potential early warning signs of cancer.
27. Describe the proper way to prepare a large (greater than 20-cm diameter) biopsy specimen prior to placing it in formalin. Three specific points must be mentioned for full credit; do *not* include comments about the formalin-to-tissue ratio.
28. An owner calls 10 days after her dog's last dose of a cancer-treatment drug to say the patient is not eating well and has diarrhea. What two critical pieces of information should you obtain from this client or from the patient's record for the veterinarian treating the patient?

CHAPTER 11

PREVENTIVE HEALTH PROGRAMS

For the next four questions, match the canine vaccine with its description.
    A. Canine distemper vaccine
    B. Canine parvovirus type 2 vaccine
    C. *Giardia* vaccine
    D. Canine leptospirosis vaccine

1. This protects against a serious, often fatal disease affecting dogs of any age that results in severe bloody diarrhea, vomiting, dehydration, fever, and a low white blood cell count. Doberman pinschers, Rottweilers, and Labrador retrievers are at higher risk for serious infection than many breeds, so they often receive an extra booster.
2. Traditionally, two serovars (*canicola* and *icterohaemorrhagiae*), which cause hepatic and renal disease, were included in this vaccine. However, new species (*grippotyphosa, pomona,* and *hardjo*) are emerging as disease-causing agents in the dog, and it is important that these serovars be included in this vaccine.
3. This vaccine, which protects against a disease characterized by recurrent diarrhea, is most effective when dogs are continuously exposed to water contaminated with the organism.
4. This vaccine can be used with a measles vaccine to increase the chance of protecting 6- to 12-week-old puppies from the respiratory, gastrointestinal, and neurologic effects of this usually fatal and extremely contagious disease.
5. Concerning rabies, which statement is most accurate?
    A. Rabies virus is transmitted by casual contact between affected and unaffected animals.
    B. The disease is characterized by altered behavior, possible aggression, progressive paralysis, and, in most species, death.
    C. Rabies commonly affects the dog, cat, skunk, raccoon, and bat, among other small carnivorous animals.
    D. B and C
6. All puppies and kittens should be vaccinated for rabies at the age of _____ and again _____ later.
    A. 12 weeks; 3 to 4 weeks
    B. 16 weeks; 3 to 4 weeks
    C. 12 weeks; 1 year
    D. 16 weeks; 1 year
7. Infectious tracheobronchitis (kennel cough) is an extremely contagious disease of dogs caused by:
    A. *Bordetella bronchiseptica*
    B. Canine adenovirus type 1
    C. A parainfluenza virus
    D. A and/or C
8. A 2-year-old Cairn terrier who has never received a kennel cough vaccination is coming in on December 21 to be boarded for 14 days. It is now November 1. When do you recommend she be immunized intranasally against kennel cough?
    A. As soon as possible but no later than November 7
    B. As soon as possible but no later than November 21
    C. As soon as possible but no later than December 10
    D. Upon admission on December 21
9. A dog exposed to _____ is a good candidate for the Lyme borreliosis vaccine.
    A. Mosquitoes
    B. Fleas
    C. Ticks
    D. Biting flies
10. Which feline disease is considered the "canine parvovirus infection" of cats?
    A. Feline infectious peritonitis
    B. Feline panleukopenia
    C. Feline chlamydiosis
    D. Feline leukemia virus

11. The feline FVRC-P vaccine can be boosted yearly or every 3 years.
    A. True
    B. False
12. For which feline disease does vaccination generally reduce clinical signs or shorten the course but not always completely prevent the disease?
    A. Feline leukemia
    B. Feline upper respiratory disease
    C. Feline panleukopenia
    D. Rabies
13. Concerning vaccination for the feline retroviruses feline leukemia (FeLV) and feline immunodeficiency syndrome (FIV), which statement is true?
    A. The FeLV and FIV vaccines should be administered to healthy kittens, two doses 3 to 4 weeks apart and then annually.
    B. The FeLV vaccine will interfere with FeLV testing in kittens or cats, sometimes causing false positive results.
    C. No vaccine is yet available for FIV.
    D. The FeLV and FIV vaccines should only be administered to indoor-only cats.
14. Feline *Bordetella bronchiseptica* is a primary respiratory pathogen in cats of all ages and breeds.
    A. True
    B. False
15. Both puppies and kittens can be started on heartworm-preventive therapy at the age of 6 to 8 weeks.
    A. True
    B. False

For the next five questions, match the horse vaccine with its description.
    A. Tetanus vaccine
    B. Equine encephalomyelitis vaccine
    C. Equine rhinopneumonitis vaccine
    D. Equine influenza vaccine
    E. Botulism vaccine
    F. Strangles vaccine

16. This vaccine protects against a viral neurologic disease transmitted by biting insects. A trivalent vaccine is commonly used for horses in states bordering Mexico to create a buffer zone that may prevent the spread of the Venezuelan strain into the United States. In areas where winter freezes are uncommon, semiannual vaccination may be advisable.
17. The most common application of this vaccine is vaccination of mares 30 days before foaling to prevent shaker foal syndrome in areas of high incidence.
18. The toxoid version of this vaccine is given to immunize horses against a disease characterized by muscle rigidity and spasms that may result in respiratory arrest and convulsions. Administration of antitoxin to unvaccinated horses induces immediate protection that lasts approximately 2 weeks.
19. The duration of protective immunity from this vaccine is short-lived, requiring vaccination every 2 to 3 months during periods of exposure. Disease outbreaks usually occur in horses 1 to 3 years of age after mixing with infected horses at the racetrack or show grounds. Infection is characterized by fever, depression, anorexia, muscle soreness, and coughing.
20. Pregnant mares should be vaccinated with this vaccine in the fifth, seventh, and ninth months of gestation to prevent a viral disease whose strains can cause upper respiratory disease, abortions, stillbirths, and weak neonatal foals that fail to survive.
21. Which disease is extremely contagious through direct contact or fomites, is caused by *Streptococcus equi*, and causes abscesses in the submaxillary, retropharyngeal, and submandibular lymph nodes?
    A. Equine viral arteritis
    B. Potomac horse fever
    C. Anthrax
    D. Strangles
22. Horses and cattle need *not* be vaccinated for rabies.
    A. True
    B. False
23. In general, pastured horses should be dewormed every _____ and have their feet trimmed every _____.
    A. 60 days; 6 weeks
    B. 30 days; 12 weeks
    C. 60 days; 12 weeks
    D. 30 days; 6 weeks
24. Venereal diseases of cattle that cause various manifestations of abortion, and for which vaccination is a basic requirement for all breeding stock, include
    A. Campylobacteriosis (vibriosis), leptospirosis, and brucellosis
    B. Leptospirosis, anaplasmosis, and *Haemophilus somnus* infection
    C. Brucellosis, *Moraxella bovis* infection, and pasteurellosis
    D. Trichomoniasis, campylobacteriosis, and *Moraxella bovis* infection
25. Accidental injection, ingestion, or exposure through broken skin or mucous membranes of the vaccine for _____ can cause serious human disease.
    A. Anaplasmosis
    B. Brucellosis
    C. Bovine respiratory disease complex
    D. Campylobacteriosis
26. Clostridial bacteria can cause which disease?
    A. Multiplication of the organisms in damaged liver tissue, subsequent release of potent toxins, and rapid death
    B. Multiplication of the organisms in bruised (anaerobic) muscles, subsequent release of potent toxins, and rapid death ("black leg" and "malignant edema")

C. Hemorrhagic, necrotic enteritis, and sudden death in young animals after overeating concentrated feed (grain)
D. All of the above

27. Which agents can cause respiratory disease in cattle?
A. *Haemophilus somnus* and *Pasteurella haemolytica*
B. Infectious bovine rhinotracheitis (IBR) and bovine viral diarrhea (BVD) viruses
C. Bovine respiratory syncytial virus (BRSV) and *Pasteurella multocida*
D. All of the above

28. Parainfluenza-3 virus causes a mild respiratory disease in cattle often associated with shipment to a feedlot and commonly called:
A. The coughs
B. Sore lung
C. Snuffles
D. Shipping fever

29. Concerning the IBR vaccine in cattle, which statement is most accurate?
A. Intramuscular, attenuated (modified live virus) IBR vaccines should never be administered to pregnant cows or to calves nursing on pregnant cows.
B. Both the intramuscular and intranasal attenuated IBR vaccines can cause abortion when administered to pregnant cows or calves nursing on pregnant cows.
C. Intranasal attenuated IBR vaccines are safe for pregnant cows and calves nursing on pregnant cows.
D. A and C

30. Oral bovine rotavirus, coronavirus, and *Escherichia coli* vaccines are administered to newborn calves on farms where there is a problem with:
A. Calf respiratory disease
B. Calf diarrhea
C. Calf conjunctivitis
D. Calf infectious hepatitis

31. The principal cause of infectious bovine keratoconjunctivitis (inflamed cornea and conjunctiva) is:
A. Bovine rotavirus
B. IBR
C. *Moraxella bovis*
D. BRSV

32. Which cattle breed may be sensitive to insecticidal products for external parasites?
A. Brahman, Brahman cross, and exotic breeds
B. Hereford
C. Aberdeen Angus
D. Holstein

33. If a calf does *not* nurse on its own shortly after birth, the most important thing the herdsman can do to ensure its survival is:

A. Call the veterinarian out to the farm to administer hyperimmune serum intravenously.
B. Administer at least 2 L of warm, high-quality colostrum to the calf within the first hour of life.
C. Manually support the calf in a standing position for 30 minutes of every hour for the first 6 hours.
D. Administer penicillin intramuscularly within the first 3 hours.

34. A good rule of thumb to follow when feeding calves manually is:
A. Feed for a weight gain of 5 kg per day.
B. Feed for a weight gain of 10 kg per week.
C. Feed 10% of the body weight twice daily.
D. Feed 10% of the body weight daily divided into two feedings (i.e., 5% twice daily).

35. Farrowing is:
A. Another term for *weaning* in pigs
B. Placing groups of pigs in pens according to their age
C. Removing a pig from the herd for slaughter
D. The term applied to a sow giving birth

36. A lactating sow nursing 10 pigs should receive at least _____ lb of feed daily.
A. 5
B. 10
C. 15
D. 20

37. *Bordetella bronchiseptica* is considered the major cause of _____ in swine.
A. Hepatitis
B. Atrophic rhinitis
C. Infectious tracheobronchitis
D. Porcine reproductive and respiratory syndrome

For the next five questions, match the swine vaccine with its description.
A. *Streptococcus suis* vaccine
B. *Erysipelothrix rhusiopathiae* vaccine
C. Transmissible gastroenteritis vaccine
D. Porcine parvovirus vaccine
E. Pseudorabies vaccine

38. This vaccine immunizes swine against a primary bacterial cause of meningitis (inflamed meninges) and septicemia (bacterial toxins in the blood) in postweaning pigs that can pose a significant human health hazard.

39. This vaccine immunizes against a viral disease that can cause fever, vomiting, encephalitis, and sudden death in nursing pigs and abortion, stillbirths, or fetal mummies in pregnant sows. Vaccines are available, but their use is limited by state regulations.

40. This vaccine protects against an extremely common disease known as *diamond skin disease* that causes acute septicemia, skin discoloration, arthritis, and heart-valve disease. Routine vaccination of gilts and sows before parturition and of pigs at weaning is highly recommended.

41. This vaccine protects against a common viral disease causing profuse and watery diarrhea, vomiting, and anorexia that can lead to death in pigs younger than 10 days old.
42. Prebreeding vaccination is recommended of swine herds experiencing infection with this virus that is the leading cause of infectious reproductive failure.
43. Pigs are generally weaned at _____ of age.
    A. 4 to 5 weeks
    B. 6 to 8 weeks
    C. 8 to 10 weeks
    D. 12 to 14 weeks
44. In general, vaccination of pregnant animals is intended to help prevent disease in their young.
    A. True
    B. False
45. Due to the limited number of vaccines licensed for use in small ruminants, products licensed for use in other species (particularly cattle) are sometimes used.
    A. True
    B. False
46. The use of vaccines depends upon the disease incidence within a given goat herd or sheep flock, but vaccination for _____ and _____ should be included in every small-ruminant health program.
    A. Bluetongue; foot rot
    B. Contagious ecthyma; tetanus
    C. Enterotoxemia (*Clostridium perfringens* types C and D); tetanus
    D. Chlamydiosis; vibriosis
47. When a sheep rancher speaks of *overeating disease*, she is referring to a condition caused by:
    A. *Campylobacter jejuni*.
    B. *Clostridium perfringens* types C and D.
    C. *Chlamydia psittaci*.
    D. *Clostridium tetani*.
48. What precaution must be taken when dealing with goat and sheep herds affected with contagious ecthyma (also called *sore mouth* or *orf*)?
    A. Wear gloves when handling affected animals.
    B. Wear gloves when administering the vaccine.
    C. Dispose of the vaccine vials in biohazard-approved containers.
    D. All of the above.
49. In general, due to the risks to developing fetuses, the vaccination of pregnant females must be undertaken with caution and only with full knowledge of the indications and contraindications of the specific vaccine.
    A. True
    B. False
50. Concerning general nutritional guidelines for the various species, which statement is most accurate?
    A. A horse's diet should contain mostly high-quality grain with just enough hay supplemented to maintain a good body weight.
    B. Pregnant sows are fed enough food to maintain their body weight at 25% above normal due to the significant unavoidable weight loss during lactation.
    C. Feeding horse or cattle feeds to small ruminants may result in zinc deficiency because the zinc levels in those feeds are much lower than required by sheep and goats.
    D. The body weight of a growing puppy fed a high-quality puppy food steadily increasing at each office visit is an indication that the puppy is receiving adequate nutrition.
51. Because clostridial infections commonly occur in cattle, routine vaccination for them is highly recommended.
    A. True
    B. False
52. Which of the following statements is *false* regarding early spay-neuter programs for puppies and kittens?
    A. Increased operative time
    B. More rapid recovery from anesthesia
    C. Pets seem to be gentler, calmer, and less likely to wander.
    D. Visibility of intraabdominal structures is improved.
53. Short, repeated groups of base pairs of DNA that can be used to track defective genes in the canine genome are called:
    A. Chromosomes
    B. Markers
    C. B and D
    D. Microsatellites
54. To ensure a reduction in the frequency of a targeted disease gene, it is best to breed:
    A. Affected dog to affected dog
    B. Clear dog to clear dog
    C. Carrier dog to clear dog
    D. Clear dog to affected dog
55. Protection against the west nile virus in previously unvaccinated horses is afforded by vaccinating with
    A. 3 doses, 2 weeks apart
    B. 2 doses, 3 weeks apart
    C. 2 doses, 4 weeks apart
    D. 2 doses, 2 weeks apart
56. Pet pigs should be vaccinated against leptospirosis and erysipelas annually.
    A. True
    B. False
57. Most pet pigs weigh approximately _____ lb when fully grown.
    A. 40 to 50
    B. 50 to 70
    C. 70 to 80
    D. 120
58. What do the letters in the canine DA$_2$PL-PC vaccine represent?

59. What do the letters in the feline FVRC-P vaccine represent?
60. Name two reasons why proper manure disposal is important to livestock health.
61. Name five procedures commonly performed with newborn pigs (not including vaccination).
62. Name three modalities that, when used in strategic combination, are effective in the control of foot rot in sheep and goats.

EXTRA CREDIT

63. In the horse, *floating* teeth refers to
    A. A routine dental cleaning and polishing with the horse under anesthesia
    B. Rasping down sharp points on the teeth, created by uneven wear, with a large file
    C. Filling and emptying the mouth repeatedly with warm water prior to a dental cleaning
    D. A bunch of extracted teeth in a bucket of water
64. "Red nose" is
    A. Severe hyperemia of the muzzle of a cow with IBR
    B. Severe hyperemia of the nasal planum of a cat with panleukopenia
    C. Hemorrhage from the nares (nostrils) of a hog with erysipelas
    D. A certain reindeer's nickname

CHAPTER 12

NEONATAL CARE OF PUPPY, KITTEN, AND FOAL

1. Puppy and kitten eyes normally open _____ after birth.
   A. Within 12 hours
   B. 12 to 24 hours
   C. 1 to 5 days
   D. 5 to 14 days
2. A litter of Boston terrier puppies is brought in at 2 weeks of age for their initial veterinary evaluation with the umbilical cords still attached.
   A. This is abnormal; the cords should have fallen off at 2 to 3 days of age.
   B. This is abnormal; the cords should have fallen off at 7 to 10 days of age.
   C. This is expected; the cords normally fall off at about 14 days of age.
   D. This is expected; the cords normally fall off at about 20 days of age.
3. For certain diagnostic procedures, ultrasonography is tolerated better by puppies and kittens and is safer for personnel than routine radiography.
   A. True
   B. False
4. Concerning radiography of young puppies and kittens, which statement is most accurate?
   A. Kilovoltage must be greatly reduced for radiography of a young puppy or kitten because of the minimal absorption of x-rays by partially mineralized bones and because of the thinness of soft tissue body parts.
   B. A general guideline for reducing kilovoltage is to reduce the radiographic exposure to about one half of that used for adults dogs and cats of the same thickness.
   C. Radiographic techniques and machine settings are generally equivalent to those used in adult animals.
   D. A and B
5. The most accurate way to evaluate a puppy with suspected congenital deafness or blindness is:
   A. By evaluating the animal's gross response to auditory or visual stimuli in the examination room
   B. With sophisticated electrical and computer equipment
   C. By owner evaluation of the puppy's responses to auditory or visual stimuli at home in comparison to those of his littermates
   D. By veterinary otoscopic or ophthalmoscopic evaluation
6. Puppies and kittens are usually mature enough to be sold at 4 to 6 weeks of age.
   A. True
   B. False
7. When mother's milk is unavailable (as with orphans), puppies are best fed:
   A. Cow's milk
   B. Goat's milk
   C. A commercial milk-replacement formula
   D. A home-prepared milk-replacement formula
8. Feed orphaned puppies and kittens to provide a weight gain of _____ g/day/kg of anticipated adult body weight and _____ g weekly, respectively.
   A. 1 to 2; 10 to 25
   B. 1 to 2; 25 to 50
   C. 2 to 4; 25 to 50
   D. 2 to 4; 50 to 100
9. When measuring and marking an infant feeding tube for use in kittens, the correct length is:
   A. From the tip of the nose to the thoracic inlet
   B. From the caudal jaw to the fourth rib
   C. From the tip of the nose to the last rib
   D. From the caudal jaw to the point of the hip (tuber coxae)
10. Start offering food to neonatal puppies or kittens when they are _____ or _____ weeks of age, respectively, and initially feed at least _____ times daily.
    A. 3; 4; 2
    B. 3; 4; 3

C. 5; 6; 2
   D. 5; 6; 3
11. One indication that a nursing puppy is receiving insufficient or inadequate milk is:
   A. Inactivity
   B. High-pitched, constant crying
   C. A weak suckling reflex
   D. All of the above
12. If diarrhea occurs in a kitten during the feeding of adequate amounts of commercial milk-replacement formula:
   A. Feed another brand of milk substitute.
   B. Dilute the formula with a mixture of equal parts Ringer solution and 5% dextrose in water.
   C. Reduce by 50% the amount of formula fed at each feeding until the diarrhea resolves.
   D. Feed a homemade formula.
13. Concerning the nursing care of severely ill neonatal puppies, which statement is most accurate?
   A. Before feeding, the neonate should be slowly rewarmed with a circulating hot-water blanket or hot-water bottle to a preferred rectal temperature of 37.7° C (100° F).
   B. Dehydration is best corrected subcutaneously with an appropriate parenteral fluid.
   C. Assessment of activity level is helpful for very early recognition of overhydration.
   D. The neonate is adequately hydrated when the urine is clear and light yellow.
14. A "high-risk" foal is best defined as:
   A. A critically ill foal younger than 3 days old
   B. A foal out of a mare whose previous foal(s) became critically ill
   C. A foal not necessarily ill but at high risk of becoming ill
   D. A foal that did not nurse in the first 6 hours of life
15. Sick foals generally appear normal for the first 24 hours of life and then quickly decompensate.
   A. True
   B. False
16. Which sign in a foal should alert the technician to the possibility of immaturity with accompanying skeletal fragility?
   A. Soft, silky hair coat
   B. Cloudy corneas
   C. White-to-yellow hooves
   D. Lethargy
17. The normal foal should nurse within _____ hours of birth.
   A. 0 to 1
   B. 2 to 3
   C. 4 to 5
   D. 6 to 7
18. The normal heart rate of a resting foal is:
   A. 50 to 60 beats per minute (bpm)
   B. 90 to 100 bpm
   C. 150 to 160 bpm
   D. 190 to 200 bpm
19. A neonatal foal's lung sounds are normally very quiet, making evaluation difficult.
   A. True
   B. False

For the next five questions, identify the finding as normal or abnormal in the 0- to 3-day-old foal.
   A. Normal
   B. Abnormal
20. A grade II to VI machinery or holosystolic heart murmur
21. Harsh lung sounds
22. Diarrhea
23. Frequent passage of dilute urine
24. A rectal temperature of 36.1° C (97° F).
25. Why is the cephalic vein the best vessel from which to draw blood for initial hematologic evaluation of the sick neonatal foal?
   A. It is the largest vein.
   B. It saves the jugular vein for intravenous catheter use.
   C. It is least likely to be contaminated with feces.
   D. It is the easiest location to place a post-draw bandage.
26. A recumbent foal should be placed in what position during and for 30 minutes after nasogastric tube feeding?
   A. Right lateral recumbency
   B. Left lateral recumbency
   C. Sternal recumbency
   D. Dorsal recumbency
27. In addition to tender loving care, the most important aspect of neonatal foal care is:
   A. Speed while treating
   B. Cleanliness
   C. Exact timing of treatments
   D. Avoiding overfeeding
28. Concerning parenteral fluid administration to critically ill neonatal foals, which statement is most accurate?
   A. Intramuscular injections should only be placed in the neck or gluteal region.
   B. Teflon intravenous catheters should be removed and new ones placed in an alternative vein every 24 hours.
   C. Intravenous catheters should be flushed with heparinized saline every 8 hours.
   D. Once disconnected, fluid lines are contaminated and should be replaced.
29. In general, one must feed significantly more than the label directions of commercial milk replacement formula to foals.
   A. True
   B. False

30. What special action should people raising orphan, neonatal puppies and kittens take to encourage normal urination and defecation? Until what age should this be done?
31. Briefly comment on the care of puppies and kittens during the first month of life regarding heat source, bedding, container, and at what rectal temperature the young should be maintained.
32. How is intravenous catheter care unique in the critically ill foal? Briefly describe the care of the equine umbilicus at birth.

EXTRA CREDIT

33. "Retrograde" is:
    A. Injecting contrast material to radiographically evaluate the urogenital system
    B. A type of ultrasonography used to detect septal wall heart defects
    C. Flowing backward or in a direction opposite to a substance's normal flow
    D. A poodle cut popular in the 1950s and 1960s
34. BAER is:
    A. An acronym for brain stem auditory-evoked response
    B. An acronym for bridging and enveloping chemical response
    C. An acronym for Billow's auditory and electrical receptor
    D. A large, brown animal that loves honey

CHAPTER 13

GERIATRIC MEDICINE IN COMPANION ANIMALS

1. Which of the following statements is *false*?
    A. Mature and giant breed dogs spend less time as young and mature adults.
    B. Care for older dogs and cats must focus on owner education and disease prevention strategies.
    C. The senior lifestyle for the average cat begins at approximately 12 years of age.
    D. Size and genetics of a dog or cat impact the onset of the animal's health decline.
2. The geriatric healthcare program should include bereavement counseling, specific disease prevention and treatment, and respite care.
    A. True
    B. False
3. Which of the following are common effects of aging?
    A. Urinary incontinence
    B. Development of dental calculus and tooth loss
    C. Decreased immune competence
    D. All of the above
4. Organ enlargement is generally an indication of inflammation, infiltrative disease, or _____.
    A. Cancer
    B. Intoxication
    C. Old age
    D. Hypoproteinemia
5. It is important to auscultate the senior animal's thorax in a quiet room to be able to detect:
    A. Heart murmurs
    B. Kidney disease
    C. Abnormal lung sounds
    D. A and C
6. Whereas ataxia is a clinical sign of a _____ problem, lameness is a clinical sign of a _____ disease.
    A. Neurologic; circulatory
    B. Neurologic; musculoskeletal
    C. Musculoskeletal; neurologic
    D. Traumatic; neurologic
7. The evaluation of joints should be performed with the animal in _____ recumbency.
    A. Lateral
    B. Ventrodorsal
    C. Dorsoventral
    D. Sternal
8. Laboratory data, including blood and urine screening tests, should be obtained for seemingly healthy geriatric animals.
    A. True
    B. False
9. Common parasites in older dogs and cats include
    A. Hookworms, fleas, and roundworms
    B. Hookworms, ticks, and malassezia pachydermatis
    C. Fleas, giardia spp., and lungworm
    D. Fleas, ticks, ear mites, and tapeworms
10. Which of the following statements are true regarding the geriatric exam?
    A. The discharge consultation after a geriatric exam should be performed without the pet present.
    B. Visual aids and written form should be used to make specific recommendations to the owner.
    C. Geriatric patients should be scheduled during less busy periods of the day.
    D. All of the above.
11. Home care for pets with untreatable disease
    A. Minimizes the quality of the pet's life.
    B. Makes the family helpless to stop procedures and practices that none of them desire.
    C. Provides respite care for primary caregivers
    D. A and B
12. Comprehensive care for geriatric pets and pets with terminal disease consists of physical, _____, and spiritual care.
    A. Emotional
    B. Psychosocial
    C. Financial

13. The first person with whom owners have control is usually the _____, so it is important that this person understands the geriatric healthcare program.
    A. Receptionist
    B. Veterinary technician
    C. Veterinarian
    D. Kennel worker
14. Name 10 commonly encountered geriatric diseases in the dog. (See Box 13-3.)
15. Name 10 commonly encountered geriatric diseases in the cat. (See Box 13-3.)

EXTRA CREDIT

16. Crepitus:
    A. Can be diagnosed on radiographs
    B. May be noted when moving a joint through a range of motion
    C. Is a degenerative disease
    D. Usually manifests as lameness

CHAPTER 14

ANIMAL BEHAVIOR

1. Components of a behavior wellness program include:
    A. Discouraging socialization of young animals
    B. Allowing owners to select a pet without providing information for them
    C. A and B
    D. Providing timely referrals when needed
2. Technicians can provide help for owners of pets with behavioral problems by:
    A. Improving their knowledge of species-specific communication signals and body postures
    B. Giving up-to-date, scientifically accurate information to owners
    C. Building their own education in behavior basics
    D. All of the above
3. By initiating questions/discussions about a pet's behavior with the owners, the technician is practicing a _____ approach.
    A. Reactive
    B. Proactive
    C. Scientific
    D. Realistic
4. Criteria for behaviorally healthy cats and dogs include adapting to _____ with minimal problems; readily relinquishing control of _____, food, toys, and other objects; _____ only in acceptable places.
    A. Change, space, elimination
    B. Space, change, elimination
    C. Change, elimination, space
    D. Change, space, elimination
5. Accusing a pet of being vindictive, spiteful, jealous, or rebellious is considered a(n) _____ explanation for unrealistic expectations.
    A. Exaggerated
    B. Alternative
    C. Anthropomorphic
    D. Self-fulfilling
6. The process by which an animal develops appropriate social behaviors toward members of its own and other species is called:
    A. Sensitization
    B. Socialization
    C. Integration
    D. Anthropomorphism
7. The appropriate time to begin socialization in horses is approximately 4 to 12 weeks of age.
    A. True
    B. False
8. Owners should use negative punishment when:
    A. Their puppy is sleeping quietly.
    B. Their kitten is resting on a chair.
    C. The foal nuzzles rather than nips at its owner's hand.
    D. Their dog will not release the toy for the owner to throw.
9. To prevent/minimize inappropriate behavior from a pet, the owners must:
    A. Play with the kitten's paws rather than its toys.
    B. Use crate training with the puppy.
    C. Allow the puppy to pull on the leash while walking as long as the leash is used.
    D. Allow the puppy or kitten to make as many mistakes as possible while they are still young.
10. Appropriate crate training includes:
    A. Increasing the length of time the dog is in the crate so that it can eventually spend most of its time there
    B. Strapping the crate to a stationary object if it is in a different location when the owner gets home from work
    C. Switching to a smaller crate if the dog soils in it
    D. Acclimating the dog very slowly to the crate
11. Positive and negative punishment refer to adding something and taking something away, in learning theory terminology.
    A. True
    B. False
12. Delivering punishment within a few minutes after the behavior refers to _____ of punishment.
    A. Immediacy
    B. Consistency
    C. Appropriateness
    D. Remoteness

13. Which of the following represents an example of appropriate remote training?
    A. Motion detectors
    B. Having neighbors come over and punish the pet while you are at work
    C. Handheld noisemakers
    D. A and C
14. Which of the following is *not* an early warning sign of potential problems that can lead to relinquishment of the pet?
    A. A cat that urinates next to the box
    B. A dog that leaves the room to avoid an infant who has been placed on the floor
    C. The dog that lies still and quiet while its nails are being clipped
    D. The dog that growls when told to move off of furniture
15. When technicians observe dangerous or threatening behavior from a pet at the clinic:
    A. The front of the pet's file should be marked with a hard to miss symbol.
    B. The veterinarian should be informed.
    C. The owners should be informed.
    D. All of the above.
16. While interviewing clients about their pet's behavior, asking open-ended questions is discouraged because this does not lead to informative answers.
    A. True
    B. False
17. The following interviewing skills are strongly encouraged:
    A. Conducting a behavior interview sitting down
    B. Standing or sitting behind a desk or counter while you ask questions
    C. Keeping arms and legs crossed
    D. B and C
18. An animal that growls or hisses, bares teeth, air-snaps, and/or lunges is exhibiting _____ behavior.
    A. Dominant
    B. Threatening
    C. Submissive
    D. Aggressive
19. During a(n) _____ visit, a pet might be placed on a scale, given a tidbit, and subjected to brief handling procedures in order to make its next visit a more pleasant experience.
    A. Socialization
    B. Geriatric assessment
    C. After hours
    D. Vaccination
20. What can be done in the waiting area to help establish a more positive experience for the pet and owner?
    A. Arrange chairs to create more space between patients and minimize face-to-face encounters.
    B. Move overly excited pets out of the waiting area as quickly as possible.
    C. Cover see-through cat carriers immediately so that the cat feels safer.
    D. All of the above.
21. Most cats prefer to be petted:
    A. On the head
    B. On their scent glands located on their cheeks and in front of their ears
    C. On the belly
    D. On the back
22. Reinforcement or punishment of emotionally induced behavior is referred to as _____ conditioning.
    A. Positive
    B. Negative
    C. Operant
    D. Counter
23. The appropriate response if a dog jumps up on you is to:
    A. Squeeze the animal's paws.
    B. Knee the dog's chest.
    C. Try to step on his/her paws.
    D. Turn away and move out of its reach.
24. The way to remove an unruly cat from a carrier is to:
    A. Tilt the carrier so that the cat slides out.
    B. Reach into the carrier and grab the cat.
    C. A and D
    D. Take the top off of the carrier.
25. The goals of animal restraint in the veterinary clinic include:
    A. Keeping personnel safe while performing necessary procedures
    B. Teaching the pet a lesson that it will remember at future visits
    C. Applying negative punishment
    D. None of the above

EXTRA CREDIT

26. Excessive barking, house soiling, and separation anxiety should be addressed in _____ classes, while pulling on the leash, not coming when called, and jumping up should be addressed in _____ classes.
    A. Behavior, obedience
    B. Socialization, obedience
    C. Behavior, socialization
    D. Obedience, behavior

CHAPTER 15

COMPANION ANIMAL CLINICAL NUTRITION

1. Which of the following statements is/are true?
    A. The goal of feeding food animals is to maximize the length of the animal's life.

B. The goal of feeding companion animals is to encourage rapid weight gain.
C. The goal of feeding food animals is to encourage rapid weight gain.
D. B and C

2. Which of the following statements is *false*?
   A. *Nutrients* can be defined as any substance which when ingested produce energy.
   B. Water, vitamins, and minerals cannot be broken down to produce energy.
   C. Proteins, fats, and carbohydrates are considered energy-producing nutrients.
   D. Animals that are exercising, reproducing, and growing have a higher requirement for energy or nutrition.

3. _____ fatty acids have no double bonds in the primary hydrocarbon chain.
   A. Monosaturated
   B. Polysaturated
   C. Long chain
   D. Saturated

4. Functions of fat include
   A. Provides fatty acids
   B. Facilitates digestion
   C. Provide palatability and texture to food
   D. All of the above

5. _____ are considered building blocks for plant and animal protein.
   A. Fatty acids
   B. Amino acids
   C. Arachidonic acids
   D. Complex carbohydrates

6. As protein quality is increased, the amount of protein needed decreases.
   A. True
   B. False

7. Regarding crude protein content on pet food labels, in order to measure the amino acid bioavailability and protein digestibility, one must:
   A. Contact the manufacturer directly.
   B. Look at the total nitrogen content.
   C. Assume that a higher crude protein content also means higher protein quality.
   D. Understand that food with low crude protein content must be supplemented with another protein source.

8. Macrominerals are:
   A. Supplied in adequate amounts in most commercial diets
   B. Harmful if consumed in excess
   C. Required by animals in relatively large amounts
   D. All of the above

For the following five statements, choose the correct response from the following choices.
   Iron
   Calcium
   Water-soluble vitamins
   Fat-soluble vitamins
   Vitamin E
   Phosphorus
   Vitamin K

9. These are depleted in the body faster because of limited storage capability, making toxicity less likely.
10. A deficiency of this can lead to clotting abnormalities and hemorrhage.
11. Excess of this in the diet may possibly lead to hip dysplasia, osteochondrosis, and wobbler syndrome.
12. A deficiency of this is not common among healthy animals fed standard commercial diets because of the high meat content.
13. Cats fed home-cooked diets rich in polyunsaturated fatty acids are at increased risk of developing yellow fat disease because of the deficiency of this in the diet.
14. The ratio of calcium to this in the body should be approximately 11.
15. Vitamins C and E are _____, respectively.
    A. Fat soluble and water soluble
    B. Fat soluble and antioxidants
    C. Water soluble and fat soluble
    D. Antioxidants and fat soluble
16. A diet adequate in dry foods and hard, baked treats can virtually eliminate the need for dental prophylaxis for most cats and dogs.
    A. True
    B. False
17. Feeding diabetic animals the following food is not recommended.
    A. Treats
    B. Semimoist food
    C. Dry food
    D. Dry food and treats
18. It is not necessary to feed _____ to a pet in addition to a balanced commercial pet food.
    A. Supplements
    B. Treats
    C. Microminerals
    D. Essential fatty acids
19. Pet food manufacturers are required by the FDA to include the following on labels:
    A. A statement that the diet is compete and balanced with respect to life stages of the animal
    B. Feeding instructions
    C. Name and address of the manufacturer or distributor
    D. Caloric content
20. Which of the following statements is/are true?
    A. Nutritional adequacy statements are required in the United States on treats or snacks intended for intermittent feeding.
    B. Heavier ingredients are listed last on pet food labels.

C. Generic and private label foods are made at contract feed mills using least-cost formulation methods.
D. In the United States, the maximum moisture content in pet food allowed is 78% as long as the words stew, gravy, and juice are not on the label and the food does not contain milk replacer.

21. A thorough nutritional assessment includes a patient's history, physical examination including body weight, body condition scoring, and _____ status.
    A. Hydration
    B. Musculoskeletal
    C. Neurologic
    D. Cardiovascular

22. It is recommended to avoid feeding dogs before exercise, particularly large and giant breed dogs, to minimize the possibility of _____.
    A. Ileus
    B. Increased energy requirements
    C. Vomiting
    D. Gastric dilatation volvulus

23. When raising puppies, the environment should be kept at _____ ° F.
    A. 95-98
    B. 84-90
    C. 80-85
    D. 99-102

24. Puppies (except for toy breeds and weak animals) should begin to eat gruel at approximately _____ weeks of age; peak lactation occurs at _____ weeks.
    A. 2, 5
    B. 3, 6
    C. 6, 8
    D. 3, 4

25. Overfeeding large and giant breed puppies can cause:
    A. Panosteitis
    B. Hip dysplasia
    C. Osteochondritis
    D. All of the above

26. Animals that undergo aerobic training should be fed _____ training to avoid the onset of _____.
    A. Before, hypothermia
    B. Before, hypoglycemia
    C. After, hypoglycemia
    D. After, gluconeogenesis

27. During lactation, _____ is/are the most important nutrient(s).
    A. Water
    B. Iron
    C. B vitamins
    D. Folic acid

28. Which of the following statements is/are true?
    A. Once formed, adipocytes are present for life.
    B. Several nutrients can slow down the process of aging.
    C. Some antioxidants can ameliorate disorientation and loss of bladder and bowel control.
    D. A and C.

29. Cats with renal insufficiency have elevated requirements for this nutrient.
    A. Protein
    B. Potassium
    C. Phosphorus
    D. Sodium chloride

30. Which of the following statements is *false*?
    A. Kittens are generally weaned at 7 to 9 weeks.
    B. Frequent administration of laxatives and/or lubricants to cats to control hairballs can interfere with nutrient absorption.
    C. Female kittens generally grow faster than male kittens.
    D. Consuming excessive amounts of liver can potentially cause hypervitaminosis A.

31. _____ is characterized by chronic weight loss despite a ravenous appetite; fasting obese cats is associated with _____ accumulation in the liver.
    A. Hepatic lipidosis, lipid
    B. Diabetes mellitus; glycogen
    C. Hyperthyroidism, lipid
    D. Hyperthyroidism, glycogen

32. Struvite crystals cannot form in the urine of cats if the urine pH is _____; however, it is not recommended to give urinary acidifiers to kittens because of the potential to form _____.
    A. <6.5; hyperthyroidism
    B. >7.5; struvite crystals
    C. <7.5; calcium oxalate crystals
    D. <6.5; bone demineralization

33. Which of the following statements is/are true?
    A. Undernourished pets are three times as likely as well-nourished pets to have major surgical complications.
    B. The enteral route of feeding is always preferred whenever possible.
    C. The brain, kidney, and red blood cells require glucose continuously for energy.
    D. All of the above.

34. While tube feeding a dog, the dog becomes restless and vomits. What should you do?
    A. Remove the tube and inform the veterinarian; the tube may have been placed inappropriately and serious complications may be occurring.
    B. Give the pet an antiemetic.
    C. Feed the animal per os instead.
    D. Try to tube feed the animal again, but only one half the amount.

35. The resting energy requirement of a 10 lb cat is approximately:
    A. 206 kcal
    B. 370 kcal

C. 2060 kcal
D. 206 cal

36. The illness energy requirement of a 50-lb dog that has suffered head trauma is approximately:
    A. 2200 kcal
    B. 800 kcal
    C. 500 kcal
    D. 1300 kcal

37. Parenteral nutrition may be offered through a central, _____, or peripheral catheter, but is typically offered through a central catheter to avoid _____ and infection.
    A. Intraperitoneal, phlebitis
    B. Intraosseous, phlebitis
    C. Intraperitoneal, overadministration
    D. Intraosseous, overadministration

38. A small portion of enteral feeding to prevent intestinal hypertrophy, intestinal mucosal deterioration, and to facilitate healing by promoting intestinal growth is encouraged, if possible, for the patient that is being fed parenterally.
    A. True
    B. False

39. Exocrine pancreatic insufficiency is typically treated by ____ dietary fiber, ____ dietary fat, and offering highly-digestible ____ such as rice (along with other dietary measures).
    A. Increasing, avoiding, proteins
    B. Restricting, avoiding, proteins
    C. Restricting, avoiding, carbohydrates
    D. Eliminating, increasing, carbohydrates

40. Which of the following statements is/are true?
    A. Birds are able to preferentially balance their diets by selecting certain foods.
    B. Fruits and vegetables dilute key nutrients present in nutritionally balanced commercially prepared foods.
    C. Birds often select food items based on water content, texture, color, or taste, resulting in imbalanced nutrient intake.
    D. B and C.

41. Seed mixtures easily provide the protein requirement of most pet birds.
    A. True
    B. False

42. Birds have no _____ and therefore water plays an important role in thermoregulation.
    A. Sweat glands
    B. Endocrine glands
    C. Exocrine glands
    D. Hypothalamus

For the following eight statements, choose the animal to which it refers.

43. Sunlight or ultraviolet light should be provided to allow cholecalciferol synthesis for shell formation and repair.

44. They preferentially eat sunflower seeds at the expense of other dietary ingredients, resulting in obesity and possible calcium deficiency.

45. They are unable to synthesize vitamin C and therefore require supplementation daily.

46. The typical diet may include rabbits, mice, rats, gerbils, chicken, and lizards.

47. The normal urine color varies from straw to reddish brown.

48. During the maintenance life stage, good quality grass or legume hay, calcium, phosphorus as needed, free-choice water, and trace-mineralized salt are the only foods needed.

49. Diets devoid of fiber can cause bloat, constipation, rectal prolapse, and diarrhea.

50. They are capable of copious sweating.

51. Which of the following statements is *false*?
    A. Despite reduced gastrointestinal motility of a horse after colic surgery, a diet rich in protein, calories, and micronutrients is still required.
    B. Molasses and other sweet feeds should be given sparingly to horses because of their high calcium content.
    C. Fence chewing in horses generally indicates the need for some long-stem or coarse chopped hay in the diet.
    D. Salt blocks are not useful for sick or depressed horses.

EXTRA CREDIT

52. An animal's energy requirement may decrease ____% after spaying and adjustments in diet may be necessary to avoid weight gain.
    A. 50
    B. 20
    C. 30
    D. 10

CHAPTER 16

CONCEPTS IN LIVESTOCK NUTRITION

1. Which ruminant disease can be directly related to nutritional causes?
   A. Bloat
   B. Milk fever
   C. Obturator nerve paralysis
   D. A and B

2. Fescue toxicosis is a nutritional disease that can involved lameness, tail-tip necrosis, abortion, and/or decreased milk production. What is fescue?
   A. A fungus
   B. A grass

C. A mineral
D. A vitamin
3. Amino acids are made up of carbon, oxygen, _____, and _____.
   A. Protein; nitrogen
   B. Phosphorus; potassium
   C. Calcium; phosphorus
   D. Nitrogen; sulfur
4. Concerning protein in plants, which statement is most accurate?
   A. A feed can possess a high protein content yet that protein's biologic value is low.
   B. Protein biologic value is the percent of total amino acids ingested that pass through the intestinal cells into the bloodstream.
   C. The protein efficiency ratio of a feed is the ratio of essential amino acids to the total number of amino acids in the feed.
   D. The biologic value of the protein in corn is comparable to that of animal-origin protein.
5. Twins or triplets are desirable in and most commonly carried by:
   A. Dairy cattle
   B. Beef cattle
   C. Horses
   D. Sheep
6. What allows the ruminant animal to convert nonprotein nitrogen sources into a significant amount of usable protein?
   A. The cecum
   B. Rumen microorganisms
   C. The reticulum
   D. Regurgitation of rumen contents and chewing their cud
7. Nonprotein nitrogen sources for ruminants include:
   A. Urea
   B. Ammonium salts
   C. Ammoniated by-products
   D. All of the above
8. Which nutrient fed in the given amount would supply the greatest weight gain?
   A. 100 g of fat or oil
   B. 100 g of pasture
   C. 100 g of hay
   D. 100 g of oats
9. Why can feeds containing low-quality protein be fed long-term to ruminants but *not* to horses?
   A. Ruminants ingest dirt and plant roots, which supplement the protein obtained from feeds.
   B. Ruminants have a much lower protein requirement than horses.
   C. On average, a ruminant will chew its feed three times longer than a horse, resulting in greater feed exposure to salivary digestive enzymes.
   D. The protein quality from moderate-to-poor feeds will usually be improved by rumen metabolism.
10. Daily-energy-requirement tables for livestock express the net-energy requirement in megacalories (Mcal). It is assumed these calories will be supplied by:
    A. Fat
    B. Protein
    C. Carbohydrates
    D. An equal mixture of all of the above
11. *Concentrates* include _____ while *forages* include _____.
    A. All feeds with more than 10 Mcal/g; all feeds with less than or equal to 10 Mcal/g
    B. Grains and high-starch compounds; grass hays and legumes
    C. Vitamin and mineral supplements; pasture grasses
    D. Vitamin and mineral supplements; all other feed sources
12. What is the difference between digestible energy and metabolizable energy?
    A. The term *digestible energy* applies to the energy available in grains, while the term *metabolizable energy* applies to the energy available in hays.
    B. Digestible energy is the total energy potentially available in a feed consumed by an animal, while metabolizable energy is the energy available after all metabolic-process energy has been subtracted.
    C. Digestible energy is the gross energy consumed minus the undigested energy lost in the feces, while metabolizable energy is the digestible energy minus the energy lost in the urine and as combustion gases.
    D. Digestible energy is calculated using the known contents of total digestible nutrients, while metabolizable energy is measured in the animal.
13. Apart from the need for fresh water continuously, what single factor most determines the productivity (i.e., how much milk is produced) of lactating dairy cows?
    A. Milking schedule
    B. Feeding
    C. Milking-parlor temperature
    D. The number of cows in the herd
14. Which vitamin can become toxic to food animals if supplied in too-high amounts?
    A. Biotin
    B. Folic acid
    C. Vitamin C
    D. None of the above
15. Vitamins and minerals need to be supplemented throughout the life of domestic:
    A. Swine
    B. Sheep
    C. Cattle
    D. Horses

16. Which livestock feed is a significant source of calcium?
    A. Grass hay
    B. Alfalfa hay
    C. Oat grain
    D. Molasses
17. In general, protein is an expensive nutrient, and care is taken not to supply it in amounts that exceed requirements.
    A. True
    B. False

For the next four questions, match the vitamin(s) with the correct description
    A. Vitamin K
    B. Vitamin A
    C. Vitamin D
    D. Thiamine, choline, and niacin

18. This is the only fat-soluble vitamin readily synthesized by rumen microorganisms; supplementation is normally not required.
19. This vitamin is synthesized through ultraviolet radiation by the skin or added to a dairy ration as sun-cured forage or a vitamin supplement; supplementation is not necessary in beef cattle.
20. Forages of good quality that are properly harvested normally contain adequate levels of the precursor for this vitamin, carotene.
21. Although these water-soluble vitamins are synthesized by the rumen microflora, some evidence indicates that supplementation may be beneficial in cows undergoing heavy stress or in various disease states.
22. Colostrum can be successfully frozen and used at a later date.
    A. True
    B. False
23. Concerning differences in the management of dairy and beef cattle, which statement is most accurate?
    A. The term *cow-calf* operation applies to the dairy cattle industry only.
    B. Beef calves are weaned at 1 to 2 months of age.
    C. Dairy calves are weaned at 7 to 8 months of age.
    D. Dairy calves are generally removed from their dams almost immediately and hand-raised, while beef calves are allowed to remain with and nurse from their dams for many months.
24. In general, a profitable cow-calf producer will produce a live calf for every _____ cow(s) per year.
    A. One
    B. Two
    C. Three
    D. Four
25. If beef cattle are losing weight on pasture, supplemental energy is usually provided in the form of:
    A. Silage (fermented green feed) or hay
    B. Oat grain
    C. Barley grain
    D. Corn oil
26. Corn cobs, straw, and corn stalks are examples of:
    A. Bedding for confined animals
    B. Roughage used to supplement vitamin A in the case of vitamin A–deficient hay
    C. High-grade roughage supplying adequate protein of high biologic quality
    D. Low-grade roughage supplying inadequate protein if fed over extended periods
27. What must always be supplemented to nonpregnant beef cattle on pasture?
    A. Minerals
    B. Energy in the form of grain
    C. Protein
    D. Fat
28. The ewes of a 50-head sheep operation are having lambing problems, low wool output, and depressed milk production. These problems are most likely due to poor care and inadequate nutrition:
    A. When the ewes are not pregnant
    B. During the first trimester of pregnancy
    C. During the second trimester of pregnancy
    D. During the third trimester of pregnancy
29. Lambs are the only domestic-animal newborns that do *not* require colostrum immediately after birth to achieve adequate immunity.
    A. True
    B. False
30. Concerning feeding lambs, which statement is most accurate?
    A. Hand-raised lambs are weaned from milk replacement formula at 8 weeks of age.
    B. Lambs can be fed a relatively low-quality feed once they reach a weight of 10 kg.
    C. Large, fast-growing lambs on high-grain rations are particularly susceptible to a bacterial "overeating disease" (enterotoxemia) that can cause death.
    D. "Grower" rations are for lambs weighing 15 to 25 kg (30 to 50 lb) and "finisher" rations are for those weighing 25 to 40 kg (50 to 85 lb).
31. Many pigs in the swine industry are raised in confinement.
    A. True
    B. False
32. Sows in production are generally allowed to nurse their litters for:
    A. 7 to 14 days
    B. 14 to 21 days
    C. 21 to 35 days
    D. 35 to 42 days
33. Sows are limit-fed (controlled calorie intake) _____ and full-fed (to achieve as much energy consumption as possible) _____.
    A. During gestation; during lactation
    B. When not pregnant; during gestation

C. During lactation; when not pregnant
D. During lactation; during gestation
34. When visiting a swine operation, you see the farmer brushing the nursing sows' teats with a solution. What is most likely in this solution?
   A. An antiseptic
   B. Iron
   C. Calcium
   D. Glucose
35. Contemporary swine nutrition does not concentrate on the total protein content of feeds, but on the:
   A. Nitrogen content
   B. Amino acid levels
   C. Source of protein
   D. Albumin content
36. Name and briefly describe each of the two feeding programs most often used in dairies.
37. Because of their importance, the daily requirements for what two macrominerals are included in the feeding tables for dairy cattle?
38. To what does "finishing" of beef cattle refer?
39. Care must be taken when feeding sheep premixed feeds and providing trace-mineral salt blocks to avoid toxicity due to an oversupply of what nutrient?

EXTRA CREDIT
40. "Creep feed" is:
   A. Feed ground to a particle size smaller than 0.5 mm in diameter.
   B. Feed to which a vitamin supplement has been added.
   C. Feed placed on one side of a barrier so only the young have access to it.
   D. Fed only on Halloween.

CHAPTER 17

ANIMAL REPRODUCTION

1. In what species is scrotal circumference, rather than a sperm count using a hemacytometer, used to estimate sperm concentration?
   A. Feline
   B. Canine
   C. Bovine, ovine, caprine
   D. Equine
2. The stages of the reproductive cycle in the correct order of occurrence are:
   A. Diestrus, estrus, proestrus, anestrus
   B. Proestrus, estrus, diestrus, anestrus
   C. Estrus, proestrus, anestrus, diestrus
   D. Anestrus, estrus, diestrus, proestrus

3. Ovulation is:
   A. The hormone that maintains pregnancy
   B. The transformation of the ovarian follicle into a corpus luteum
   C. The term applied to the reproductive cycle in the female
   D. The release of the oocyte from the ovarian follicle
4. Veterinarians will sometimes give prostaglandins to synchronize the estrous cycles of groups of females, to bring a female into estrus (heat), or to terminate pregnancy. How do prostaglandins accomplish these tasks?
   A. Prostaglandins cause ovulation.
   B. Prostaglandins stimulate the development of the ovarian follicle.
   C. Prostaglandins lyse (rupture) the corpus luteum, thus reducing progesterone concentrations.
   D. Prostaglandins cause the release of gonadotropin-releasing hormone from the anterior pituitary gland.

For the next four questions, match the species with its length of gestation.
   A. Queen
   B. Cow
   C. Mare
   D. Sow
5. 65 days
6. 114 days
7. 330 days
8. 283 days

Use the following scenario to answer the next three questions. Mrs. Jones wants to breed her male and female Pembroke Welsh Corgi dogs. She calls to say that "Corky," the female, has had a bloody vaginal discharge for 2 days but is not letting "Mikey," the male, breed.
9. Are Corky and Mikey exhibiting normal canine breeding behavior and physical signs?
   A. Yes
   B. No
10. In what stage of the estrous cycle is Corky?
   A. Proestrus
   B. Estrus
   C. Diestrus
   D. Anestrus
11. What is the best advice to give Mrs. Jones?
   A. Bring Corky in for a vaginal smear.
   B. Corky should let Mikey mate sometime in the next 20 days when the bleeding stops, so put the dogs together every other day as long as she lets him mate.
   C. Corky is showing abnormal breeding behavior and signs and should be brought in for a breeding-soundness examination.
   D. A and B
12. Owners who use artificial insemination and have limited access to a male dog or own bitches with

erratic estrus behavior will need to be told exactly when to breed. The exact day of ovulation is best predicted by:
A. Daily, in-house serum luteinizing-hormone assays
B. Every-other-day, in-house serum progesterone assays
C. A or B
D. None of the above

13. In the bitch, vaginal cultures are best performed with:
A. A sterile culture swab
B. A sterile, microsized culture swab
C. A guarded, sterile, culture swab
D. A nonsterile swab, the tip of which is then placed in a new red-top Vacutainer tube

14. Pregnancy diagnosis in the bitch can be performed as early as about _____ days after breeding using ultrasound.
A. 28
B. 21
C. 14
D. 7

15. A client wishing to know the number of pups in utero (in the uterus) should be told to make an appointment for _____ at least _____ days after breeding.
A. Ultrasound; 20 to 25
B. Radiography; 30 to 35
C. Radiography; 40 to 45
D. Ultrasound; 50 to 55

16. Anxious owners can be advised that the bitch is unique in that _____ signals parturition will occur in the next 24 hours.
A. Colostrum leaking from her nipples
B. Nesting behavior
C. A rise in body temperature above 38.8° C (102° F)
D. A drop in body temperature below 37° C (98.6° F)

For the next four questions, match the species with its estrous-cycle characteristics.
A. Feline
B. Canine
C. Equine
D. Bovine

17. Estrus occurs two times per year with ovulation 3 to 4 days after the onset of cytologic estrus.

18. She cycles all year round, the estrous cycle is 21 days long, and ovulation occurs 12 to 18 hours after the end of estrus.

19. She is seasonally polyestrous (spring, summer, and fall), the estrous cycle is 21 days long, and ovulation occurs 1 to 2 days before the end of estrus.

20. She is seasonally polyestrous (spring) and an induced ovulator, and the estrous-cycle length depends on whether ovulation occurs.

21. In the queen, abdominal palpation can be used to diagnose pregnancy on days _____ postbreeding and by ultrasound on days _____ postbreeding.
A. 7 to 15; 10+
B. 7 to 15; 14+
C. 16 to 30; 14+
D. 20+; 15 to 25

22. What is often used to induce estrous activity in the mare during the winter months?
A. Increasing the day length with artificial light
B. Increasing stall temperature with heaters
C. Melatonin supplementation
D. Placing mares in groups together

23. What two preparatory actions are often taken prior to performing reproductive procedures on the mare?
A. Withhold food for 12 hours and water for 6 hours.
B. Wrap the tail and aseptically scrub the vulva and perineal area.
C. Draw 5 cc of blood and place it in an EDTA tube and place hobbles on her hind legs.
D. Clip the perineal area and clean it three times with water.

24. Equine pregnancy diagnosis is usually done with the aid of ultrasonography 2 weeks after ovulation.
A. True
B. False

25. Clients breeding their mares for the first time should be counseled that:
A. The placenta should pass out of the vagina within 3 to 6 hours after birth or a veterinary visit is warranted.
B. A "red bag" protruding from the vulva just prior to parturition is normal.
C. Parturition should be a very rapid process.
D. A and C

26. Are there any pharmaceutical options available to prevent or control estrous behavior in performance mares?
A. Yes, altrenogest
B. Yes, deslorelin
C. Yes, estrone sulfate
D. No

27. In the cow, pregnancy is most frequently diagnosed using:
A. Rectal palpation or ultrasound
B. Serum progesterone
C. The failure to return to estrus 21 days after behavioral estrus
D. The appearance of the vulva

28. The period of no ovarian follicular activity is known as:
A. Metestrus
B. Proestrus
C. Anestrus
D. Diestrus

29. The normal onset of puberty is _____ in the heifer and _____ in the sow.
    A. 10 to 12 months; 10 to 12 months
    B. 16 to 18 months; 6.5 to 8 months
    C. 12 to 14 months; 3 to 4 months
    D. 9 to 10 months; 4.5 to 6 months
30. Estrus can be detected in swine by:
    A. Observing dramatic changes in behavior including panting, rolling, and vocalizing
    B. Placing pressure on the pig's back and her responding by standing still and quietly and passively assuming a mating position
    C. Observing her response to a boar's approach
    D. B and C
31. It is important to assist sows during delivery, because early detection and correction of potential problems during parturition prevents piglet losses.
    A. True
    B. False
32. Which statement concerning artificial insemination is true?
    A. Sperm in frozen or refrigerated semen are equally as viable (able to fertilized an egg) as those in fresh semen.
    B. Artificial insemination is common in the dairy cattle and swine industries.
    C. Deposition of semen into the uterus using laparoscopic procedures is most common in the beef cattle industry.
    D. All of the above
33. What stimulates sheep and goats to start cycling (come out of estrus)?
    A. Cool weather
    B. Decreasing day length
    C. Geographic origin of a specific breed
    D. All of the above
34. Estrus detection in ewes and does is accomplished by:
    A. Vaginal cytology
    B. Observing the females seeking out a male, wagging their tails, and standing immobile in his presence
    C. Abdominal palpation
    D. Ultrasound
35. What species, when in estrus, will simultaneously squat, urinate, lift her tail, and "wink" in the presence of a male?
    A. Pig
    B. Horse
    C. Sheep or goat
    D. Alpaca or llama
36. Llamas cycle _____, and their ovulation time resembles that of _____.
    A. In the spring and summer; horses
    B. In the summer and fall; cows
    C. In the fall and winter; sows
    D. All year round; cats
37. Sperm-cell production is dependent on:
    A. Testosterone
    B. Testis temperature
    C. Follicle-stimulating hormone
    D. All of the above
38. Unlike oocyte release, sperm-cell production is relatively constant.
    A. True
    B. False
39. When evaluating semen in the laboratory, it is important to have all equipment:
    A. Cooled to freezer temperature
    B. Cooled to refrigerator temperature
    C. At body temperature
    D. Hot to the touch
40. Complete semen analysis involves examining what three characteristics?
    A. pH, sperm motility, and concentration
    B. Color, pH, volume
    C. Sperm motility, concentration, and morphology
    D. Color, pH, specific gravity
41. Semen collection from the bull, ram, and buck is performed using an artificial vagina and:
    A. A female in estrus
    B. An ovariectomized female
    C. A castrated male
    D. An electroejaculator
42. When collecting semen from stallions using an artificial vagina, it is critical to precisely control the:
    A. Internal temperature of the artificial vagina
    B. Angle at which the artificial vagina is held during collection
    C. Internal pressure of the artificial vagina
    D. A and C
43. When adding an extender to stallion semen prior to cooling and shipping, the final concentration should be:
    A. 5 to 10×10^6 sperm cells/ml
    B. 15 to 20×10^6 sperm cells/ml
    C. 25 to 50×10^6 sperm cells/ml
    D. 75 to 100×10^6 sperm cells/ml
44. A boar's semen is collected by manual pressure on the distal penis as long as pressure is applied to the penile tip, the boar will continue to ejaculate.
    A. True
    B. False

For the next nine questions, match the term with its definition.
    A. "Boar" effect
    B. Estrus
    C. Pyometra
    D. Cria
    E. Pseudopregnancy in the canine or feline

F. "Ram" or "buck" effect
G. "Foal" heat
H. "Standing" heat
I. Pseudopregnancy in the caprine
45. Mammary development, lactation, and maternal behavior in a nonpregnant female in diestrus
46. The period when the female is sexually receptive enough to the male to allow him to mount and copulate
47. Purulent material in the uterus due to a uterine infection
48. The term applied to the time during which a cow will brace herself while standing to be mounted by a bull or another cow
49. The first estrus in a mare after foaling, usually occurring about 9 days after parturition
50. The pheromones in the male's salivary glands stimulate pubertal females to start cycling sooner
51. A baby camelid
52. The introduction of a new, mature, odoriferous male during the transition from the anestrus season into the breeding season induces estrus in most females
53. A collection of fluid in the uterus without pregnancy (If not treated with prostaglandin, the natural expulsion of the fluid is called *cloudburst*.)
54. When should a mare inseminated with frozen semen?
    A. Within 12 hours before and 12 hours after ovulation
    B. Within 24 hours before and 24 hours after ovulation
    C. Within 12 hours before and 6 hours after ovulation
    D. Within 24 hours before and 6 hours after ovulation
55. When should pubertal ewes and does be bred?
    A. If they have attained 65% of their adult body weight
    B. If they have attained 50% of their adult body weight
    C. If they have attained 75% of their adult body weight
    D. In the spring
56. Which of the following can be done to help stimulate uterine clearance in the mare after breeding?
    A. Uterine lavage
    B. Give oxytocin or cloprostenol
    C. Intrauterine infusion of antibiotics
    D. All of the above
57. A nonodorous, hemorrhagic postpartum discharge lasting ____ is normal in the bitch.
    A. 6-8 months
    B. 8-10 weeks
    C. 2 weeks
    D. 6-8 weeks
58. Describe the appearance and percentages of cells seen on a canine vaginal smear during estrus.
59. A client calls to say her 8-month-old, unspayed, female cat is rolling around, vocalizing, and arching her back when petted and is "driving [her] crazy." What do you tell her is wrong? What do you recommend she do to stop the behavior?
60. Your best dairy-operation client calls to say one of his cows, which just calved, has "something large with big bumps all over it" protruding from her vulva. What is wrong with this cow and how soon should you schedule a veterinary visit?
61. When visiting a sheep operation, you see groups of ewes in pens with an occasional ram wearing a body harness in with them. What is the purpose of this harness?
62. When collecting canine semen for breeding-soundness evaluation or artificial insemination, which part of the ejaculate need *not* be collected?

EXTRA CREDIT

63. The "ampulla" is:
    A. The hole left on a follicle after oocyte release
    B. An accessory sex gland in the male
    C. Part of the oviduct
    D. The instrument a ram plays to attract ewes
64. "Whelping" is:
    A. Parturition in a canine
    B. Parturition in a feline
    C. Parturition in a caprine
    D. The sound a dog makes when left in the backyard alone

CHAPTER 18

CARE OF BIRDS, REPTILES, AND SMALL MAMMALS

1. Which species is very social and requires additional attention from its owners to meet its psychological needs?
   A. Mouse
   B. Hedgehog
   C. Guinea pig
   D. Sugar glider
2. Approximately ____ of the problems seen in exotic pet medicine can be attributed to a lack of information on the basic husbandry of these species among pet stores, pet owners, veterinarians, and veterinary technicians.
   A. 10%
   B. 35%
   C. 50%
   D. 85%

3. Which statement is most accurate concerning the technician's instructions to a bird owner calling about a sick bird?
   A. The bird should be brought to the hospital in a thick, corrugated cardboard box with tiny holes punched in the top.
   B. The bird's container should be lined with fresh, clean newsprint.
   C. The owner should bring in a 3-day supply of food for the bird including all commercial and home-prepared foods.
   D. Most sick-avian telephone inquiries should be considered emergencies.
4. Which of the following make up the majority of species seen on a normal avian fecal Gram stain?
   A. Gram-positive organisms
   B. Gram-negative organisms
   C. Motile protozoa
   D. Club-shaped, gram-positive clostridial species of bacteria
5. What is the normal body temperature of most psittacine species?
   A. 35.5° C to 36.6° C (96° F to 98° F)
   B. 36.6° C to 38.3° C (98° F to 101° F)
   C. 38.3° C to 39.4° C (101° F to 103° F)
   D. 38.8° C to 40.0° C (102° F to 104° F)
6. Which statement concerning radiography of the avian patient is true?
   A. Lateral views are not part of the standard radiographic series in avian patients.
   B. Sedation or anesthesia and a restraint board are recommended in patients capable of tolerating them.
   C. Contrast agents such as iohexol and barium sulfate are toxic to birds and should never be used.
   D. A and C
7. Injections of drugs into birds are best done in the pectoral muscles, because drugs injected into the caudal half of the animal may result in the drug being shunted toward the kidneys by way of the renal portal system.
   A. True
   B. False
8. Concerning wing trimming, which statement is most accurate?
   A. An asymmetrical result is desirable; therefore only one wing should be clipped.
   B. Typically the primary flight feathers are cut for heavier birds, and both the primary and secondary feathers for lighter birds, to achieve maximal flight restriction.
   C. Wing clipping prevents flight completely.
   D. The final "look," or cosmetic result, of the trim is not important as long as flight restriction is achieved.

9. A large macaw is being brought in for a beak and nail trim. What basic tools should you set out for the procedure?
   A. Small garden shears and a towel
   B. Rescoe nail trimmers, silver nitrate, and a towel
   C. A rotary grinding tool and a towel
   D. Human nail clippers, powder cauterizer, and a towel
10. Sick, anorexic birds and reptiles are hospitalized and nutrition is usually provided:
    A. Enterally by a tube placed into the crop or esophagus through the glottis
    B. Enterally by syringe feeding into the commissures (corners) of the mouth
    C. Enterally by a percutaneously placed gastric tube
    D. Parenterally
11. The gastrointestinal zoonosis of greatest concern in birds is _____, which is caused by _____.
    A. Visceral-larval migrans; *Toxocara* spp.
    B. Tuberculosis; *Mycobacterium* spp.
    C. Clostridial diarrhea; *Clostridium perfringens*
    D. Psittacosis; *Chlamydia psittaci*
12. How is the gender of a snake best determined?
    A. With a metal probe inserted into the cloaca
    B. By the skin color and markings
    C. By the overall size of the animal
    D. By examining the retina with an ophthalmoscope
13. What information is critical to obtain when taking an environmental history on a reptilian patient?
    A. Cage temperature and humidity level
    B. Photoperiod and light source
    C. Type of heat source and temperature gradient in the cage
    D. All of the above
14. Hospitalized birds are best kept in a room at:
    A. 15.5° C to 21.1° C (60° F to 70° F).
    B. 21.1° C to 26.6° C (70° F to 80° F).
    C. 26.6° C to 32.2° C (80° F to 90° F).
    D. 32.2° C to 37.7° C (90° F to 100° F).
15. A lizard with suspected gastrointestinal disease has an appointment today. The owner was instructed to bring in a fresh fecal sample and calls to say one is unavailable. What do you tell him?
    A. Let's reschedule the appointment for the day after tomorrow because most lizards defecate at least every other day.
    B. Come in at the scheduled time. Your lizard will be examined, nonfecal tests will be performed, and he will be hospitalized until he defecates.
    C. Come in at the scheduled time. A fecal sample can be obtained by colonic wash during the appointment.
    D. Place the lizard in warm water. He should defecate 30 to 60 minutes after being submerged. Call us back if he does not defecate.

16. Many turtles and lizards have urinary bladders, and a routine urinalysis may be performed on fresh urine samples.
    A. True
    B. False
17. Sites commonly used for venipuncture in snakes include:
    A. The caudal or coccygeal tail vein, cardiac puncture, ventral abdominal vein, or palatine vessels
    B. The jugular veins or coccygeal tail vein
    C. The occipital sinus or palatine vessels
    D. The peribulbar or retrobulbar plexus
18. Why is it important to house avian and reptilian patients in separate rooms?
    A. They have dramatically different temperature requirements.
    B. Infected birds can easily transmit tuberculosis to reptiles.
    C. Avian vocalizations place undue stress on convalescing reptiles.
    D. The normal gram-negative fecal flora of most reptiles can infect the birds.
19. It is important to remember to give nephrotoxic drugs in the cranial third of the reptile's body.
    A. True
    B. False
20. Why must reptiles be exposed to full-spectrum artificial light during normal daylight hours?
    A. To enable proper elimination cycles
    B. To aid in regular shedding cycles
    C. To help prevent metabolic bone disease due to lack of vitamin D_3 and calcium
    D. To help prevent skin infections
21. The zoonotic microorganisms of greatest concern when handling reptiles are _____, which are found primarily in the _____.
    A. Gram-positive, rod-shaped bacterial species such as *Bacillus anthracis;* blood
    B. Protozoa; respiratory secretions
    C. Gram-negative, enteric bacteria such as *Salmonella* spp.; feces and saliva
    D. Gram-negative, enteric bacteria such as *Salmonella* spp.; blood
22. Blood samples from the ferret can be obtained from the:
    A. Cranial vena cava
    B. Jugular vein
    C. Cephalic vein
    D. Any of the above
23. Which statement concerning ferret-owner counseling is most accurate?
    A. Female ferrets not intended for breeding need not be spayed, because there is little risk of complications if the uterus and ovaries are left intact.
    B. Owners calling with a complaint of a female ferret with hair loss and/or vulvar swelling should be instructed that she is in estrus and need not be seen by a veterinarian.
    C. Ferrets exposed to mosquitoes require heartworm preventative.
    D. Nonlactating, nonpregnant ferrets can be maintained on high-quality dog food.
24. Flea-infested ferrets are best treated with feline flea-control products.
    A. True
    B. False
25. Which statement concerning ferret diseases is true?
    A. Ferrets are susceptible to human influenza and can catch this virus from infected owners.
    B. Ferrets are susceptible to feline panleukopenia and require vaccination for this disease.
    C. Ferrets are susceptible to canine distemper and can be vaccinated using a canine distemper vaccine.
    D. No vaccines are yet approved specifically for use in ferrets, so canine and/or feline vaccinations must be used.
26. A life span of _____ is expected in a rabbit maintained with proper husbandry.
    A. 2 to 3 years
    B. 5 to 6 years
    C. 7 to 9 years
    D. 11 to 13 years
27. The rabbit that is a candidate for anesthesia should have food withheld for 8 to 12 hours and be free from respiratory disease.
    A. True
    B. False
28. Intravenous injections are generally given to rabbits in the:
    A. Jugular vein
    B. Medial saphenous vein
    C. Central ear artery
    D. Marginal ear vein
29. Guinea pigs, rabbits, and hamsters are extremely sensitive to _____, which can cause severe illness in these species.
    A. Ivermectin
    B. Penicillin antibiotics
    C. Ketamine
    D. Barbiturates
30. A client wishing to breed his 1-year-old female guinea pig must be counseled that:
    A. If she has a litter of more than two pigs, they will have to be hand-raised because she has only two mammary glands.
    B. Female guinea pigs over 10 months of age are infertile.

- C. In general, breeding after the age of 7 months is not recommended because pubic-symphysis fusion can lead to dystocia and death during parturition. If he does choose to breed his pet, cesarean section may be required.
- D. The babies should be removed from the sow after 5 days to prevent her from cannibalizing them.

31. Which small mammal requires vitamin C supplementation?
    A. Gerbils
    B. Guinea pigs
    C. Mice
    D. Rabbits

32. Hamsters live an average of _____ and have a gestation length of _____.
    A. 1 year; 16 days
    B. 3 years; 16 days
    C. 5 years; 25 days
    D. 7 years; 25 days

33. Zoonotic diseases transmitted by poor hygiene are of greatest concern in the:
    A. Rat
    B. Hamster
    C. Guinea pig
    D. Hedgehog

34. The ideal hamster or gerbil habitat will include:
    A. Cedar shavings, an exercise wheel, and a nonwood cage with a tight-fitting lid
    B. Aromatic pine shavings and a wooden cage with a tight-fitting lid
    C. Hardwood shavings, an exercise wheel, and a nonwood cage with a tight-fitting lid
    D. Cedar shavings, a place to hide, and a nonwood cage with a loose-fitting (or no) lid

35. The sex of mice and gerbils can be determined by:
    A. Visualizing a prepuce and scrotum in males
    B. Identifying the presence of a hairless patch on the abdomen of males
    C. Noting the greater relative urogenital distance in males than in females
    D. Noting the presence of an oily tail head in males

36. It is legal to keep the black-tailed prairie dog (*Cynomys ludovicianus*) in captivity as a pet.
    A. True
    B. False

37. _____ usually require anesthesia in order for a close physical examination to be performed on them.
    A. Hedgehogs
    B. Sugar gliders
    C. Prairie dogs
    D. Hamsters

38. Rabbits are susceptible to ear mites.
    A. True
    B. False

39. An ideal diet for a sugar glider consists of:
    A. High-quality cat food
    B. A commercial diet formulated specifically for sugar gliders
    C. A handmade diet consisting of a zoo-formula insectivore diet, apples, grapes, carrots, sweet potatoes, cooked egg yolks, mealworms, and vitamin/mineral powder
    D. B or C

40. Which of the following is/are true regarding restraint of the avian patient during the examination process?
    A. Examination, diagnostic sample collection, and treatment should be performed slowly and take as long as necessary so as not to unduly stress the bird.
    B. Capture and restraint should be done with a hand that is covered by a towel.
    C. All diagnostic testing materials should be ready before the bird is restrained.
    D. All of the above.

41. You are asked to obtain a cloacal swab on a cockatoo. Briefly explain how this procedure is performed.

42. Name four common venipuncture sites used in the avian species.

43. A client brings in a rat that is having trouble breathing and has a red nasal discharge. Assuming the discharge is not blood-tinged, why is it red in color?

EXTRA CREDIT

44. Define *scutes*.
    A. Any scalelike structures
    B. A main component of aquatic frog diets
    C. The clear membranes covering the eyes of snakes
    D. How a dog attempts to empty his impacted anal glands

45. Snuffles is:
    A. A respiratory disease in mice caused by mycobacterial species
    B. A respiratory disease in snakes caused by subnormal cage temperatures
    C. A respiratory disease in rabbits caused by *Pasteurella multocida*
    D. A Sesame Street character

CHAPTER 19

VETERINARY ANESTHESIA

1. General anesthesia:
    A. Describes the loss of sensation to all or part of the body.

B. Refers to drug-induced unconsciousness and is controlled and reversible.
C. Can be induced via injectable or inhaled drugs.
D. B and C

2. Induction and maintenance of general anesthesia through a mask is preferable to injectable anesthesia and much safer.
   A. True
   B. False

3. A balanced anesthetic protocol might include a(n)
   A. Analgesic
   B. Sedative
   C. Tranquilizer
   D. All of the above

4. An intravenous catheter:
   A. Provides a route for the administration of fluids.
   B. Should never be used to administer anesthetic drugs.
   C. Provides a route for the administration of drugs required in case of emergency.
   D. A and C

5. The endotracheal tube should not be inflated in birds because:
   A. They can bite it off and swallow it.
   B. They have complete tracheal rings, making the trachea less compliant when the endotracheal tube cuff is inflated.
   C. The inflated cuff becomes easily lodged in air sacs.
   D. Their trachea is soft and may be traumatized.

6. A(n) _____ should be used to intubate any animal with an upper airway obstruction.
   A. Laryngoscope
   B. Mouth gag
   C. Local anesthetic
   D. Inflated endotracheal

7. Cylinders containing _____ are white or green and cylinders containing _____ are blue.
   A. Nitrous oxide; oxygen
   B. Oxygen; nitrous oxide
   C. Liquid nitrogen; nitrous oxide
   D. Nitrous oxide; helium

8. Which of the following statements is false?
   A. The bain coaxial system is a commonly used nonrebreathing system in veterinary medicine.
   B. In the circle breathing circuit, the animal rebreathes some previously exhaled gases.
   C. The appropriate size rebreathing bag is determined by multiplying the animal's tidal volume by 6.
   D. The oxygen flush valve delivers high flows of oxygen to the fresh gas outlet just before entering the vaporizer.

9. Preanesthetic thoracic radiographs are indicated in animals with:
   A. Pulmonary disease
   B. Cardiac disease
   C. History of trauma
   D. All of the above

10. Prior to the induction of anesthesia, small animals should have food and water withheld for _____ and _____, respectively.
    A. 6 hours, 24 hours
    B. 10 hours, 12 hours to 14 hours
    C. 12 hours, 8 to 10 hours
    D. 24 hours, 10 hours

11. The anesthetic record is used to:
    A. Help recognize gradual changes over a period of time (trends)
    B. Help plan subsequent anesthetic procedures
    C. Record heart rate, respiratory rate, and blood pressure
    D. All of the above

12. An esophageal stethoscope is used to monitor:
    A. Respiratory rate
    B. Heart rate and rhythm
    C. The strength of peristalsis
    D. Pulse quality

13. An electrocardiogram yields information about:
    A. The heart's electrical activity
    B. Myocardial contractility
    C. Tissue perfusion
    D. Regurgitation

14. Respiratory rate and adequacy of ventilation may be measured using:
    A. A pulse oximeter
    B. An arterial blood sample
    C. An electrocardiogram
    D. A capnometer

15. In horses, what are indications of light anesthesia?
    A. Decreased heart rate
    B. Nystagmus
    C. Lacrimation
    D. B and C

16. Excessive anesthetic depth may be indicated by:
    A. Sluggish palpebral reflex
    B. Loss of anal tone
    C. Lacrimation
    D. Increased heart rate

17. The normal inspiratory to expiratory ratio in small animals is:
    A. 2 seconds to 1 second
    B. 15 ml/kg to 20 ml/kg
    C. 12
    D. 31

18. Which of the following can be administered epidurally?
    A. Alpha$_2$ agonists
    B. Local anesthetics such as lidocaine or bupivacaine
    C. Opioids
    D. All of the above

19. Which of the following statements is false regarding epidural anesthesia?
    A. The animal should be placed in a head-down position.
    B. The dosage should be increased by 50% if cerebrospinal fluid is observed in the hub of the needle during injection.
    C. To avoid hypotension, the animal must be adequately volume-expanded before injection.
    D. A and B
20. After intubation, what must be done before inflating the cuff to its proper level?
    A. Check that the tube is properly placed.
    B. Desensitize the larynx with 2% lidocaine.
    C. Close the pop-off valve.
    D. A and C
21. When total protein falls below 35 g/dl during the anesthetic period, the animal can develop _____.
    A. Pulmonary edema
    B. Ascites
    C. Hypertension
    D. Urticaria
22. For most elective surgical procedures, intravenous fluids should be given at a rate of _____ ml/kg/hr in small animals.
    A. 5 to 10
    B. 10 to 20
    C. 15 to 20
    D. None of the above
23. For approximately 3 to 5 minutes after induction, after the tube is properly inflated, the fresh gas flow rate should be:
    A. 10 ml/kg/min
    B. 500 ml/kg/min
    C. 50 ml/kg/hr
    D. 100 ml/kg/min
24. If the vaporizer must be filled during the anesthetic period, the _____ must be turned _____.
    A. Vaporizer; on
    B. Pop-off valve; on
    C. Vaporizer; off
    D. Fresh gas flow; off
25. The halter must be removed from horses during the anesthetic period to avoid damage to the _____.
    A. Facial nerve
    B. Nares
    C. Eyes
    D. Jugular vein
26. An animal's endotracheal tube may be removed once the _____ reflex returns.
    A. Pupillary light
    B. Pharyngeal
    C. Anal
    D. Patellar
27. Most animals are _____ following general anesthesia.
    A. Hypothermic
    B. Volume-overloaded
    C. Hyperthermic
    D. Volume-depleted
28. Which of the following should be done for horses recovering from general anesthesia?
    A. Cover the eyes.
    B. Administer a sedative or tranquilizer if rough recovery is anticipated.
    C. Replace the halter for horses recovering in the field.
    D. All of the above
29. While ruminants are recovering from anesthesia, they should be placed in ____ recumbency to minimize ____.
    A. Left lateral; regurgitation
    B. Sternal; regurgitation
    C. Right lateral; regurgitation
    D. Left lateral, atelectasis
30. A body temperature below ___° F predisposes an animal to life-threatening ventricular arrhythmias.
    A. 95
    B. 88
    C. 90
    D. 86
31. Fluid containing _____ should not be given during CPR because it can exacerbate cerebral damage.
    A. Potassium
    B. Calcium
    C. Magnesium
    D. Dextrose
32. A preanesthetic agent is used to:
    A. Facilitate animal restraint in overly excited or aggressive patients.
    B. Minimize autonomic reflex activity such as salivation and bradycardia.
    C. Reduce the dose of potentially more severe cardiopulmonary-depressant drugs used in the anesthetic protocol.
    D. All of the above
33. When are atropine or glycopyrrolate included in a preanesthetic regimen?
    A. In small animals and swine when bradycardia or excessive salivation are anticipated
    B. In fractious horses and cattle for sedation
    C. When cardiac arrhythmias are anticipated
    D. A and C
34. Why should the use of acepromazine be avoided in geriatric and pediatric patients?
    A. It has a long duration of action and is dependent on metabolism by the liver.
    B. It can cause excitement in the very young and very old.

C. It causes tachycardia.
D. It causes significant respiratory depression.
35. One advantage to using ____ or ____ is that their effects can be reversed by administration of a specific reversal agent.
   A. Guaifenesin; dissociative agents
   B. Propofol; barbiturates
   C. Benzodiazepine tranquilizers; dissociative agents
   D. Opioids; alpha$_2$-adrenergic agonists
36. *Induction* is best defined as:
   A. The administration of any injectable anesthetic agent
   B. The administration of an anesthetic agent that provides a rapid transition from consciousness to unconsciousness
   C. The administration of the first injectable anesthetic agent of the anesthetic protocol
   D. Causing unconsciousness with gas anesthetics only, using a mask or chamber
37. When monitoring anesthesia, vital signs are generally assessed and recorded every:
   A. Minute
   B. 5 minutes
   C. 10 minutes
   D. 15 minutes
38. If a patient is hypoventilating (not breathing deeply and/or frequently enough to remove carbon dioxide [CO_2] from the body), ____ readings will be abnormal.
   A. Capnometry and blood CO_2
   B. ECG
   C. Ultrasonic Doppler
   D. All of the above
39. You are monitoring anesthesia for a miniature schnauzer undergoing radial fracture repair. The surgeon asks you to "sigh" the patient. What do you do?
   A. Place slight pressure on the lateral thorax once with your hand during patient expiration.
   B. Assist ventilation once using a slightly higher than normal peak inspiratory pressure.
   C. Remove the Y-piece from the endotracheal tube, place your mouth over the tube, and breathe once into the tube to slightly expand the dog's chest.
   D. Depress the oxygen flush valve for 5 seconds.
40. What agent is used to desensitize the larynx for endotracheal tube placement?
   A. Atropine
   B. Epinephrine
   C. 2% lidocaine
   D. Heparinized saline
41. Away from the animal hospital, surgical procedures requiring general anesthesia in horses and cattle are best performed in a grassy area.
   A. True
   B. False

EXTRA CREDIT
42. A "stylet" is:
   A. A rigid structure placed inside an endotracheal tube to aid in the tube's placement in the trachea
   B. A device screwed onto an inhalant-anesthetic jar to keep the liquid from spilling while filling a vaporizer
   C. A device used to visualize the larynx during endotracheal tube placement
   D. A young and very beautiful miniature horse actress
43. Atelectasis is:
   A. A rapid respiratory rate
   B. A collapsed or airless state of the lung
   C. Blue mucous membranes
   D. Rapid horizontal eye movement

CHAPTER 20

PAIN MANAGEMENT

1. Which statement concerning pain in animals is most accurate?
   A. In general, pain in animals is beneficial, especially postoperatively, because it provides a constant reminder to the patient to avoid movement that might cause further injury.
   B. Controlling pain in animals may lead to prolonged hospitalization, poor wound healing, and an increased rate of complications.
   C. The transmission of a painful sensation involves the stimulation of receptors and peripheral nerves in the traumatized tissue with subsequent conduction through the spinal cord to multiple areas in the brain.
   D. A and B
2. What chemical substance produced by the body contributes to the intense pain associated with inflammation?
   A. Prostaglandins
   B. Histamine
   C. Proteolytic (protein-digesting) enzymes
   D. All of the above
3. Thoracic or visceral pain is more vague and difficult to localize than skin or muscle pain because:
   A. The localization of pain to a particular part of the body is the responsibility of the central nervous system.
   B. There are few sensory nerves in the viscera and thorax.
   C. Pain from internal organs is perceived by the thalamus, while skin or muscle pain is perceived locally where the pain occurs.

D. Visceral pain fibers are classified as A-delta and those in skin and muscle as C fibers.
4. _____ tissue is one of the most important pain-free regions in the body.
   A. Arterial-wall
   B. Brain
   C. Joint-capsule
   D. Tendon
5. One common physiologic response to pain is
   A. Increased heart rate and blood pressure.
   B. Pupillary constriction.
   C. Decreased respiratory rate.
   D. Warm (not hot) extremities.
6. Behavioral signs of discomfort tend to be species-specific and vary also between breeds and individuals.
   A. True
   B. False
7. A new horse owner calls to say her 6-year-old quarter horse gelding is sweating, kicking at his abdomen, pawing, and rolling. This horse is exhibiting signs of:
   A. Lameness (leg pain)
   B. Neck pain
   C. A headache
   D. Abdominal pain (colic)
8. A 2-year-old Bernese mountain dog is biting, licking, and scratching at the bandage placed over the site of a recent surgical cranial cruciate-ligament repair. The best way to handle him is to:
   A. Punish him remotely (such as with a squirt gun) when he disturbs the bandage.
   B. Evaluate him for pain, treat him for pain if necessary, then restrain him from chewing, such as with an Elizabethan collar.
   C. Administer the correct dose of oxymorphone subcutaneously every hour until he stops chewing.
   D. Spray a chew-deterrent, such as bitter apple, on the bandage.
9. _____ are the most commonly used analgesics for postoperative patients, while _____ are predominately used for mild-to-moderate chronic musculoskeletal pain.
   A. Nonsteroidal antiinflammatory drugs (NSAIDs); narcotics
   B. Tranquilizers; narcotics
   C. Narcotics; NSAIDs
   D. NSAIDs; tranquilizers
10. In small animals, loud, persistent vocalizing immediately after an operation is generally considered:
    A. A sign of significant pain and/or anxiety that needs treating
    B. A sign of moderate pain that may or may not need treating
    C. A sign of mild pain not necessary to treat
    D. A normal response to awakening from anesthesia not requiring treatment
11. Which aspect of nursing care will best soothe and relieve most animals in pain?
    A. Frequent moving
    B. Gently talking to and stroking the animal
    C. Frequent administration of medications
    D. Frequent monitoring
12. The analgesic effect of opioids is due to their:
    A. Interaction with specific opioid receptors in the brain and spinal cord
    B. Inhibition of cyclooxygenase
    C. Interaction with alpha$_2$ receptors in the central nervous system
    D. Interaction with histamine receptors
13. Common side effects of narcotics in dogs include:
    A. Panting, respiratory depression, and bradycardia
    B. Gastrointestinal ulceration
    C. Vocalization and hypertension
    D. Salivation, mydriasis (dilated pupils), and diarrhea

For the next four questions, match the narcotic drug with its description.
   A. Oxymorphone
   B. Butorphanol
   C. Buprenorphine
   D. Naloxone

14. This narcotic agonist/antagonist is effective for mild-to-moderate pain; however, its short duration of action requires frequent redosing.
15. This pure narcotic antagonist is used to rapidly reverse the effects of morphine, it lasts 1 to 4 hours, and it is not a controlled substance.
16. This narcotic agonist/antagonist is effective for mild-to-moderate pain and has a longer duration of action than similar drugs.
17. This semi-synthetic narcotic analgesic is considered excellent for moderate-to-intense pain because of its potency and duration of action.
18. At high doses, narcotics can cause excitement in:
    A. Cats
    B. Horses
    C. Swine and cattle
    D. All of the above
19. The analgesic effect of NSAIDs is due to:
    A. Interaction with specific opioid receptors in the brain and spinal cord
    B. Inhibition of cyclooxygenase
    C. Interaction with alpha$_2$ receptors in the central nervous system
    D. Interaction with histamine receptors
20. *Antipyretic* means relieves:
    A. Fever
    B. Headache
    C. Inflammation
    D. Pain

21. When administering aspirin to cats for pain relief, it is important to remember:
    A. To give it no more frequently than every other day.
    B. It can also cause sedation.
    C. It can also cause diarrhea.
    D. They can only tolerate the children's liquid formulation.
22. _____ refers to an increased response to a stimulus that is normally painful, whereas _____ refers to the production of pain due to a stimulus that does not normally provoke pain.
    A. Analgesia; hyperalgesia
    B. Hyperalgesia; allodynia
    C. Allodynia; hyperalgesia
    D. Nociception; analgesia
23. Which tissues contain a high concentration of nociceptors?
    A. Periosteum and muscle
    B. Skin and cornea
    C. Dental pulp and arterial walls
    D. All of the above
24. The use of _____ is *not* recommended in dogs.
    A. Meclofenamic acid
    B. Ketoprofen
    C. Ibuprofen
    D. Phenylbutazone
25. Phenylbutazone is commonly used in horses for relief of musculoskeletal pain; however, lower daily doses should be administered to _____ because some breeds exhibit acute toxicity to the drug.
    A. "Gaited" horses such as Andalusians
    B. Warm-blooded horses such as Hanoverians
    C. Draft horses such as Clydesdales
    D. Ponies such as Shetland and Welsh ponies
26. It is inappropriate to use tranquilizers alone for postoperative pain control.
    A. True
    B. False
27. The effects of alpha$_2$-andrenergic agonists (e.g., xylazine) can be reversed with _____ or _____.
    A. Atipamezole; yohimbine
    B. Detomidine; corticosteroids
    C. Flunixin meglumine; nalorphine
    D. Naloxone; nalorphine
28. You are unsure whether a ferret that has received an adrenalectomy is experiencing a significant amount of pain. What is the best way to determine whether this patient needs analgesics?
    A. Check the body temperature; if more than 2° F above normal less than 12 hours after the surgery, administer analgesics.
    B. Check the heart rate; if greater than two times normal, administer analgesics.
    C. Check the respiratory rate; if greater than two times normal, administer analgesics.
    D. Rule of thumb if a procedure would be painful for you to endure, it is likely that is painful for the animal.
29. In the horse and dog, what is the most commonly encountered adverse reaction to NSAIDs?
    A. Gastrointestinal ulceration
    B. Constipation
    C. Diarrhea
    D. Low blood pressure
30. Detomidine is classified as a(n) _____ and therefore _____ a controlled substance.
    A. Narcotic; is
    B. Alpha$_2$-andrenergic agonist; is not
    C. NSAID; is not
    D. Corticosteroid; is
31. Concerning the use of corticosteroids in the treatment of pain, which statement is most accurate?
    A. Corticosteroids are very effective analgesics because they actually treat the cause of pain rather than just mask the symptoms of the underlying disease.
    B. Corticosteroids should not be used with NSAIDs due to the increased risk of gastrointestinal ulceration.
    C. Significant impairment of wound healing and masking of the underlying disease can occur with prolonged high doses of corticosteroids.
    D. B and C

For the next two questions, use the information provided in the following scenario. While working with an equine veterinarian, you visit a farm with a 3-year-old Thoroughbred stallion exhibiting signs of colic. His vital signs are as follows: temperature, 39.0° C (102.2° F); pulse, 60; respiratory rate, 30; mucous membranes, muddy; and capillary refill time, 3 to 4 seconds. He is showing violent signs of abdominal pain and is sweating.

32. What drug will the veterinarian likely use to treat this horse's pain?
    A. Phenylbutazone
    B. Xylazine
    C. Flunixin meglumine
    D. B or C
33. What two vital signs given above are frequently used to assess the severity and prognosis of colic in horses?
    A. Temperature and pulse
    B. Mucous membrane color and capillary refill time
    C. Pulse and respiratory rate
    D. Mucous membrane color and temperature
34. How do sodium hyaluronate and polysulfated glycosaminoglycans work to reduce the pain of degenerative joint disease (arthritis)?
    A. They reduce inflammation, but their exact mechanism of action is unknown.
    B. They inhibit cyclooxygenase.

Copyright © 2006 by Elsevier, Inc. All rights reserved.

C. They return the joint capsule to normal, and some inhibit the enzymes involved in cartilage degeneration.
D. They prevent white blood cells from releasing inflammatory mediators such as kallikreins and bradykinins.
35. At clinical doses, deracoxib is a COX-2 inhibitor.
A. True
B. False
36. When morphine is administered epidurally, its latency of onset is approximately ___ minutes and the duration of analgesia is approximately ___ hours.
A. 10 to 20; 2 to 4
B. 30 to 60; 12 to 18
C. 5 to 10; 6 to 8
D. 30 to 60; 4 to 6
37. The amount of fentanyl taken up from a patch is decreased by:
A. Anesthesia
B. Hyperthermia
C. Low blood pressure
D. A and C
38. Briefly describe how to apply a fentanyl transdermal skin patch.
39. A client asks you why he should use carprofen, more expensive and available by prescription only, instead of aspirin for his dog's arthritic hip pain. What do you tell him?
40. Why might a veterinarian elect to use a local or regional analgesic technique, such as an epidural infusion or an intercostal nerve block, in addition to standard oral or parenteral administration of analgesia?
41. Which dog breed has shown a potentially serious, although sporadic and uncommon, reaction to carprofen? What is this reaction?

EXTRA CREDIT

42. *Kappa* and *mu* are:
A. Adjectives used to differentiate classes of NSAIDs
B. Adjectives used to describe the different locations at which epidural anesthesia is performed
C. Types of opioid receptors in the central nervous system
D. Bovine-only sororities

CHAPTER 21

PHARMACOLOGY AND PHARMACY

1. A drug's site of action is termed its:
A. Active site
B. Target tissue
C. Receptor zone
D. Active location
2. In general, the absorption rate of a drug is slower when the drug is given _____ and more rapid when given _____.
A. Subcutaneously; intramuscularly
B. Intravenously; intramuscularly
C. Intramuscularly; subcutaneously
D. Intravenously; subcutaneously
3. In order for many drugs to be effective, their concentration at the site of action must be maintained above a certain level at all times. How is this generally achieved?
A. The drug is administered concurrently with a second drug that has a stronger affinity for the plasma protein to which both drugs are bound.
B. The drug is administered parenterally.
C. The drug is given frequently, at least three times daily.
D. Another dose is administered before the complete removal of the previous dose.
4. A drug that exactly produces the actions of a natural body substance when it binds to its receptor is called:
A. A biotransformer
B. An inhibitor
C. An agonist
D. An antagonist
5. What two organs are most often involved in deactivating drugs and eliminating them from the body?
A. Small intestine and lung
B. Liver and kidney
C. Liver and lung
D. Brain and small intestine
6. Which method of oral administration should be used only if there is no other feasible route?
A. Administration in the drinking water
B. Liquid
C. Tablet
D. Paste
7. Meticulous technique and needle placement are essential when giving intramuscular injections because of the risk of:
A. Accidental injection into a blood vessel
B. Accidental injection into a nerve
C. Introduction of infection into the animal
D. All of the above
8. Injecting certain drugs too rapidly into a vein can lead to death.
A. True
B. False
9. Concerning the autonomic nervous system, which statement is true?
A. The neurotransmitter norepinephrine is degraded by the enzyme acetylcholinesterase.
B. Acetylcholine produced by the parasympathetic nervous system produces a fight-or-flight response

that increases the heart rate and dilates the bronchioles.
C. Alpha and beta receptors are part of the parasympathetic nervous system.
D. Drugs affecting the autonomic nervous system may mimic or block all or selected effects of the neurotransmitter, or they may alter the synthesis, storage, release, degradation, or uptake of the transmitter.

10. Which pair of agents has the most similar effects?
    A. Anticholinergics and sympathomimetics
    B. Anticholinergics and cholinomimetics
    C. Sympathomimetics and sympatholytics
    D. Sympatholytics and anticholinergics

11. The common signs of organophosphate overdose in animals—miosis, salivation, breathing difficulties, vomiting, defecation, and muscle fasciculations—are due to the chemical's:
    A. Anticholinergic effects
    B. Anticholinesterase effects
    C. Sympathomimetic effects
    D. Beta-receptor effects

For the next 10 questions, classify each autonomic drug according to its function. A classification can be used more than once.
    A. Anticholinergic
    B. Neuromuscular blocker
    C. Sympathomimetic
    D. Tranquilizer
    E. Alpha$_2$-andrenergic agonist
    F. Opioid analgesic
    G. Corticosteroid
    H. Diuretic
    I. Cardiac glycoside
    J. Nonsteroidal antiinflammatory drug
    K. Angiotensin-converting enzyme (ACE) inhibitor
    L. Antiarrhythmic
    M. Anticonvulsant

12. Prednisone
13. Acepromazine
14. Butorphanol
15. Furosemide
16. Digoxin
17. Atropine
18. Flunixin meglumine
19. Diltiazem
20. Guaifenesin
21. Phenylbutazone
22. A popular anti-motion-sickness agent for dogs and cats is _____, which is classified as a(n) _____.
    A. Xylazine; alpha$_2$-andrenergic agonist
    B. Xylazine; sympathomimetic
    C. Acepromazine; phenothiazine tranquilizer
    D. Acepromazine; alpha$_2$-andrenergic agonist

23. Concerning the narcotic agonists, which statement is true?
    A. Their pharmacologic effects can be reversed by administration of a narcotic antagonist.
    B. They are the most potent analgesic drugs available.
    C. They can cause excitement in cats and horses.
    D. All of the above

24. Immunizations should *not* be given during corticosteroid therapy due to the potential for inadequate immune response.
    A. True
    B. False

25. Antiinflammatory agents:
    A. Reduce pain caused by inflammation.
    B. Increase blood pressure.
    C. Stop seizures.
    D. A and C

26. As a veterinary technician, you must be especially vigilant with a patient taking _____ because even slight carelessness in calculations, administration, or observation of the patient can lead to death.
    A. Prednisone
    B. Furosemide
    C. Enrofloxacin
    D. Digoxin

27. Toxicities, sometimes fatal, have occurred with higher doses of this drug in pure Collie breeds.
    A. Ivermectin
    B. Pyrantel
    C. Milbemycin
    D. Piperazine

28. In dogs, _____ can be used once monthly to prevent heartworm infestation, while _____ is an injectable agent used to treat existing heartworm disease.
    A. Milbemycin; melarsomine dihydrochloride
    B. Melarsomine dihydrochloride; milbemycin
    C. Diethylcarbamazine; doramectin
    D. Doramectin; diethylcarbamazine

29. Concerning the treatment of tapeworms in dogs and cats with praziquantel and epsiprantel, which statement is most accurate?
    A. These are currently the most popular drugs used to treat tapeworms.
    B. Both drugs are relatively toxic.
    C. Both drugs have a narrow margin of safety, and even minor overdoses can cause severe liver toxicity.
    D. B and C

30. These topical insecticides, whose natural compound originates from the extract of a flower, come in a variety of formulations, are relatively nontoxic to pets, and are known for their quick "knockdown" effect.
    A. Cephalosporins
    B. Chlorinated hydrocarbons
    C. Pyrethrins
    D. Calcium-channel blockers

Copyright © 2006 by Elsevier, Inc. All rights reserved.

For the next four questions, classify each of the following once-a-month agents according to the description given.
- A. Lufenuron
- B. Imidacloprid
- C. Selamectin
- D. Fipronil

31. Topical formulation that kills only adult fleas and ticks
32. Topical flea larvicide and adulticide; shampooing may shorten the duration of flea protection
33. Oral and injectable insect-development inhibitor that controls flea populations by breaking the life cycle at the egg stage
34. Topical agent for use in the prevention of heartworm disease and in the control of fleas, ear mites, sarcoptic mange, canine tick infestation, and feline intestinal hookworm and roundworm infections
35. Which statement concerning antibiotic therapy is most accurate?
    - A. Indiscriminate choice of antibiotics and inadequate doses or treatment lengths can lead to microbial resistance to the antibiotic used.
    - B. Each antibiotic is effective against specific groups of organisms.
    - C. Antibiotics are substances that kill or inhibit the growth of microorganisms, including bacteria.
    - D. All of the above
36. Bacteria are classified as either gram positive or gram negative based on their ability to absorb gentian violet dye into their cell walls.
    - A. True
    - B. False

Listed below are the names of six antibiotics followed by the group in which they belong. For the next six questions, match each antibiotic with its characteristics.
- A. Gentamicin (aminoglycosides)
- B. Enrofloxacin (quinolones)
- C. Chloramphenicol
- D. Tetracycline (tetracyclines)
- E. Tilmicosin (macrolides)
- F. Nitrofurazone (nitrofurans)

37. This antibiotic is potentially ototoxic (disturbs hearing or balance) and nephrotoxic (toxic to kidneys).
38. This agent can cause a rare but potentially fatal blood disease in humans; therefore, direct contact with the drug should be absolutely avoided.
39. This agent should *not* be administered to young animals because it can cause tooth discoloration.
40. Administration of this antibiotic to rapidly growing animals should be limited due to this drug's potential ability to disrupt cartilage formation.
41. This bovine-only antibiotic should be administered only by subcutaneous or intramuscular routes because intravenous dosing has caused fatalities.
42. Due to this drug's potential carcinogenicity, the U.S. Food and Drug Administration has restricted its use in food animals to topical only.
43. Insulin doses must be measured and administered with the utmost care because an overdose can lead to life-threatening hyperglycemia.
    - A. True
    - B. False
44. Antiemetics:
    - A. Induce vomiting.
    - B. Prevent vomiting.
    - C. Soften the stool.
    - D. Treat diarrhea.
45. Sucralfate and omeprazole are both used in the treatment of gastric ulcers. Which statement is true concerning their mode of action?
    - A. Sucralfate works much like antacids by neutralizing stomach acid to increase gastric pH, while omeprazole adheres to damaged mucosa and creates a protective, adhesive-bandage-like barrier.
    - B. Sucralfate adheres to damaged mucosa and creates a protective, adhesive-bandage-like barrier, while omeprazole works much like antacids by neutralizing stomach acid to increase gastric ph.
    - C. Sucralfate adheres to damaged mucosa and creates a protective, adhesive-bandage-like barrier, while omeprazole acts on parietal cells to directly inhibit gastric acid secretion.
    - D. Sucralfate acts on parietal cells to directly inhibit gastric acid secretion, while omeprazole adheres to damaged mucosa and creates a protective, adhesive-bandage-like barrier.
46. A 10% concentration of solution contains:
    - A. 10 g of drug per 100 ml of solution
    - B. 1 g of drug per 100 ml of solution
    - C. 100 g of drug per 1000 ml (1 L) of solution
    - D. A and C
47. What will the units of your final answer be for the following problem: How much of a 5% solution can be prepared from 100 ml of a 10% solution?
    - A. g (grams)
    - B. % (percent)
    - C. ml (milliliters)
    - D. g/ml
48. If 480 ml of 0.9% sodium chloride is to be infused intravenously over 24 hours, what is the correct infusion rate if the set delivers 60 drops/ml?
    - A. 20 drops/min
    - B. 200 drops/min
    - C. 480 drops/min
    - D. 1200 drops/min

49. Concerning the veterinary hospital's pharmacy, which statement is most accurate?
    A. Ideally, the quantities of each item stocked should be as large as possible but still fit into the space allocated.
    B. One may purchase supplies through veterinary-wholesale suppliers (distributors) or directly from manufacturers.
    C. Using the services of a retail, human pharmacy is seldom required in the practice of high-quality veterinary medicine.
    D. Borrowing seldom-used drugs from another veterinary clinic in an emergency is not only discouraged as unprofessional, it can be illegal in some instances.
50. Which statement is true concerning veterinary use of controlled substances?
    A. A controlled substance is a substance of high abuse potential for which detailed written records of amounts used and amounts on hand are required.
    B. The law states that controlled substances must be kept in a "securely locked, substantially constructed cabinet or safe."
    C. The controlled substances used medically are designated on the label by the letter C with a roman numeral inside the C.
    D. All of the above
51. Certain states mandate the use of childproof containers to dispense oral pharmaceuticals.
    A. True
    B. False
52. Concerning the Occupational Safety and Health Administration's requirement for Material Safety Data Sheets (MSDS) for the chemicals to which workers are exposed, which statement is most accurate?
    A. MSDS are only available for hazardous chemicals.
    B. Only veterinary hospitals with more than 10 employees are required MSDS on file.
    C. Hazardous ingredients, flammability, and explosive- and health-hazard data are among the essential parts of an MSDS.
    D. All of the above.
53. Placing the expiration date on medications is optional for the manufacturer but strongly recommended by the FDA.
    A. True
    B. False
54. Which of the following statements is true?
    A. Although the veterinarian makes the decision to use a compounded product, it is the manufacturer of the individual drug components who is responsible for the safety of animals that take the compounded drugs.
    B. No written prescription is required by pharmacists who compound drugs.
    C. When drug products are compounded, distributed, and used, there is a possibility of harm to public health and animals if there is no adequate and well-controlled safety and effectiveness data.
    D. Veterinarians may not compound medications for their own patient use.
55. Examples of nutraceuticals used in veterinary medicine include:
    A. Omega-3 fatty acids
    B. Glucosamine/chondroitin sulfate
    C. Antioxidants
    D. All of the above
56. Which of the following statements is/are true?
    A. The FDA requires that manufacturers of nutraceuticals provide evidence that their products are stable enough to withstand extreme temperatures and prolonged storage.
    B. A number of side effects of their use has been identified, but not passed on to the consumer.
    C. Some nutraceuticals are naturally toxic to certain species and breeds of animals.
    D. All of the above.
    E. B and C
    F. A and C
57. Medications dispensed that are considered unsafe for laypersons to administer without monitoring by a licensed veterinarian are called _____ drugs and bear the "caution" sign, which restricts the use of the drug.
    A. Controlled
    B. Compounded
    C. Counterfeit
    D. Legend
58. This certification identifies to the public those online pharmacy sites that are appropriately licensed and legitimately operating over the Internet.
    A. FDA
    B. NABP
    C. VIPPS
    D. USP
59. When should the consumer suspect that an Internet pharmacy is illegitimate?
    A. If it contacts the prescriber to obtain a valid verbal prescription
    B. When it does not have a toll-free number and street address posted to the Web site
    C. If it does not advertise the availability of a registered pharmacist for consultation
    D. B and C
60. At work, you notice that the veterinarian often doses geriatric pets only once a day with a drug that is given twice daily to most other patients. What is the most likely reason she does this? Be specific.

61. List three common uses for the drug atropine.

Use the following drug-dosage problem to answer the next two questions. A 2-lb ferret is to receive a drug dosage of 10 mg/kg body weight. The drug is supplied at a concentration of 30 mg/ml.

62. What is the approximate weight of the ferret in kilograms?
63. How many milliliters of the supplied drug are required?
64. List the information required on a prescription label for a legend (prescription) drug in your state.

EXTRA CREDIT

65. *Syncope* is:
    A. A sympathomimetic agent
    B. Breathing deeply
    C. Fainting
    D. A tranquilizer commonly used in show horses to help them cope with the stress in the judging arena

CHAPTER 22

SURGICAL INSTRUMENTS AND ASEPTIC TECHNIQUE

1. *Trocar, sleeve, blunt obturator, triangulation,* and *light cable* are all terms used in:
    A. Orthopedic surgery
    B. Ophthalmologic surgery
    C. Arthroscopic surgery
    D. Dermatologic surgery
2. Which of the following are heavy operating scissors with a straight or curved blade used to cut tough tissue?
    A. Metzenbaum
    B. Bard-Parker
    C. Lister
    D. Mayo
3. Needle holders are designed for:
    A. Holding curved suture needles
    B. Performing instrument suture ties
    C. Bending or twisting wire suture
    D. A and B
4. _____ thumb forceps do not have teeth and are used exclusively for applying and removing dressings.
    A. Brown-Adson
    B. Dressing
    C. Cooley and DeBakey
    D. Adson
5. You are assisting a bovine practitioner with the repair of a left-displaced abomasum. He asks you to hand him the Rochester-Ochsner forceps. You hand him:
    A. A large, crushing forceps with longitudinal grooves along its length and cross-grooves at the tips
    B. A large, transversely grooved forceps
    C. A large, transversely grooved forceps with interdigitating teeth at the tips
    D. A small, curved, transversely grooved forceps
6. Dr. B asks you to hand her the "Gelpi's" while surgically repairing a diaphragmatic hernia. What is she asking for?
    A. Retractors
    B. Scissors
    C. Stapler
    D. Electrocautery
7. The major disadvantage of using stapling devices to cut or close tissue edges is they are much slower than traditional methods.
    A. True
    B. False
8. How are Michel skin clips removed?
    A. With wire-cutting suture scissors
    B. With a Senn retractor
    C. With rongeurs
    D. With the opposite end of the special forceps used to apply them

For the next four questions, match the piece of equipment used in orthopedic surgery with its description.
    A. External fixator
    B. Trephine
    C. Osteotome
    D. Rongeurs

9. This T-shaped, tubular instrument with a cylindrical cutting blade is usually used to remove a core of bone for biopsy.
10. This is a means of stabilizing a fracture using pins placed through the skin and bone.
11. This is a straight instrument with a blade on one end used to cut bone by pounding on the flared end of the handle with a mallet.
12. This has sharp, cupped tips used to cut small pieces of dense tissue such as bone, cartilage, or connective tissue.
13. Arthroscopy requires absolute asepsis, sterile technique, and a surgical scrub prior to the procedure.
    A. True
    B. False
14. Arthroscopy is used in veterinary medicine to examine and perform surgery on the:
    A. Joints of horses
    B. Sinuses of horses
    C. Joints of dogs
    D. All of the above

15. What type of fluid is most often used for arthroscopic procedures?
    A. Any sterile, balanced electrolyte solution
    B. 5% dextrose in water
    C. 50% dextrose in water
    D. 0.45% sodium chloride with 10 ml/L of chlorhexidine added
16. Which statement concerning instrument-pack preparation is true?
    A. After being rinsed, each instrument is scrubbed with an alkaline-pH instrument detergent.
    B. Instruments are placed in instrument "milk" for disinfection prior to sterilization.
    C. Each type of pack should be organized such that items are always placed in the same location in the tray.
    D. To allow for adequate steam penetration, packs should never be double-wrapped.
17. How do you tell the difference between a no. 3 and a no. 4 scalpel handle?
    A. Color
    B. Material from which it is made
    C. Size
    D. One is grooved and the other is smooth.
18. Most surgical instruments are made of
    A. Titanium
    B. Silver
    C. Chrome
    D. Stainless steel
19. Concerning drapes and gowns used in surgery, which statement is most accurate?
    A. Cloth drapes and gowns should be folded accordion style.
    B. Paper drapes and gowns are designed to be disposable and should be used only once.
    C. Cloth drapes and gowns are usually double-wrapped in paper or cloth prior to sterilization.
    D. All of the above.
20. Aseptic technique:
    A. Includes all steps taken to prevent contamination of the surgical site by infectious agents.
    B. Requires all people involved in patient care wash their hands thoroughly with an antibacterial soap between patients.
    C. Requires that all cages be cleaned and thoroughly disinfected between patients.
    D. B and C
21. Heat destroys bacteria through protein denaturation.
    A. True
    B. False
22. Dry heat kills by _____ and moist heat kills by _____.
    A. Coagulation of critical cellular proteins; damaging cellular DNA
    B. Coagulation of critical cellular proteins; protein oxidation
    C. Damaging cellular DNA; protein oxidation
    D. Protein oxidation; coagulation of critical cellular proteins
23. How does an autoclave raise the temperature of steam to the high levels required for sterilization?
    A. Increased time of exposure
    B. Increased pressure
    C. Liquid chemicals added to the steam
    D. Gaseous chemicals added to the steam
24. Which practice helps ensure adequate steam penetration in the autoclave?
    A. Stacking packs on top of each other
    B. Keeping pack size smaller than 30 × 30 × 50 cm
    C. Keeping pack weight below 5 kg
    D. Leaving less than 2 cm of space between packs and between the packs and autoclave walls
25. The safe, minimal standard for autoclave sterilization is:
    A. 101° C (213.8° F) for 9 minutes
    B. 121° C (249.8° F) for 13 minutes
    C. 141° C (285.8° F) for 15 minutes
    D. 161° C (321.8° F) for 19 minutes
26. The "flash" sterilization setting on the autoclave is used for:
    A. Emergency (very rapid) sterilization of instruments
    B. Items sensitive to heat, such as rubber and some plastics
    C. Motorized equipment such as orthopedic drills
    D. Cleaning the autoclave
27. After ethylene oxide sterilization, materials should be:
    A. Rinsed well in sterile, distilled water
    B. Quarantined in a well-ventilated area for at least 24 hours
    C. Packed closely in an air-tight cabinet
    D. Placed in an autoclave at 131° C (267.8° F) for 3 minutes
28. How is an antiseptic different from a disinfectant?
    A. The former is used in consumer cleaners and the latter in cleaners intended for hospital use only.
    B. The former kills only growing bacteria, while the latter kills growing bacteria, bacterial spores, and viruses.
    C. The former kills or inhibits infectious agents on living tissues and the latter on inanimate objects.
    D. The former is used only in soaps and the latter only in foams or liquids.

For the next four questions, match the chemical agent with its description.
    A. Alcohol
    B. Quaternary ammonium
    C. Chlorhexidine
    D. Povidone-iodine

29. One of the most popular agents used in veterinary medicine as a surgical scrub, this agent kills bacteria, viruses, fungi, protozoa, and yeast; yet it can be irritating to tissues.
30. This antiseptic and disinfectant is effective against bacteria, viruses, fungi, and yeast. It has a rapid onset and 2-day residual activity unaffected by organic matter and is nonirritating to tissues.
31. This disinfectant is effective against bacteria but not spores or some viruses and is very bland and nontoxic.
32. This antiseptic and disinfectant is bactericidal but does not kill spores or fungi, it has no residual effects, and it is both painful and cytotoxic when used in open wounds.
33. Which statement concerning cold sterilization is most accurate?
    A. Chloride compounds (bleach) are the most popular agents used for cold sterilization.
    B. Since sterility cannot be guaranteed, most cold-sterilized instruments should be used only for minor procedures.
    C. Exposure times should always exceed 30 minutes (except for arthroscopic equipment).
    D. Cold-sterilized instruments should never be rinsed prior to use.
34. _____ systems use a gas to sterilize items.
    A. Gas plasma sterilization
    B. Phenolic
    C. Ethylene oxide
    D. A and C
35. _____, the operating room should undergo a thorough cleaning that includes all permanent structures, floors, cabinets, and movable equipment.
    A. At the beginning of the surgery day
    B. At the end of the surgery day
    C. Once a week
    D. Once a month
36. A surgical site should be scrubbed and rinsed a minimum of _____ times.
    A. One
    B. Two
    C. Three
    D. Four

Use the information provided in the following scenario to answer the next two questions. You are asked to prepare "Brownie," a 6-month-old, brown-tabby domestic shorthair cat, for castration. He will be restrained in dorsal recumbency with his hind legs tied cranially to expose the scrotal region.

37. How do you prepare his scrotum?
    A. Shave with a No. 40 clipper blade and perform a surgical scrub.
    B. Shave with a safety razor and perform a surgical scrub.
    C. Pluck hair and perform a surgical scrub.
    D. Leave hair on the scrotum and perform a surgical scrub.
38. *Dorsal recumbency* means Brownie is:
    A. On his back (face up)
    B. On his sternum (face down)
    C. On his head
    D. On his tail
39. Surgical caps and masks should always be worn during surgery.
    A. True
    B. False
40. A surgeon's or surgical assistant's initial surgical scrub _____ their hands and arms and should involve a skin-soap contact time of _____ minutes.
    A. Disinfects; 10
    B. Sterilizes; 10
    C. Disinfects; 5
    D. Sterilizes; 5
41. Which of the following statements is true?
    A. Disadvantages of using surgical lasers include some hemostasis and possibly less postoperative swelling and pain.
    B. Special glasses must be worn by everyone in the room and care must be taken to avoid ignition of combustible materials.
    C. Advantages include shorter healing times.
    D. Surgical lasers should not be used to ablate (destroy) tissue.
42. The total hip prosthesis consists of a long stem that fits inside the proximal _____; a special cup replaces the _____.
    A. Femur; femoral head
    B. Humerus; acetabulum
    C. Femur; greater trochanter
    D. Femur; acetabulum
43. Gloved hands may be rested on a sterile drape or clasped in front of the body in the zone between the _____ and _____.
    A. Chin; waist
    B. Shoulders; hips
    C. Shoulders; waist
    D. Armpits; waist
44. Which of the following statements is false?
    A. Draping must be performed by personnel who have scrubbed in
    B. Draped tables and instrument trays are considered to be sterile only on top of the draped surface.
    C. The first layer of draping can be performed by nonsterile assistants.
    D. It is recommended to use two layers of drapes—four quarter drapes and a large drape that covers the entire animal and instrument table.

45. The outer wrap of an instrument pack may be opened by the surgeon or a nonsterile assistant.
    A. True
    B. False
46. The inner wrap of an instrument pack may be opened by the surgeon or a nonsterile assistant.
    A. True
    B. False
47. You are asked to order four pairs of new towel clamps and have a choice between two types. Name the type you choose and give one reason for your choice.
48. What is the difference between sterilization and disinfection?
49. List four types of sterilization indicators used in autoclaves.
50. Name the two methods of gloving for surgery.
51. Why are masks worn during surgery? Be specific.

EXTRA CREDIT

52. The term *scrub in* refers to:
    A. The process of clipping and washing a site on an animal in preparation for surgery at that site
    B. Preparing oneself to perform or assist in surgery
    C. The process of sterilizing instruments
    D. What a technician is doing while washing a dirty animal
53. In arthroscopic surgery, "burrs" are:
    A. The pumps used to deliver fluids to the surgical site
    B. Used to grasp and remove osteochondral chip fragments
    C. Often referred to as a *motorized arthroplasty system*
    D. Removed from the animal's coat before the procedure

CHAPTER 23

SURGICAL ASSISTANCE AND SUTURE MATERIAL

1. The veterinary technician's role in surgery can include:
   A. Monitoring anesthesia
   B. Manipulating the instrumentation and tissues into position as a sterile assistant
   C. Performing minor surgical procedures such as castrations under direct veterinary supervision
   D. A and B
2. Sterile towels are attached around an incision, or sterile, plastic, adherent drapes are applied to the skin after the surgical scrub, to prevent contamination of deeper tissues from the nonsterile:
   A. Skin
   B. Surgical instruments
   C. Laparotomy sponges
   D. Surgeon's gloves
3. A skin incision made with _____ results in the most rapid healing and the least amount of scar formation.
   A. Sharp Metzenbaum scissors
   B. Sharp Mayo scissors
   C. A sharp scalpel blade
   D. An electroscalpel
4. Concerning assisting in hollow-organ surgery, which statement is most accurate?
   A. Doyen intestinal forceps are specifically designed to not damage the intestines regardless of how much they are tightened or how long they are left in place.
   B. When handling hollow organs, always use dry fingers to increase your grip strength and prevent the tissues from sliding through your fingers.
   C. The surgeon places "stay" sutures and the suture ends are held up by the assistant to prevent the leakage of inner-organ contents.
   D. All of the above
5. One of the most important things to remember as a sterile surgical assistant is to handle tissues as gently as possible because they are very fragile.
   A. True
   B. False
6. For which procedure would it be most beneficial to count the gauze sponges used for hemostasis (stopping bleeding)?
   A. Feline declawing procedure
   B. Adult canine tail amputation
   C. Equine castration
   D. Adult canine ovariohysterectomy (spay)
7. The correct technique to use when clamping bleeding vessels with hemostatic forceps is tips _____ initially, then direct the concave surface _____ for ligation (tying a knot with suture around the vessel).
   A. Horizontal; up
   B. Horizontal; down
   C. Vertical; up
   D. Vertical; down
8. Always use the _____ of the scissors when cutting suture ends for the surgeon.
   A. Tips
   B. Middle
   C. Deepest portion
   D. Any of the above
9. To prevent patient injury, it is critical to _____ when the surgeon will be using electrosurgery with a unipolar handpiece.
   A. Not place a circulating warm-water pad under the patient
   B. Place a lubricated ground plate under the patient

C. Attach electrocardiographic leads to the patient
D. Monitor the patient's body temperature every 3 minutes

10. During surgery, the veterinarian asks you to remove the carbon built up on the tip of the electroscalpel. How is this done?
    A. It is rubbed off with sterile steel wool.
    B. It is wiped off with a solution specifically designed for that purpose.
    C. It is rubbed off with an alcohol-moistened gauze sponge.
    D. It is scraped off with a hard metallic edge such as a scalpel handle.

11. How can you tell by looking at an electroscalpel handpiece whether it is unipolar or bipolar?
    A. It is written on the handpiece.
    B. The former has a shiny metal surface and the latter a dull metal surface.
    C. The latter is shaped like thumb forceps.
    D. The former has two cords exiting it and the latter has one.

12. Gelatin sponge and cellulose gauze are used for:
    A. Hemostasis
    B. Bandaging
    C. Wound dressing
    D. Packing around cut skin edges during surgery

13. To make up an antiseptic irrigation solution for surgical lavage, add:
    A. 10 ml of chlorhexidine scrub to 1 L of normal saline (NS) or lactated Ringer solution (LRS)
    B. 10 ml of povidone-iodine solution to 100 ml of NS or LRS
    C. 10 ml of chlorhexidine solution to 1 L of NS or LRS
    D. B or C

14. Concerning irrigation solutions and suction during surgery, which statement is most accurate?
    A. Periodic suction of a clean irrigation solution during the surgical procedure will reduce the incidence of suction-tube plugging and will make cleaning the tube much easier.
    B. Multiple-fenestrated suction tips are used for small volumes of fluid, and single-orifice tips are used for large volumes of fluid.
    C. The irrigation solution should be at room temperature (21.1° C, or 70° F).
    D. Always apply the irrigation solutions with very little pressure, as when squeezing out a solution-soaked gauze sponge.

15. Penrose drains are thick-walled tubes made of hard rubber or Silastic.
    A. True
    B. False

16. Which element of proper operating-room conduct is designed specifically to reduce bacterial contamination of the incision?
    A. Placing the saline bowl either inside a sterile tray or on waterproof draping
    B. Anticipating the surgeon's needs
    C. Placing frequently used instruments on the front of the tray
    D. "Snapping" the instruments into the surgeon's open palm

17. The various types of suture materials are designed with specific characteristics, and the surgeon carefully chooses each according to its intended use.
    A. True
    B. False

18. Which suture material is least expensive?
    A. Surgical gut (catgut)
    B. Vicryl
    C. PDS
    D. Monocryl

19. One advantage of monofilament over multifilament suture is
    A. Better knot security
    B. Better handling characteristics
    C. Less chance of infection due to bacterial "wicking"
    D. The former is harder to pull through tissues

For the next five questions, place the suture material into the appropriate category.
    A. Synthetic absorbable
    B. Synthetic nonabsorbable
    C. Natural absorbable
    D. Natural nonabsorbable

20. Polymerized caprolactum (Vetafil)
21. Nylon
22. Surgical gut (catgut)
23. Stainless steel
24. Polydioxanone
25. The scientific name for Vicryl is:
    A. Polyglycolic acid
    B. Silk
    C. Polypropylene
    D. Polyglactin 910

26. Place the various sizes of suture in order from the smallest to the largest diameter:
    A. 1-0 < 6-0 < 1 < 2
    B. 6-0 < 1-0 < 1 < 2
    C. 1 < 2 < 1-0 < 6-0
    D. 2 < 1 < 1-0 < 6-0

27. Generally, _____ cannot tolerate autoclaving because it destroys the suture's strength.
    A. Surgical gut
    B. PDS
    C. Vicryl
    D. All of the above

28. You will be assisting in a cystotomy surgery during which bladder stones will be removed. Dr. S asks for 3-0 Dexon to suture the bladder but does not specify the type or shape of needle. What needle would be the least traumatic for suturing the bladder closed?
    A. Swaged reverse cutting
    B. Swaged taper
    C. French-eyed cutting
    D. Round-eyed reverse cutting
29. Cut skin-suture ends to _____ in length.
    A. 3 to 5 mm
    B. 5 to 10 mm
    C. 10 to 20 mm
    D. 20 to 30 mm
30. Which of the following precautions must the veterinary technician or surgical assistant take before and during surgery?
    A. In patients with intravenous/arterial catheters or blood pressure monitoring devices, ensure that adequate flow of fluids is maintained.
    B. Ensure that securing devices do not restrict respiratory function or apply excessive pressure on peripheral nerves, vessels, or muscles.
    C. Ensure that the surgical site is accessible for the surgeon and assistant.
    D. All of the above
31. Which of the following statements is/are *false*?
    A. Backhaus towel clamps are considered unsterile once they have penetrated the skin.
    B. For orthopedic or neurologic surgeries, spray adhesives should never be applied to skin because of the increased risk of joint infection.
    C. The assistant performing the draping procedure should stand at lease 15 inches away from the table border.
    D. A and C
32. For contaminated or oncologic surgeries, it is important to remember that:
    A. The surgeon might change gloves during the surgery.
    B. Suction devices should never be used.
    C. It is not necessary to use sterile instruments.
    D. Drapes should never be changed during surgery.
33. The sleeves of gowns are sterile from ___ cm above the ___ to the level of the ___.
    A. 3; elbow; shoulder
    B. 5; elbow; cuff
    C. 5; cuff; shoulder
    D. 3; cuff; elbow
34. After high-energy cutting, skin sutures or staples should remain in place 2 to 3 days longer compared to convention scalpel incisions.
    A. True
    B. False
35. Which of the following statements is true?
    A. Bipolar coagulation only works in a dry surgical field.
    B. Most electrosurgical units allow only coagulation functions.
    C. For a truly bloodless incision, using the monopolar mode, the handpiece is held in a modified pencil grip at an angle of approximately 30 degrees to the skin.
    D. Monopolar cautery only works in a dry surgical field.
36. How does bovine collagen provide hemostasis?
    A. It functions as a mechanical plug when pressed into bleeding body surfaces.
    B. It provides a lattice to which forming clots can adhere.
    C. It triggers clot formation via platelet aggregation and release of coagulation factors.
    D. It degrades platelets that aggregate at the site of clot formation.
37. What technique should always be used when applying gauze sponges for hemostasis?
38. List three reasons why a surgeon would place a drain to provide postoperative drainage of a surgical area.
39. List two reasons why the tissues surrounding a Penrose drain must be kept scrupulously clean.

EXTRA CREDIT

40. "Catgut" is suture material made from:
    A. Sheep intestines
    B. Plastic
    C. Cat whiskers
    D. Cat intestines
41. *Dehiscence* is:
    A. The removal of suture material from its sterile package
    B. The splitting open of a surgical wound
    C. The removal of a surgical drain
    D. The sound a snake makes as it's being anesthetized

CHAPTER 24

SMALL ANIMAL SURGICAL NURSING

1. An animal that has not been eating or drinking for some time before surgery may require a(n) ____ after rehydration because ____ of the cell volume occurs with rehydration.
    A. Splenectomy; sequestration
    B. Blood/plasma transfusion; dilution
    C. Upper gastrointestinal study; dilution
    D. Blood/plasma transfusion; hemoconcentration

2. Which of the following must be done before elective surgery can be performed on a small animal?
   A. Confirm that the patient has not eaten for 12 hours before surgery.
   B. Obtain the results of all preanesthetic screenings.
   C. Place a circulating, heated water blanket on the operating table.
   D. All of the above
3. Patients scheduled to under toe or ear surgery should never be given prophylactic antibiotics.
   A. True
   B. False
4. What procedure might be done if a patient that has undergone a spay procedure is suspected of hemorrhaging from the surgery site?
   A. Thoracocentesis
   B. Serum chemistry profile
   C. Abdominocentesis
   D. Complete blood count with differential
5. Which of the following statements is true?
   A. Electric heating pads are the most appropriate means of warming anesthetized patients.
   B. When the postoperative patient's body temperature approaches 95° F, heating sources can be discontinued.
   C. Heating lamps can cause thermal burns, especially in anesthetized patients who cannot respond to painful, concentrated heat.
   D. Heated circulating water blankets should never be used to warm anesthetized animals.
6. Indications of intra- and postoperative pain include:
   A. Decreased appetite
   B. Decreased blood pressure
   C. A and D
   D. Elevated heart rate
7. As a general rule in small animals, pain lasts for approximately ____ days after most soft tissue surgeries, and for approximately ____ days after bone or joint surgery.
   A. 4 to 5; 8 to 10
   B. 8 to 10; 4 to 5
   C. 1 to 2; 2 to 4
   D. 5 to 10; 10 to 20
8. Seromas and hematomas that form postoperatively can be treated with:
   A. Drainage
   B. Warm compresses
   C. Hydrotherapy
   D. All of the above
9. Postoperative incision infections and cellulitis can be treated with:
   A. Aspiration
   B. Ice packs
   C. Systemic antibiotics
   D. Bandaging
10. Using inappropriate suture to close a wound, inappropriate suture techniques, incision infection, seroma formation, tension on the incision line, and disease or drug therapy leading to delayed wound healing can all contribute to ____ after abdominal surgery.
    A. Wound dehiscence
    B. Evisceration
    C. Pneumothorax
    D. A and B
11. ____ is/are caused by serum seeping through a bandage on a limb and extending to the external environment and can bead to wound ____.
    A. Strike-through; infection
    B. Strike-through; evisceration
    C. Cellulitis; infection
    D. Seromas; infection
12. Passive drains have an exit port for fluid to the environment.
    A. True
    B. False
13. Animals undergoing routine spay/neuter surgical procedures usually require ____ days of restricted activity.
    A. 5 to 7
    B. Approximately 21
    C. 10 to 14
    D. 30 to 35

Choose the surgical procedure to which each of the statements 14 to 35 refers. Procedures may be selected more than once, but each statement has only one correct answer.
   A. Onychectomy
   B. Pelvic limb amputation
   C. Enterotomy
   D. Diaphragmatic hernia
   E. Inguinal hernia
   F. Feline castration
   G. Cystotomy
   H. Resection and anastomosis
   I. Dewclaw removal
   J. Long bone fracture repair
   K. Ovariohysterectomy
   L. Urethrostomy
   M. Caesarean section
   N. Gastric-dilatation volvulus
   O. Neurologic procedures
   P. Canine castration
   Q. Mammary neoplasia
14. This procedure is performed during the first week of life and is beneficial to hunting dogs that run over densely shrubbed terrain.
15. This is performed when a devitalized section of intestine is removed.
16. This is often performed for abdominal masses of unknown origin.

17. As much preoperative work as is possible should be done before the patient is anesthetized and while the patient is in lateral recumbency.
18. Scrotal swelling is a major concern and castration and scrotal ablation are recommended in intact dogs.
19. Pyometra, metritis, and endometrial hyperplasia may be treated with this procedure.
20. Some dogs experience infertility after this procedure because of scar formation.
21. The goal of surgery is to have permanent adhesions between the stomach and the body wall.
22. Severe respiratory compromise may result when the animal is placed in dorsal recumbency; sometimes holding the animal gently with the head up and the rear legs hanging down will allow some abdominal contents to shift back into the abdomen.
23. The most common late postoperative complication is stricture, generally manifested as stranguria.
24. Owners should be told that these can develop bilaterally even if the condition is not present yet on the opposite side at the time of presentation.
25. Approximately 80% to 90% are malignant in cats and these tend to metastasize to the lungs and lymph nodes.
26. The tourniquet must be placed distal to the elbow.
27. Scrotal hairs are gently plucked from the scrotum with thumb and finger.
28. Postoperatively, decubital ulcers, urinary bladder infections, muscle atrophy, pneumonia, and gastrointestinal ulceration are possible complications.
29. Trocharization may need to be performed behind the last rib on the right.
30. This procedure can be performed to treat perianal and anal tumors, perineal hernias, and testicular tumors.
31. Some animals experience renal dysfunction secondary to accidental ureteral ligation.
32. During the first 48 to 72 hours postoperatively, a mild hematuria with or without clots and frequent urination can be expected.
33. The surgical assistant helps by performing muscle retraction, muscle fatigue, alignment and reduction, and suction of the field.
34. The stomach must be decompressed to help stabilize the animal and decrease the chance of gastric wall necrosis.
35. This is often done to remove a foreign body from the intestines.
36. If an intervertebral disk has already ruptured, this procedure might be performed to alleviate compression on the spinal cord.
    A. Intervertebral disk fenestration
    B. Decompression
    C. Ankylosis
    D. Traction and reduction
37. At the end of most fenestration procedures, bone is placed over the spinal cord in the defect to prevent restrictive scar formation.
    A. True
    B. False
38. Vomitus that contains coffee-grounds-like material is indicative of ____.
    A. Dehydration
    B. Diaphragmatic hernia
    C. Pyloric outflow obstruction
    D. Gastric bleeding secondary to ulcer formation
39. What is the best form of therapy for pressure sores?
    A. Prevention
    B. Antibiotics
    C. Massages
    D. Surgical debridement
40. Generally, the patient is placed in ____ for repair of tibia-fibula fractures.
    A. Lateral recumbency, affected leg up
    B. Ventral recumbency, affected leg up
    C. Dorsal recumbency, affected leg down
    D. Lateral recumbency, affected leg down

EXTRA CREDIT

41. Explain why retractors should not directly contact cartilage during joint surgery.
42. Name three procedures that require the use of shredded paper instead of litter for several days postoperatively.

CHAPTER 25

SMALL ANIMAL MEDICAL NURSING

1. A low-sodium diet is most often indicated in the treatment of:
    A. Bladder disease
    B. Pancreatic disease
    C. Liver disease
    D. Heart disease
2. An animal with decreased skin turgor (skin "tents" when pinched), eyes sunken into its orbits, prolonged capillary refill time, and dry mucous membranes is:
    A. Mildly dehydrated (5% to 6%)
    B. Moderately dehydrated (6% to 8%)
    C. Severely dehydrated (10% to 12%)
3. When evaluating an adult feline admitted with an upper respiratory infection, you discover a low body temperature of 36.6° C (98° F). Yesterday it was 38.8° C (102° F). The first thing to do is:
    A. Tell the veterinarian.
    B. Take his temperature again to verify the reading.

    C. Fill some examination gloves with warm water and place them, along with some extra blankets, around him.
    D. Place him on a heating pad.
4. For which procedure is it important to obtain the owner's permission?
    A. Clipping or removing hair for medical reasons
    B. A cleanup bath prior to sending the animal home after prolonged boarding or hospitalization
    C. Supplementing an animal showing respiratory distress with oxygen in order to save her life
    D. Trimming the nails while a pet is anesthetized or sedated
5. A 10-year-old boarding cat does not eat her breakfast on the first day of her stay. What is an appropriate first action to take?
    A. Try force-feeding her.
    B. Tell the veterinarian.
    C. Try talking to her to encourage her to eat or hand-feed her.
    D. Remove the food from the cage for the day and refeed her in the evening when she is hungrier.
6. Force-feeding an adult patient is usually accomplished with:
    A. A red rubber feeding tube and a commercial puppy or kitten milk-replacement formula
    B. A syringe and prescription diet specifically formulated for hospitalized pets
    C. Boluses of a high-calorie supplement (such as Nutri-Cal) placed on the roof of the patient's mouth with the finger
    D. A syringe and canned version of the patient's regular diet
7. Which statement concerning nail trimming is most accurate?
    A. It is never necessary to trim a cat's nails.
    B. Nail trimming in dogs and cats is considered a medical procedure, and therefore should not be performed by owners at home.
    C. Place a pressure bandage on the paw for 5 to 10 minutes to stop bleeding from a nail cut too short.
    D. To avoid cutting pigmented canine nails too short, hold the cutting surface of the nail trimmer parallel to the palmar (or plantar) surface of the digital footpad.
8. Place the following steps of a basic ear cleaning in the correct order: (1) apply ceruminolytic; (2) pluck hair; (3) lavage with a bulb syringe; and (4) dry ear.
    A. 4, 1, 3, 2
    B. 4, 3, 2, 1
    C. 2, 1, 3, 4
    D. 1, 3, 2, 4

9. If the tympanic membrane (eardrum) cannot be visualized, clean and flush the ears only with:
    A. Povidone-iodine diluted with sterile saline and warmed
    B. Chlorhexidine diluted with sterile saline and warmed
    C. Normal saline
    D. Any of the above
10. Normal anal sac secretions are:
    A. Off white or brown and foul smelling
    B. Clear mucus without odor
    C. Brown with red streaks or reddish-brown and foul smelling
    D. White or cream colored without odor
11. Cat litter in pans of hospitalized patients should be changed:
    A. Once a week
    B. Every 3 days
    C. Every other day
    D. Every day
12. Hospitalized or boarding dogs should generally be exercised or walked at least:
    A. Every other day
    B. Once a day
    C. Twice a day
    D. Three times a day
13. Scalding due to urine or diarrhea is best prevented by:
    A. Application of a protective compound such as petroleum jelly
    B. Frequent sponging with diluted povidone-iodine
    C. Frequent washing with water and a gentle cleanser
    D. Placing absorbent padding under the patient
14. Geriatric patients acting aggressively should be evaluated for:
    A. Chronic pain
    B. Decreased hearing
    C. Decreased vision
    D. All of the above
15. How often should orphaned puppies and kittens be fed in the first 2 to 3 weeks of life?
    A. Every 2 hours
    B. Every 4 to 8 hours
    C. Two times daily
    D. Once daily
16. Which statement concerning obtaining a body temperature is true?
    A. Human thermometers will give inaccurate readings in the dog and cat.
    B. Placing the thermometer in the axilla or ear canal for several minutes will give a reading equal to a rectal temperature.
    C. Mercury glass thermometers should always be cleaned in hot water.

D. Thermometers using an infrared beam focused on the eardrum give accurate (rectal temperature) readings.

17. The feline pulse is most commonly palpated over the:
    A. Proximal, medial thigh
    B. Ventral jaw
    C. Tongue
    D. Central pinna (ear flap)
18. Which finding is normal in the dog?
    A. Sinus arrhythmia
    B. Pulse deficit
    C. Hyperpnea
    D. Tachycardia
19. A vomiting patient generally should *not* receive medication:
    A. Intravenously
    B. Intramuscularly
    C. Subcutaneously
    D. Orally
20. The amount of fluids needed by an adult dog not losing extra fluid due to any disease is:
    A. 120 ml/kg/day
    B. 60 ml/kg/day
    C. 30 ml/kg/day
    D. 15 ml/kg/day
21. Which parameters can aid in assessing the hydration status (degree of hydration or dehydration) of a patient? (Select all that apply.)
    A. Body temperature
    B. Serum glucose
    C. Packed cell volume
    D. Total protein
    E. Body weight
    F. Urine specific gravity
    G. Liver enzymes (ALT, ALP, GGT)
    H. Central venous pressure
22. Which agent should never be given subcutaneously?
    A. Dextrose solutions with a concentration of greater than 2%
    B. Lactated Ringer's solution
    C. 0.9% sodium chloride
    D. 0.45% sodium chloride
23. How many units of heparin would you add to a 1-L bag of saline to prepare a standard solution of "heparinized saline"?
    A. 100
    B. 5000
    C. 10,000
    D. 20,000
24. Concerning the measurement of central venous pressure (CVP), which statement is most accurate?
    A. The CVP value is obtained with the animal in three standard positions.
    B. The three standard positions used for each CVP measurement are lateral and sternal recumbency and sitting.
    C. Suspect obstruction of the catheter if the manometer does not fluctuate 2 to 5 mm with respiration.
    D. A and B
25. Which of the following are examples of canine blood types?
    A. A, B, AB, O
    B. APB-1, APC-1, APD-1
    C. CEA-1, CEA-2, CEA-3
    D. None of the above because all dogs have the same blood type
26. Which statement concerning small-animal blood transfusions is true?
    A. Blood-borne parasites cannot be transmitted during blood transfusions.
    B. If multiple blood transfusions are required, blood-type cross-matching should be performed to determine donor-recipient compatibility.
    C. About 100 ml of blood can be safely drawn from a feline every 3 weeks.
    D. About 30 to 40 ml blood/kg body weight can be safely drawn from a 25-kg dog every 3 weeks.

For the next four questions, use the information provided in the following scenario. A 2-year-old Skye terrier needs a blood transfusion immediately to save his life. The hospital where you work maintains a nonpremise, canine universal blood donor. You find a previously obtained, unused bag of blood in the 5° C (41° F) refrigerator, collected using ACD anticoagulant, and dated "November 1." It is now November 10.

27. What do you do with the refrigerated blood?
    A. Discard it. It is outdated.
    B. Prepare to administer it as is.
    C. Warm it slowly to 37° C (98.6° F) in a warm-water bath.
    D. Heat it slowly to 50° C (122° F) in a hot-water bath.
28. How do you administer blood?
    A. Slowly and intravenously through a sterile blood-administration kit
    B. Rapidly and intravenously through a sterile blood-administration kit
    C. Slowly and intramuscularly through a sterile blood-administration kit
    D. Slowly and intravenously through a regular intravenous drip set
29. If you have to draw blood from the donor, from where will you draw it?
    A. Cephalic vein
    B. Femoral artery
    C. Cranial vena cava
    D. Jugular vein

30. If you used the bag of blood and had some left over, could you reuse the remaining blood on another day?
    A. Yes
    B. No
31. Which recipient of incompatible blood is most likely to have the most severe hemolytic (rupture of red blood cells) transfusion reaction?
    A. A first-time recipient
    B. A second-time recipient
    C. A third-time recipient
    D. A fourth-time recipient
32. Possible signs of a negative blood-transfusion reaction include:
    A. Vomiting, fast heart rate, and low blood pressure
    B. Salivation, muscle tremors, and fever
    C. Dry cough and respiratory distress
    D. All of the above
33. In the case of a mild transfusion reaction, the first thing to do is slow down the administration rate.
    A. True
    B. False
34. What should the owner of a diabetic patient receiving insulin be instructed to do if her pet has a seizure?
    A. Administer another dose of insulin and call the hospital immediately.
    B. Reduce the dose of insulin by half for the next dose.
    C. Administer corn syrup orally and call the clinic or emergency hospital immediately.
    D. Rush the animal to the emergency clinic without taking time to call first.
35. Use _____ for the early treatment of traumatic injuries, such as sprains, and _____ for the reduction of peripheral edema (limb swelling).
    A. Cold; massage
    B. Heat; cold
    C. Cold; heat
    D. Massage; heat
36. A treatment sheet states to "hot pack" an area twice daily. What is the best way to do this?
    A. Soak a cloth in very hot water, wring lightly, apply until it cools, and repeat. Treat for up to 20 minutes.
    B. Fill an examination glove with water as hot as you can stand, apply it to the area until it cools, and repeat. Treat for up to 20 minutes.
    C. Place a 1-L bag of intravenous fluids heated to body temperature on the area until it cools.
    D. Place a heating pad set on "medium" heat on or around the affected area for 20 minutes.
37. Therapeutic exercise of a weak or nonambulatory patient can be provided by:
    A. Assisted walking using a towel or sling around the abdomen to help support the body's weight
    B. A treadmill
    C. Swimming
    D. A and C
38. What term is applied to an animal needing oxygen supplementation?
    A. Anemic
    B. Hypoxic
    C. Hypoventilating
    D. Bradycardic
39. *Hypertrophic, dilated,* and *restrictive* are all forms of:
    A. Canine heart disease
    B. Feline heart disease
    C. Canine liver disease
    D. Feline liver disease
40. On an oxygen cage, the inspired oxygen concentration should be set at:
    A. 0.5 L/min
    B. 4 L/min
    C. 10% to 20%
    D. 30% to 40%
41. Percussion (coupage) is a technique that involves striking the animal's chest to loosen bronchial secretions and thus facilitate drainage.
    A. True
    B. False
42. Whenever possible, animals with lung problems should be maintained in:
    A. Sternal recumbency
    B. Right lateral recumbency
    C. Left lateral recumbency
    D. B or C

For the next three questions, match the shampoo ingredient with its common usage.
    A. Benzoyl peroxide
    B. Sulfur plus salicylic acid
    C. Tar plus sulfur
    D. Colloidal oatmeal
43. Treating oily, flaky seborrhea (dandruff)
44. Soothing skin and reducing pruritus (itching)
45. Treating dry, flaky seborrhea
46. How is a medicated bath performed differently from a cleansing bath?
    A. In the former, leave the shampoo on at least 15 minutes.
    B. In the former, cover more of the body, such as between the toes and on the face.
    C. Rinse more completely in the former.
    D. Do not dry with a towel in the former; place the pet directly in the cage under a dryer or in an outdoor run.
47. When treating ear mites with nonivermectin, topical, otic (ear) preparations, which statement is most accurate?
    A. All animals in the house must be treated.
    B. Treatment should continue for at least 3 weeks.

C. Gloves must be worn when instilling the medication into the ears.
D. A and B
48. "Yeast" are _____ often found on microscopic examination of ear wax.
A. Parasites
B. Fungi
C. Bacteria
D. Protozoa
49. The appetite can be enhanced in patients whose eyes and nose are obstructed with discharge by:
A. Frequent walking
B. Clearing the accumulated discharge from the eyes and nose
C. Placing them in an isolated ward
D. A and C
50. What measures will help prevent the spread of infectious respiratory disease in the hospital? (Select all that apply.)
A. Isolating affected (coughing, sneezing) animals
B. Using disposable food trays and litter boxes
C. Using autoclavable water bowls
D. Cleaning cages thoroughly with a dilute bleach solution
E. Moving animals frequently between cages
F. Having all personnel maintain meticulous hygiene of clothing and hands
51. Which often fatal canine infectious disease often begins with mucoid eye and nose discharge?
A. Parvovirus
B. Kennel cough
C. Canine distemper
D. Rabies
52. Feline leukemia is spread between cats primarily by _____ and feline immunodeficiency virus by _____.
A. Close contact; bite wounds
B. Scratches; bite wounds
C. Copulation; nursing
D. Nursing; close contact
53. As in large animals, kittens and puppies rely heavily on the ingestion of colostrum (first milk) to obtain protection from infectious diseases.
A. True
B. False
54. Vaccines given by the _____ route can produce mild clinical disease.
A. Subcutaneous
B. Intramuscular
C. Intranasal
D. A and C
55. Healthy geriatric dogs need *not* continue to be vaccinated yearly for certain diseases.
A. True
B. False

56. A vaccination may *not* protect a patient that has already been exposed to the disease.
A. True
B. False
57. Because corticosteroids suppress the immune system, vaccination of animals receiving them is usually ineffective.
A. True
B. False
58. What disease can infect personnel who accidentally ingest the urine of an infected dog even if the dog is vaccinated and showing no clinical signs of the disease?
A. Plague
B. Leptospirosis
C. Visceral larval migrans
D. Cutaneous larval migrans
59. In general, zoonotic diseases that cause diarrhea are spread to humans by accidental ingestion of infected
A. Feces
B. Urine
C. Blood
D. Saliva
60. There is a possibility that a cat with ___ is carrying a zoonotic disease; therefore, meticulous hygiene should be practiced when handling a cat with this problem.
A. Infected, draining lymph nodes
B. Vomiting
C. Otitis interna (inner ear infection)
D. An upper respiratory infection
61. Glaucoma is diagnosed with _____ that measures _____.
A. An ophthalmoscope; the density of the lens
B. A Schirmer tear strip; tear production
C. A tonometer; the pressure inside the eyeball
D. A slit lamp; anterior-chamber clarity
62. What is a cataract?
A. A focal or diffuse opacity within the lens
B. A normal aging change that decreases the clarity of the nucleus of the lens
C. A scratch on the cornea
D. An inward rolling of the eyelid
63. Fluorescein dye is most often used to diagnose:
A. Cataracts
B. Glaucoma
C. Nuclear sclerosis
D. Corneal ulcers or scratches
64. Eye pain or corneal cloudiness should be considered a medical emergency.
A. True
B. False

For the next three questions, match the dermatologic test with the equipment required to perform it.
A. Fungal culture
B. Deep skin scraping for mites
C. Superficial skin and hair scraping for dermatophytes (ringworm)

65. Saline, scalpel blade, microscope slide, coverslip, potassium hydroxide (KOH), a heat source, microscope
66. Mineral oil, scalpel blade, microscope slide, coverslip, microscope
67. Sterile scalpel blade, sterile forceps, alcohol swab, dermatophyte test medium (DTM)
68. *Congestive heart failure* is the clinical term used to describe:
    A. A heart that beats with an irregular rhythm
    B. A heart unable to maintain adequate cardiac output
    C. A heart that has stopped beating
    D. A build-up of fluid in the lungs due to heart disease
69. The most frequently diagnosed form of heart disease in the dog is:
    A. Mitral valve insufficiency (leakage)
    B. Tricuspid valve insufficiency
    C. Aortic valve insufficiency
    D. Pulmonary valve insufficiency.

For the next two questions, use the information provided in the following scenario. "Lulu," a 6-year-old, recently adopted stray poodle was found to have heartworm disease. One week after adulticide treatment, her owner called to say she was coughing a lot, sometimes coughing up blood, and her appetite was down.

70. What is the most likely cause of Lulu's symptoms?
    A. Ineffective treatment (Some live heartworms still exist.)
    B. An allergic reaction to the treatment drug
    C. Pneumonia
    D. Dead heartworms lodging in the pulmonary arteries
71. What is the best way to prevent these symptoms?
    A. Treatment with ivermectin prior to adulticide treatment
    B. Exercise restriction 3 to 4 weeks after adulticide treatment
    C. Treatment with aspirin prior to adulticide treatment
    D. Steam or vaporizer treatment twice daily for 2 weeks after adulticide treatment
72. What two breeds of dogs are prone to their own breed-specific form of dilated cardiomyopathy (weak, diseased heart muscle)?
    A. Australian cattle dogs and Great Danes
    B. Kerry blue terriers and Skye terriers
    C. Doberman pinschers and boxers
    D. English pointers and German shorthair pointers

For the next three questions, match the endocrinologic disease with its description as given below.
    A. Hyperthyroidism
    B. Hypothyroidism
    C. Hyperadrenocorticism (Cushing disease)

73. This disorder results from the excessive production of cortisol by the adrenal cortex and is diagnosed using dexamethasone-suppression tests and adrenocorticotropic hormone (ACTH)-stimulation tests.
74. This disease is common in dogs, and the signs include oily seborrhea, hair loss, thickened skin, weight gain, lethargy, and cold intolerance. It is treated with oral thyroxine supplementation.
75. This is the most common endocrine disease affecting cats older than 8 years of age, and the signs include weight loss in spite of a good appetite, hyperactivity, restlessness, and diarrhea.
76. Cough, ascites (excess fluid in the abdominal cavity), crackles heard on lung auscultation, and pleural effusion (excess fluid in the thoracic cavity) are all common signs of:
    A. Renal failure
    B. Congestive heart failure
    C. Pancreatic failure
    D. B and C
77. Glucosuria (glucose in the urine) is normally seen in:
    A. Cats
    B. Dogs
    C. Cats and dogs
    D. None of the above
78. Ketonuria (ketones in the urine) is normally seen in:
    A. Cats
    B. Dogs
    C. Cats and dogs
    D. None of the above
79. Always administer insulin:
    A. Immediately after a meal
    B. Immediately before a meal
    C. Intramuscularly
    D. A and C
80. One sign of diabetes mellitus is _____, which is caused by a lack of _____ in the bloodstream.
    A. Weight gain; glucose
    B. High blood sugar; insulin
    C. Low blood sugar; glucagon
    D. Hair loss; cortisol
81. Which sign is considered normal in the postpartum bitch?
    A. Enlarged, painful mammary glands
    B. Weakness and trembling
    C. A foul-smelling, brown or reddish-brown vaginal discharge
    D. A greenish vaginal discharge without an odor
82. Pyometritis (pus in the uterus) is a cause of illness in the unspayed dog or cat.
    A. True
    B. False
83. Because dogs do *not* possess a prostate gland, prostatic disease is not seen in this species.
    A. True
    B. False

84. Concerning the feeding of a canine patient recovering from diarrhea, which statement is most accurate?
    A. Feed frequent, small meals for 2 to 3 days.
    B. Feed a commercial diet specifically formulated for gastrointestinal disease.
    C. Feed a bland, homemade diet consisting of one carbohydrate and one protein source, such as hamburger and rice.
    D. All of the above.
85. Which medication causes black stools?
    A. Metamucil
    B. Kaopectate
    C. Pepto-Bismol
    D. Imodium
86. A client treating her pet symptomatically for diarrhea at home should be encouraged to make an appointment if the signs persist longer than:
    A. 2 days
    B. 5 days
    C. 7 days
    D. 10 days
87. Which statement concerning canine parvovirus is most accurate?
    A. Parvovirus is easily diagnosed with an in-house test performed on feces.
    B. Puppies with parvovirus are not contagious and need not be isolated.
    C. Because parvovirus is very persistent in the environment, an agent with strong virucidal properties, such as diluted bleach, should be used for cleanup.
    D. A and C.
88. Bladder stones are treated with:
    A. Surgery
    B. Diet
    C. Nuclear medicine
    D. A and B
89. _____ is of the utmost importance when maintaining indwelling urinary catheters.
    A. Aseptic technique
    B. Suturing the catheter in so it does not fall out
    C. Placing an Elizabethan collar
    D. All of the above
90. _____ is one of the most important ways to prevent the recurrence of feline lower urinary tract disease.
    A. Chronic antibiotic administration
    B. Keeping cats indoors
    C. Increasing a cat's water intake
    D. Castration or ovariohysterectomy
91. Commercially prepared diets for severe renal disease are restricted in
    A. Protein
    B. Fat
    C. Carbohydrates
    D. Calcium
92. Hip dysplasia is:
    A. Hip pain caused by a fractured femoral neck
    B. A condition in which abnormal hip-joint development leads to hip pain and, later, hip arthritis
    C. A congenital disease in which puppies are born with abnormally formed hips and hip arthritis
    D. A bacterial arthritis of the hip caused by *Staphylococcus intermedius* that leads to chronic hip pain and joint stiffening later in life.
93. _____ can help prevent hip dysplasia in large breed dogs prone to the disease.
    A. Feeding puppies a lower-calorie diet
    B. Feeding puppies a high-calcium diet
    C. Administering corticosteroids
    D. Nothing
94. Treatment of hip dysplasia can include:
    A. Surgical repair
    B. Nontraumatic exercise, such as swimming
    C. Pain-reducing medications
    D. All of the above
95. It is best *not* to breed dogs with hip dysplasia because they can pass the disease on to their offspring.
    A. True
    B. False
96. Prior to cleaning the ears, a small amount of debris should be mixed in ____ and examined under low power magnification for the presence of *Otodectes*. Likewise, a small amount of debris should be smeared on a dry slide, stained, and examined for ____.
    A. Mineral oil; yeast and bacteria
    B. Diff-Quik solution; ear mites
    C. Mineral oil; ear mites
    D. Diff-Quik solution; yeast and bacteria
97. Signs of volume overload include:
    A. Pitting edema
    B. Chemosis
    C. Hyperpnea
    D. All of the above
98. How can inadvertent fluid overload be reduced?
    A. By using rapid bolus techniques so that the patient is observed during the whole course of fluid administration
    B. By using syringe pumps with cats and very small dogs
    C. By reassessing the patient frequently and adjusting the fluid rate as needed
    D. B and C
99. It is generally acceptable to mix multiple drugs in a syringe or intravenous fluid bag as long as precipitation is not noted.
    A. True
    B. False

100. Polyarthritis that occurs in cats after vaccination may be due to the ____ vaccine, and neurological signs such as seizure that occurs in dogs within a few weeks after vaccinations may be due to the ____ vaccine.
    A. Calicivirus; distemper
    B. Distemper; feline immunodeficiency virus
    C. Feline leukemia; rabies
    D. Calicivirus; bordetella
101. If severe, life-threatening reactions to vaccines occur, then the animal should never be vaccinated again.
    A. True
    B. False
102. List five basic necessities that the veterinary technician as nurse should provide for all animal inpatients.
103. You are asked to obtain vital signs on the cat in room. What do you obtain?
104. What should be recorded in the patient's record every time a drug is administered?
105. Why are a series of vaccinations provided to puppies and kittens, with the last dose no earlier than 16 weeks in dogs?
106. List two signs of hypoglycemia (low blood sugar).

EXTRA CREDIT

107. A three-way stopcock is:
    A. A valve that allows fluid or air to be directed three separate directions
    B. A type of syringe
    C. A device often used to aid in flushing ears
    D. Three ways to stop a rooster from crowing
108. A dog is experiencing "distichiasis" when she:
    A. Has ear mites
    B. Has reduced vision because of cataracts
    C. Has a double row of eyelashes that are turned against and irritating the eyeball
    D. Can't find the stick you threw for her
109. *Melena* is:
    A. Black stool caused by digested blood
    B. Inflamed mammary glands
    C. Diarrhea with mucus present
    D. A Portuguese watermelon

CHAPTER 26

EMERGENCY AND CRITICAL CARE NURSING

1. How often should inventory be taken of emergency drugs and equipment?
    A. Once a day
    B. Once a month
    C. Whenever someone has time to do it
    D. At each shift change
2. The ideal way to supply oxygen is with a flowmeter and Ambu bag.
    A. True
    B. False
3. What supplies must also be stored and used with endotracheal tubes?
    A. Supplies needed to secure the tube in place
    B. A clean, empty syringe to inflate the cuff
    C. Intravenous catheters
    D. A and C
    E. A and B
    F. All of the above
4. Although commercial bone marrow catheters are available, ___ and ___ can also be used for the same purpose.
    A. Red rubber catheter; 18- to 20-gauge hypodermic needle
    B. Spinal needle; 18- to 20-gauge hypodermic needle
    C. Small diameter polypropylene catheter; spinal needle
    D. Spinal needle; red rubber catheter
5. Examples of synthetic colloids include:
    A. Hetastarch; oxyglobin
    B. Oxyglobin; 0.9% saline solution
    C. Lactated Ringer's; hetastarch
    D. 0.9% saline solution; oxyglobin
6. What information can a blood smear provide?
    A. Platelet count estimate
    B. Packed cell volume
    C. Blood glucose
    D. Red cell morphology
    E. A, B, and D
    F. A and D
    G. B and D
7. Which of the following statements is *false*?
    A. The hemodynamic effects of crystalloids last longer than those of colloids.
    B. Approximately 25% of colloid fluids remain in the vascular space after 1 hour.
    C. Crystalloids are more expensive to use than colloids.
    D. Colloids are primarily isotonic and contain primarily water and sodium or glucose.
    E. All of the above.
    F. None of the above.
8. If a patient's total protein decreases by ___ or more of the initial value, or if hematocrit decreases to less than ___, a change in fluid type or rate of administration is warranted.
    A. 25%; 10%
    B. 50%; 20%
    C. 50%; 30%
    D. 30%; 20%
9. Calculate the replacement fluid volume for a 12-pound cat that is 5% dehydrated.
    A. Approximately 2.7 L
    B. Approximately 27 ml

C. Approximately 270 ml
D. Approximately 3 ml
10. The condition in which air becomes trapped between the body wall and the lung is called:
    A. Flail chest
    B. Subcutaneous emphysema
    C. Hemothorax
    D. Pneumothorax
11. Mannitol and furosemide are both ___ that are used to reduce increased intracranial pressure in the patient with head trauma.
    A. Diuretics
    B. Volume expanders
    C. Antiinflammatory agents
    D. Preload reducers
12. An animal that assumes a praying or play bowing position most likely has ___ pain.
    A. Musculoskeletal
    B. Thoracic
    C. Abdominal
    D. Neurologically induced
13. Untreated pain causes further stress and harmful physiologic changes.
    A. True
    B. False
14. Disseminated intravascular coagulation is primarily a disorder of the body's ___ function.
    A. Coagulation
    B. Neurological
    C. Hepatic
    D. Renal
15. Possible indicators of DIC include:
    A. Schistocytes and decreased platelet counts
    B. Petechiae and/or ecchymoses
    C. Edema and pale mucous membranes
    D. All of the above
    E. A and B
16. Transfusing whole blood is an excellent way to provide a large quantity of long-lasting platelets to a patient with DIC.
    A. True
    B. False
17. The most recognizable clinical signs of hyperdynamic shock include ___ and ___.
    A. Increased heart rate and increased cardiac contractility
    B. Increased respiratory rate and rapid capillary refill time
    C. Ischemia and increased heart rate
    D. Bounding pulses and brick-red (injected) mucous membranes
18. During the hypodynamic phase (uncompensated) of shock, blood flow is preferentially distributed to:
    A. Skin
    B. Brain and heart
    C. Kidneys and liver
    D. Muscles
    E. All of the above

For questions 19 through 24, indicate the category of shock being described by each statement. There is only one answer for each statement.
    A. Cardiogenic
    B. Septic
    C. Distributive
    D. Hypovolemic
    E. Obstructive

19. Blood pools in capillaries and veins and results in a decrease in effective blood volume.
20. Bacterial toxins escalate the inflammatory response and exacerbate tissue damage.
21. Common causes include heartworm disease, pulmonary thromboembolism, pulmonary hypertension, and pericardial disease.
22. A reduction in circulating blood volume may result from bleeding, dehydration, or effusive fluid loss (abdominal fluid accumulation).
23. Hyperglycemia may occur in the early stages due to the effects of stress hormones on metabolism.
24. This may result from valvular disease, cardiomyopathy, and cardiac arrhythmias.
25. Vasopressor drugs that may be used with caution in patients with refractory hypotension include:
    A. Dilantin
    B. Dopamine
    C. Diltiazem
    D. Dobutamine
    E. B and D
    F. A and C
    G. All of the above
26. When performing chest compressions on an animal that weighs greater than 15 lb, the animal should be placed in ___ recumbency.
    A. Lateral or ventral
    B. Dorsal or ventral
    C. Lateral or sternal
    D. Dorsal or lateral
27. When performing cardiac compressions on a dog that weighs 9 lb, what is the point of compression?
    A. Directly over the heart
    B. Over the eighth rib
    C. Over the widest part of the chest
    D. Directly over the sternum
28. What is the treatment of choice for ventricular fibrillation?
    A. Atropine and/or epinephrine with repeated doses
    B. Electrical defibrillation
    C. Lidocaine
    D. Atropine

29. What is the ideal route of drug administration when performing advanced life support?
    A. Intracardiac
    B. Intratracheal
    C. Jugular catheter or central vein catheter
    D. Peripheral
30. Which drugs can be administered via the intratracheal route?
    A. Atropine, lidocaine
    B. Dopamine, epinephrine
    C. Epinephrine, naloxone
    D. Corticosteroids, atropine
    E. None of the above
    F. A and B
    G. A and C
    H. B and D
31. Crystalloid or colloid fluids must always be administered during cardiopulmonary cerebrovascular resuscitation.
    A. True
    B. False
32. If a patient does not respond to CPCR within ___, continuation of the resuscitation effort is unlikely to succeed.
    A. 30 minutes
    B. 20 minutes
    C. 2 minutes
    D. 10 minutes
33. After performing CPCR on a dog, the animal develops opisthotonus with rigidity in all four limbs. Where is the lesion and what is the prognosis?
    A. Intervertebral disk; fair
    B. Cerebrum; poor
    C. Brainstem; fair
    D. Brainstem; grave

For questions 34 through 40, choose the drug that is described by each statement. There is only one correct answer for each statement.

34. At low doses, this drug increases renal perfusion in dogs; at high doses, it increases systemic blood pressure in dogs.
35. This drug is a used to manage acute renal failure and cerebral edema; it is a free-radical scavenger that may be useful to treat reperfusion injury.
36. This drug is used to treat severe acidosis.
37. These drugs may inhibit the release of arachidonic acid in cell membranes, thereby preventing inflammation.
38. This drug is used to treat ventricular tachycardia.
39. This diuretic may improve renal blood flow; it is used to treat kidney failure and pulmonary edema.
40. This synthetic catecholamine may maintain mean arterial blood pressure.
    A. Glucocorticoids
    B. Lidocaine
    C. Dopamine
    D. Dobutamine
    E. Sodium bicarbonate
    F. Mannitol
    G. Furosemide
41. Which of the following statements is/are true?
    A. Many variables affect the outcome and management of an arrested patient, including the underlying diseases and reason for arrest and the experience and equipment available to the resuscitation team.
    B. All body systems are affected by cardiopulmonary arrest.
    C. The postresuscitation patient requires tremendous nursing care and 24-hour monitoring.
    D. Successful resuscitation rates in veterinary medicine are approximately 10%.
    E. None of the above.
    F. All of the above.
42. _____ provides a means to measure the expired dioxide concentration of expired air, while _____ indicates a noninvasive measurement of the hemoglobin-oxygen saturation.
    A. Blood gas analysis; capnography
    B. Capnography; pulse oximetry
    C. Pulse oximetry; capnography
    D. Capnography; blood gas analysis
43. Arterial blood samples should be drawn from the femoral, dorsal pedal, or ___ artery.
    A. Cephalic
    B. Lingual
    C. Saphenous
    D. Caudal
44. Which of the following is not a clinical sign of hypoxemia?
    A. Decreased respiratory effort
    B. Cyanosis
    C. Hyperactivity
    D. Tachycardia
45. As a general rule of thumb, the Pa_{O_2} should be approximately ___ times the Fi_{O_2}.
    A. 10
    B. 250
    C. 3
    D. 5
46. When monitoring the critically ill patient, it is imperative to perform serial assessments and monitor trends.
    A. True
    B. False
47. Systolic values more than ___ mm Hg and diastolic values greater than ___ mm Hg are required to maintain adequate perfusion of vital organs (namely the kidneys and brain).
    A. 100; 70
    B. 80; 60

C. 120; 70
D. 90; 60
48. When selecting a cuff to use to indirectly measure a cat or dog's blood pressure, the ___ of the cuff should be approximately ___% of the circumference of the limb at the site of cuff placement.
   A. Length; 40
   B. Width; 30
   C. Diameter; 40
   D. Circumference; 30
49. Which of the following statements is/are false?
   A. Arterial catheters are flushed slowly and regularly to prevent clot formation.
   B. Common arteries catheterized to assess blood pressure are the femoral and dorsal pedal arteries.
   C. A systolic blood pressure over 150 mm Hg indicates hypertension.
   D. No medications should be administered through intraarterial catheters.
50. What is the most common use of the buccal mucosal bleeding time in small animals?
   A. To diagnose disseminated intravascular coagulation (DIC)
   B. To diagnose von Willebrand disease
   C. To determine the severity of heartworm disease
   D. To determine if a platelet transfusion is needed
51. The normal urine production for cats and dogs is
   A. 1 to 2 ml/kg/hr
   B. 2 to 4 ml/kg/hr
   C. 3 to 4 ml/kg/hr
   D. 5 ml/kg/hr
52. Early signs of increased intracranial pressure include:
   A. Bradycardia
   B. Fixed pinpoint pupils
   C. Seizures
   D. Coma
   E. Death
   F. All of the above
   G. None of the above
53. Before thoracocentesis can be performed, hair on the chest over ___ must be clipped and cleaned with surgical scrub.
   A. Rib spaces 7 through 9
   B. Rib spaces 4 through 10
   C. Rib spaces 5 through 10
   D. The sternum and xiphoid

EXTRA CREDIT

54. Name four ways to administer oxygen to an animal in an emergency situation.
55. A patient's blood pressure is 120/90. Ninety is the _____ and 120 is the _____.
   A. Systolic pressure; mean arterial pressure
   B. Diastolic pressure; systolic pressure
   C. Mean arterial pressure; systolic
   D. Diastolic; systolic

CHAPTER 27

TOXICOLOGY

1. The Internet is a safe, reliable source of information on toxicants and treatment of intoxications.
   A. True
   B. False
2. Drugs used in decontamination include:
   A. Apomorphine and xylazine
   B. Activated charcoal and syrup of ipecac
   C. Hydrogen peroxide and sorbitol
   D. All of the above
3. It should be assumed that any ___ is highly toxic until a mycologist identifies it.
   A. Plant
   B. Bean
   C. Mushroom
   D. Tree bark
4. Stabilizing a patient that has ingested a toxin may include artificial respiration if the patient is _____.
   A. Tachycardic
   B. Dyspneic
   C. Vomiting
   D. Having a seizure
5. Emesis is only productive within _____ of ingestion and is contraindicated in _____.
   A. 20 minutes; rabbits
   B. 1 hour; ferrets
   C. 3 hours; birds
   D. 2 hours; pigs
6. What treatment is recommended for animals that may have ingested corrosives?
   A. Give diluted milk or water in combination with demulcents and gastrointestinal protectants.
   B. Induce emesis with hydrogen peroxide.
   C. Induce emesis with syrup of ipecac.
   D. Administer a cathartic such as activated charcoal.
7. The maximum dosage of 3% hydrogen peroxide (used as an emetic) in dogs is:
   A. 2 tbsp
   B. 3 tsp
   C. 1 oz
   D. 3 tbsp
8. Why is activated charcoal contraindicated in animals that have ingested caustic materials?
   A. It can cause diarrhea and dehydration.
   B. It causes emesis and possible severe irritation of the esophagus.
   C. It may make visualizing oral and esophageal burns difficult.
   D. It inactivates diluted milk, which is the treatment of choice.

9. Cathartics should never be used in patients:
   A. With diarrhea
   B. Who have been given activated charcoal
   C. With dehydration
   D. A and C
10. Lead, estrogen, and antineoplastic medications can cause ____, and iron, copper, and acetaminophen can cause ____.
    A. Kidney failure; liver damage
    B. Liver damage; tachycardia
    C. Liver damage; anemia
    D. Anemia; liver damage
11. Ethylene glycol antifreeze, zinc, mercury, nonsteroidal antiinflammatory drugs, and others may cause ___, requiring treatment with ___.
    A. Cardiotoxicity; diuretics
    B. Kidney damage; diuresis
    C. Liver damage; diuretics
    D. Neurologic disease; anticonvulsants

For questions 12 through 26, choose the household item that is being described. There is only one answer for each statement.
   A. Pennies
   B. Glow necklaces
   C. Ant baits
   D. Bleaches
   E. Acids
   F. Silica gel packets
   G. Liquid potpourri
   H. Detergents
   I. Cigarettes/nicotine products
   J. Mothballs
   K. Alkali
   L. Batteries
   M. Ice or snow melts
   N. Toilet water with tank cleaning drop-in tablets
   O. Moldy food

12. If these are chewed, burns can result; they can result in gastrointestinal obstruction if swallowed.
13. Naphthalene causes hemolysis, heinz bodies, and occasionally methemoglobinemia.
14. These are used in hair relaxers, some oven cleaner pads, dishwasher soaps, denture cleaners, and oven cleaners; a pH greater than 14 can cause esophageal perforation.
15. These cause the pet to foam at the mouth and drool in response to the bitter taste.
16. This desiccant may cause signs of gastrointestinal upset such as nausea, vomiting, and inappetence.
17. Ingestion may cause tremors and seizures by altering neurotransmitter levels, neurotransmitter action, and nerve action potentials.
18. Signs develop quickly (within 15 to 45 minutes) and include excitation, tachypnea, emesis, diarrhea, salivation, and possibly collapse, coma, and cardiac arrest following the period of excitation.
19. At higher concentrations, corrosive effects can be seen; this is used in oxidizing agents, deodorants, and disinfectants.
20. When diluted (have a higher pH), these agents are only irritants and not corrosives; they are found in drain openers, gun barrel cleaners, and pool sanitizers.
21. These contain cationic detergents and essential oils, both of which can be harmful.
22. Sodium ion toxicosis is possible after ingesting these, and clinical signs may include vomiting, increased thirst, fine muscular fasciculation, and metabolic acidosis.
23. Zinc toxicosis causes intravascular hemolysis.
24. If the product is actually chewed, corrosive effects could be seen; however, this is most commonly ingested after dilution in water.
25. These contain insecticides such as fipronil, avermectin, sulfluramid, and boric acid.
26. Anionic and nonionic forms are found in shampoos, laundry detergents, and electric dishwashing detergents; the cationic form is found in hair mousse, conditioners, disinfectants, and sanitizers.
27. All parts of this plant are toxic, the seeds contain the highest concentration of the toxic principal, and it is often used in jewelry.
    A. *Rhododendron* spp.
    B. Lily
    C. Onion
    D. Castor bean
28. What treatment is recommended for cats that have ingested lilies?
    A. Emesis, oral activated charcoal, and cathartic
    B. Close observation because ingestion usually causes a mild irritation
    C. Intravenous fluid therapy
    D. A and C
29. Baby food that contains this should never be fed to cats.
    A. Garlic powder
    B. Onion powder
    C. Grapes/raisins
    D. Green beans

For questions 30 through 41, choose the toxin that is being described. There is only one answer for each statement.

30. Kidney failure arises from the deposition of calcium in the kidney and aggressive decontamination is required with repeated doses of activated charcoal, prednisone, furosemide, and possibly pamidronate.
31. Phosphine gas released in the stomach causes severe respiratory distress and death occurs secondary to respiratory failure.
32. Acute renal failure can occur within 18 to 36 hours of ingesting this form of antifreeze.

33. Cats are considered to be twice as sensitive as dogs because they have a limited glucuronyl-conjugating capacity.
34. Exposure to this toxin can cause salivation, lacrimation, urinary incontinence, diarrhea, gastrointestinal cramping, and emesis (sludge syndrome).
35. A single toxic dose or cumulative dosages can lead to methemoglobinemia and liver damage.
36. This contains ephedrine and pseudoephedrine and can lead to increased blood pressure, tachycardia, ataxia, mydriasis, tremors, and seizures.
37. Used to treat psoriasis in humans, an overdose in animals can increase serum calcium levels within 12 to 72 hours.
38. Cats should be dosed cautiously because of their inability to metabolize and excrete salicylates.
39. Onset of clinical signs is within 30 minutes to 3 hours after ingestion of this pesticide and signs include nervousness, drooling, incoordination, tremors, and seizures.
40. Found in windshield washer fluid, this chemical can cause retinal toxicity in humans and mild gastric upset in dogs and cats after small exposures.
41. Clinical signs develop within 1 hr of ingestion in dogs and are life threatening; they include cardiac arrhythmia, respiratory distress, and hemorrhagic gastroenteritis.
    A. Fly bait
    B. Ethylene glycol
    C. Acetaminophen
    D. Gopher or mole bait
    E. Aspirin
    F. Ma huang
    G. Methanol
    H. Ibuprofen
    I. Cholecalciferol
    J. Calcipotriene–vitamin D derivatives
    K. 5-Fluorouracil
    L. Snail or slug bait

EXTRA CREDIT

42. What is an antidote for ingestion of anticoagulants?
    A. Vitamin B_6
    B. Vitamin K_1
    C. Naloxone
    D. Xylazine
43. What anticoagulant generally requires the longest duration of therapy?
    A. Brodifacoum
    B. Bromadiolone
    C. Warfarin
    D. Ethylene glycol

CHAPTER 28

VETERINARY DENTISTRY

1. The common term for *gingiva* is:
   A. Cavity
   B. Palate
   C. Gums
   D. Tongue
2. A normal depth for the gingival sulcus is _____ in dogs and _____ in cats.
   A. 1 to 3 mm; up to 1 mm
   B. 3 to 5 mm; 1 to 3 mm
   C. 5 to 8 mm; 3 to 5 mm
   D. 8 to 10 mm; 5 to 6 mm
3. Periodontitis is a relatively _____ disease caused by _____.
   A. Common; dental caries
   B. Common; plaque
   C. Rare; dental caries
   D. Rare; plaque
4. What is the relationship between plaque and calculus?
   A. Bacteria cause plaque; calculus is caused by harmful by-products from white blood cells as they attempt to destroy the bacteria.
   B. *Plaque* is another word for *calculus*.
   C. Plaque is a white, slippery film that collects around the gingival sulcus and later mineralizes on the tooth to become calculus.
   D. *Plaque* refers to subgingival food debris and *calculus* to supragingival food debris.
5. Gingivitis is characterized by inflammation (swelling) and hemorrhage (bleeding).
   A. True
   B. False
6. What causes gingivitis?
   A. Plaque
   B. Bacterial endotoxins
   C. Harmful by-products of white blood cells
   D. All of the above
7. The ultimate result of untreated periodontal disease is:
   A. Loose teeth that eventually fall out
   B. Dental caries
   C. Odontoclastic resorptive lesions
   D. All of the above
8. Other than seeing gingivitis, how does a veterinary technician performing dental scaling determine whether a pet has early periodontal disease?
   A. A calculus buildup greater than 2 mm wide along parts of the gum line is present.
   B. An abnormally deep gingival-sulcus depth around one or more teeth is present.
   C. Halitosis (bad breath) is present.
   D. One or more teeth, normally white, are a pinkish-brown color.

9. In the treatment of periodontal disease, a curette is used to remove calculus and dead cementum from the diseased tooth roots, using multiple overlapping strokes, until the root surface is as smooth as glass. This procedure is known as:
   A. A root canal
   B. Exodontics
   C. Subgingival curettage
   D. Root planing
10. A cat with reversible gingivitis that requires only routine dental cleaning for treatment is categorized as having grade _____ periodontal disease.
    A. I
    B. II
    C. III
    D. IV
11. How often do the teeth of pets with advanced periodontal disease require professional cleaning?
    A. Every 2 months
    B. Every 3 to 4 months
    C. Every 6 months
    D. Every 12 months
12. Sodium hexametaphosphate (HMP) and sodium tripolyphosphate are listed as the active ingredients in a preventative-dental product for dogs and cats. How do they function?
    A. They kill bacteria.
    B. They reduce calculus buildup.
    C. These ingredients physically scrape debris and plaque off teeth.
    D. They harden tooth enamel.
13. Mrs. G is calling to find out ways to reduce the need for professional dental care for her dog. Her question is, "Does the food Napoleon eats make a difference? If so, what type of food should I feed?" You reply:
    A. Yes, feed him dry food.
    B. Yes, feed him a semimoist food.
    C. Yes, feed him canned food.
    D. No, the type of food does not make a difference in the rate of plaque accumulation.
14. Chew toys should *not* be recommended for dogs because they can damage the teeth and periodontia.
    A. True
    B. False
15. Prior to professional dental cleaning, the veterinarian will often have the owners of patients with moderate-to-advanced periodontitis:
    A. Brush the pet's teeth twice daily for 7 days.
    B. Feed three tartar-control treats to the pet daily for 3 days.
    C. Administer antibiotics for at least 3 days.
    D. Rub 0.1% chlorhexidine solution on the gums twice daily for 7 days.
16. Position patients in _____ recumbency with the nose _____ for dental cleaning.
    A. Right lateral; up
    B. Right lateral; down
    C. Left lateral; down
    D. B or C
17. Proper technician attire when performing a dental cleaning includes (select all that apply):
    A. Mask over nose and mouth
    B. Gloves
    C. Eye protection
    D. Hair cap
    E. Laboratory coat
18. In the modified triadan system of teeth numbering, adult teeth in the maxillary right quadrant are assigned the:
    A. 100 series
    B. 300 series
    C. 500 series
    D. 700 series
19. A mechanical tooth scaler should never be used continuously on one tooth for more than:
    A. 5 seconds
    B. 15 seconds
    C. 30 seconds
    D. 45 seconds
20. During a dental cleaning, a hand scaler is most often used:
    A. To remove large pieces of calculus initially
    B. For the majority of calculus removal
    C. For subgingival curettage
    D. To reach those areas that are inaccessible to the mechanical scaler
21. Your dental tray will include both scalers and curettes. How do they differ in appearance?
    A. Curettes have a round tip and scalers a pointed tip.
    B. Curettes have an angled shank and scalers a straight shank.
    C. Curettes are labeled with a *C* and scalers with an *S*.
    D. Curettes are made of stainless steel and scalers of disposable plastic.
22. Polishing is *not* absolutely essential for oral health; it is performed for cosmetic reasons because it makes the teeth extra shiny.
    A. True
    B. False
23. Concerning tooth polishing after scaling, which statement is most accurate?
    A. Do not polish a tooth continuously for more than 15 seconds.
    B. Never insert the flared edge subgingivally.
    C. Use a slow-speed handpiece with a prophy cup attached and filled with prophy paste.
    D. Polish only the outside (adjacent to the lips or cheeks) surfaces of the teeth.

24. _____ can be used to rinse the mouth after polishing.
    A. 0.1% chlorhexidine
    B. Zinc ascorbate
    C. 3% hydrogen peroxide
    D. All of the above
25. Gingival recession should be measured from the level of the gingival margin to the
    A. Tip of the crown
    B. Base of the crown (cementoenamel junction)
26. What instrument is used to measure the gingival-sulcus depth?
    A. Hand scaler
    B. Dental explorer
    C. Periodontal probe
    D. Curette
27. For the best results, owners should brush their pets' teeth:
    A. Daily
    B. Every other day
    C. Twice weekly
    D. Once a week
28. In general, pets with mild dental disease require professional dental cleanings:
    A. Every 3 to 4 months
    B. Every 6 to 8 months
    C. Once a year
    D. Every 16 to 18 months
29. Mrs. G is calling about her dog again. "Napoleon will absolutely not let me put my fingers in his mouth to brush his teeth! I can lift his lip, but then he runs away!" What do you recommend she try next?
    A. A mouth rinse or spray
    B. A bioadhesive pellet
    C. No home care and increased frequency of professional cleanings
    D. A or B
30. Human or pet-formula toothpastes are acceptable for use on pets.
    A. True
    B. False
31. _____ is used in veterinary radiography to minimize distortion and produce an accurate image of the tooth on the dental film.
    A. The buccal object rule
    B. The tube shift technique
    C. The bisecting angle technique
    D. A shorter focal-film distance
32. When one is learning the positioning techniques for intraoral dental radiographs, it is easiest to place the dog or cat in _____ recumbency for views of the maxillary dentition, in _____ recumbency for views of the anterior mandible, and in lateral recumbency for views of the mandibular premolars and molars.
    A. Sternal; dorsal
    B. Lateral; sternal
    C. Dorsal; lateral
    D. Dorsal; sternal
33. Teeth with the dental pulp exposed cannot be saved and should be extracted to prevent infection and pain.
    A. True
    B. False
34. Endodontic files with endodontic stops, gutta-percha, and paper points are all used in:
    A. Tooth extractions
    B. Root planing
    C. A root canal
    D. Orthodontics
35. Prior to tooth extraction, owners should be counseled about possible complications, including:
    A. Jaw fracture
    B. Eye trauma
    C. Anesthetic risks
    D. All of the above
36. With orthodontic treatment, the dental problems of many patients who present with malocclusions can be corrected.
    A. True
    B. False
37. When pouring stone into an alginate impression to make a dental model, it is critical to:
    A. Place the impression in a vice to hold it as still as possible.
    B. Not hold the impression in your hands to avoid getting burned.
    C. Fill the incisors first, then work caudally toward the molars.
    D. Hold the impression on a laboratory vibrator while small amounts of stone are placed on the impression and allowed to run into the teeth.
38. Dental caries is _____ in dogs and cats.
    A. Rare
    B. Somewhat common
    C. Extremely common
39. What common feline oral disease affects 20% of cats?
    A. Retained deciduous teeth
    B. Feline odontoclastic resorptive lesions
    C. Fractured, brittle teeth
    D. Malocclusions

For questions 40 to 50, place the following activities in the order they are performed in a routine dental cleaning.
   A. Remove small-to-moderate remaining calculus with a mechanical scaler.
   B. Use dental explorer to check for subgingival pathology.
   C. Perform thorough examination of oral cavity.
   D. Educate client on home care of pet's teeth.
   E. Rinse patient's mouth.
   F. Extract tooth or make model, if necessary.
   G. Anesthetize patient.
   H. Remove large pieces of calculus with forceps.

I. Record findings such as loose or fractured teeth.
J. Polish teeth.
K. Hand scale difficult-to-reach teeth.

40. _____
41. _____
42. _____
43. _____
44. _____
45. _____
46. _____
47. _____
48. _____
49. _____
50. _____

51. Adult cats have the following mandibular dental formula:
    A. Three incisors, one canine, three premolars, one molar
    B. Three incisors, one canine, two premolars, two molars
    C. Three incisors, one canine, four premolars, one molar
    D. Three incisors, one canine, two premolars, one molar

52. The first set of teeth in mammals are called:
    A. Diphyodonts
    B. Deciduous
    C. Carnassial
    D. Brachydont

53. An animal with a class I malocclusion (neutroclusion) may have:
    A. Oronasal fistula
    B. An abnormally short maxilla
    C. Base narrow canines
    D. An abnormally long maxilla
    E. A and B
    F. A and C
    G. A and D

54. The terms *brachygnathic* and *prognathic* refer to the length of the ___ in relation to the ___.
    A. Maxilla; mandible
    B. Mandible; maxillary canines
    C. Maxilla; mandibular incisors
    D. Mandible; maxilla

55. What patient care is required after advanced periodontal procedures such as a gingival flap procedure?
    A. The owner should start brushing the teeth 1 week postoperatively and be very gentle around the surgery site.
    B. The patient should be placed on a soft food diet for 1 week.
    C. The mouth should be rinsed daily with a 0.2% chlorhexidine solution for 2 weeks.
    D. All of the above.
    E. None of the above.

56. Regarding nomenclature for dental instruments, which of the following is/are true?
    A. Supragingival scalers are not to be used subgingivally because they have a pointed tip that could damage the gingival sulcus.
    B. All curettes can be used subgingivally because they have a round toe and back to help prevent damage to the gingival tissue.
    C. Supragingival scalers are often referred to as curettes.
    D. Subgingival scalers are often referred to as scalers.
    E. B and C
    F. A and b
    G. All of the above

57. What are the three basic aspects of preventing periodontal disease?

58. Overinflated endotracheal-tube cuffs have been shown to cause tears in the feline trachea, most of which occur during dental procedures. List three ways for the technician to reduce the incidence of tracheal tears.

59. List three abnormal findings that should be recorded on a patient's dental chart if found during cleaning.

60. List three reasons why polishing pastes containing fluoride are preferred over those without fluoride.

61. What is the purpose of a root canal?

EXTRA CREDIT

62. In veterinary dentistry, a "shepherd's hook" is:
    A. A dental explorer commonly used in dogs
    B. A brand of mechanical scaler
    C. A scaler designed for use in the cat
    D. Used to capture dogs and cats who don't want to have their teeth brushed

CHAPTER 29

EQUINE MEDICAL AND SURGICAL NURSING

1. Which group of signs of respiratory disease in the horse should be considered an emergency?
    A. Flared nostrils, forced expiration, and a "heave" line
    B. Flared nostrils and rapid, shallow breathing
    C. Nasal discharge with mucus and pus
    D. Watery nasal discharge

2. The normal rectal temperature of adult horses is approximately:
    A. 36.3° C to 37° C (97.3° F to 98.6° F)
    B. 37° C to 38.5° C (98.6° F to 101.3° F)
    C. 38.9° C to 39.7° C (102° F to 103.4° F)
    D. 39.7° C to 40.5° C (103.4° F to 104.9° F)

3. What technique is often used to increase the depth of equine breathing to accentuate lung sounds during thoracic auscultation (listening with a stethoscope)?

A. Administration of doxapram
B. Mild exercise
C. Application of a rebreathing bag
D. Application of a mildly noxious stimulus such as a skin pinch

4. Petechiation (pinpoint, red spots of hemorrhage on a mucous membrane) is normal in:
   A. Neonatal (newborn) foals
   B. The first 24 hours after colic surgery
   C. Mares in late pregnancy
   D. None of the above

5. Equine gastrointestinal sounds are evaluated with auscultation over the:
   A. Right and left dorsal and ventral abdomen
   B. Right and left ventral abdomen
   C. Right ventral abdomen
   D. Left ventral abdomen

6. In the healthy horse, digital pulses are _____ and hoof temperature is _____.
   A. Absent; cool
   B. Palpable; cool
   C. Bounding; warm
   D. Absent; warm

For the next two questions, use the information provided in the following scenario. You are nursing "Solitaire," a horse recovering from small-intestinal surgery performed yesterday. You know she may become violently ill and have been told to contact the attending clinician if this occurs. At 10 PM on Saturday night, you discover Solitaire covered in sweat with evidence of frequent rolling in her stall. You cannot reach the veterinarian.

7. Why does a horse like Solitaire, with a buildup of fluid in her stomach, experience such pain?
   A. Horses cannot vomit to relieve the gastric pressure.
   B. Horses are especially sensitive to pain.
   C. The fluid buildup begins to cause laminitis, which is very painful.
   D. B and C

8. How can you best treat Solitaire until the veterinarian returns your call?
   A. Administer an analgesic such as flunixin meglumine intravenously.
   B. Pass a nasogastric tube to decompress her stomach.
   C. Get her up and walk her continuously.
   D. Run cold water on her front feet.

9. What needs to be more closely evaluated in the sick foal than in the sick adult horse?
   A. Scleral color
   B. Leg joints for swelling and heat
   C. Umbilicus for swelling, heat, and discharge
   D. All of the above

10. Fractious, anxious, or untrained horses are often most safely restrained by:
    A. Stocks
    B. A handler holding a halter with a lead rope or chain
    C. Cross-ties
    D. A twitch

11. Which statement concerning lip twitching a horse is most accurate?
    A. If a twitched horse becomes anxious, tighten the twitch slightly.
    B. The twitch should not be placed on the lip until immediately before it is needed.
    C. The twitch is ideal for lengthy procedures of greater than 30 minutes.
    D. All of the above

12. _____ can cause permanent penile paralysis in stallions.
    A. Acepromazine
    B. Xylazine
    C. Detomidine
    D. Butorphanol

13. In an adult horse, never administer more than _____ L of fluids by nasogastric tube.
    A. 5
    B. 8
    C. 11
    D. 15

14. A nasogastric tube is properly placed in the esophagus when:
    A. Negative pressure is obtained when one sucks on the tube's end.
    B. The tube is visually observed within the esophagus on the left side of the neck.
    C. The tube is palpated in the esophagus on the left side of the neck.
    D. All of the above.

15. Blowing into a nasogastric tube can cause accidental rupture of a neonatal foal's stomach.
    A. True
    B. False

16. Abdominal distention in sick neonatal foals is most accurately determined by:
    A. Quantifying the amount of gastric reflux (fluid) produced per hour
    B. Visual inspection of the abdomen
    C. Abdominal auscultation and percussion
    D. Measuring abdominal girth in the same location with a tape measure hourly

17. What protective gear is required in a standard equine isolation ward? (Select all that apply.)
    A. Face mask
    B. Eye protection
    C. Gloves
    D. Coveralls or bodysuit
    E. Caps
    F. Disinfectant foot dip
    G. Air-filtering device
    H. A separate place to walk isolated horses
    I. A separate place to dispose of isolated-horse feces

18. Which foodstuff has a laxativelike effect useful for constipated or recumbent horses?
    A. Oats
    B. Bran mash (wheat bran plus warm water)
    C. Fresh grass
    D. B and C
19. How are tablets usually administered to horses in the clinical setting?
    A. Balling gun
    B. By crushing the tablets, mixing the powder with a sweet substance such as molasses, adding water, and administering the mixture orally with water
    C. By crushing the tablets and mixing the powder with the horse's feed
    D. B and C
20. The volume of medication injected intramuscularly at a single site in the adult horse should *not* exceed:
    A. 5 ml
    B. 10 ml
    C. 15 ml
    D. 20 ml
21. What situation is potentially life threatening in the horse? (Select all that apply.)
    A. Accidental injection of medication into the carotid artery
    B. A bleeding rectal tear
    C. Accidental administration of fluids or medication into the lungs via nasogastric tube
    D. Bacteria in the bloodstream secondary to an infected intravenous catheter
22. What commonly used equine sedative has no analgesic properties?
    A. Butorphanol
    B. Acepromazine
    C. Xylazine
    D. Detomidine
23. Dimethyl sulfoxide (DMSO) functions as:
    A. An antiparasitic agent
    B. An antiarrhythmic agent
    C. An antiinflammatory agent
    D. A diuretic agent
24. _____ is a respiratory condition unique to horses.
    A. Guttural pouch empyema
    B. Allergic airway disease
    C. Pleuritis
    D. Maxillary sinusitis
25. Remove a horse's shoes and pack the frog area with Play-Doh when radiographing the _____ bone.
    A. Short pastern
    B. Coffin
    C. Navicular
    D. B and C
26. The standard focal spot-to-film distance using portable radiographic units is:
    A. 40 cm
    B. 65 cm
    C. 85 cm
    D. 100 cm
27. Echocardiography is:
    A. Plain-film radiography of the heart
    B. Ultrasound examination of the heart
    C. Radiologic examination of the heart using a contrast agent
    D. Endoscopic examination of the heart
28. How is nuclear scintigraphy used most often in horses?
    A. To treat hyperthyroidism
    B. To localize the site of lameness when limb x-rays are normal
    C. To diagnose early pregnancy
    D. To treat laryngeal weakness
29. Increased serum _____ is a normal physiologic response in the fasted horse.
    A. Sorbitol dehydrogenase
    B. Creatine phosphokinase
    C. Bilirubin
    D. Gamma-glutamyl transferase
30. An equine veterinarian (but *not* a dog veterinarian) will request what test when bacterial infection and inflammation is suspected?
    A. White blood cell count
    B. Platelet count
    C. Fibrinogen level
    D. B and C
31. What crystal is normally present in large numbers in equine urine?
    A. Magnesium ammonium phosphate (struvite)
    B. Calcium carbonate
    C. Calcium oxalate
    D. Urate
32. How is a carpus (knee) prepared for arthrocentesis (joint tap)?
    A. Clip hair and perform a surgical scrub.
    B. Wipe well with alcohol-moistened gauze.
    C. Wash with a cleansing shampoo and dry.
    D. Remove visible dirt, brush well, and vacuum dust.
33. All horses in the United States, regardless of geographic location or function, must be vaccinated against:
    A. Influenza
    B. Tetanus
    C. Eastern and Western encephalitis
    D. B and C
34. Young horses and performance horses (engaged in racing, showing, or off-site training) are at high risk of contracting _____ and should be vaccinated every 3 to 4 months for these diseases.
    A. Equine viral arteritis and Potomac horse fever
    B. Botulism and strangles
    C. Influenza and rhinopneumonitis
    D. A and C

35. Broodmares should be vaccinated for _____ in the fifth, seventh, and ninth month of pregnancy to prevent abortion caused by this disease.
    A. Potomac horse fever
    B. Rhinopneumonitis
    C. Rabies
    D. Botulism
36. In general, nasogastric-tube deworming is more effective than oral-paste deworming.
    A. True
    B. False
37. Weight loss and abnormal eating habits such as dropping feed from the mouth and excessive salivation are most often indications of:
    A. Blindness
    B. Abdominal pain
    C. Dental problems
    D. Respiratory disease
38. Which statement is true concerning enamel "points" in horses?
    A. Points are sharp edges that develop on teeth and are treated by filing or "floating."
    B. Points develop only in horses with an abnormal bite known as *parrot mouth*.
    C. Points can develop in all horses because their lower jaw is wider than their upper jaw.
    D. A and C.
39. Equine infectious anemia:
    A. Produces diarrhea, fever, abortion, and laminitis. It is caused by *Ehrlichia risticii*, is seen primarily in the eastern United States, and should be vaccinated for in horses at risk.
    B. Is a viral disease carried by large biting flies. Horses must have a negative Coggins test for this disease within 1 year for issuance of health certificates for interstate travel, international travel, show, and sale. If infected, horses become permanently infected and are therefore carriers of the virus.
    C. Is a contagious viral disease causing limb swelling, abortion, and respiratory disease. Stallions can transmit it to mares during breeding. A vaccine is only available for stallions and nonpregnant mares, and its administration must be supervised by the USDA.
    D. Is a fatal neurologic disease causing profound weakness and an inability to swallow. The organism, if ingested, produces a neurotoxin. A vaccine is available.
40. Horses affected with _____ must be maintained under a strict isolation protocol.
    A. Equine protozoal myelitis (EPM) and equine degenerative myelopathy
    B. Gastric ulceration and botulism
    C. Strangles and diarrhea
    D. Moldy corn toxicity and dermatophilosis
41. Owners of horses diagnosed with chronic obstructive pulmonary disease (COPD) need to be counseled that the most important aspect of treatment is:
    A. Regular vaccination
    B. Removal of the offending allergens (usually hay or straw) from the horse's environment
    C. Lifelong corticosteroid administration
    D. Lifelong antibiotic administration
42. Gastric ulcers are a common occurrence in stressed, young horses and horses receiving high doses of nonsteroidal antiinflammatory drugs such as phenylbutazone.
    A. True
    B. False
43. What equine neurologic disease is also known as *wobbles?*
    A. Rabies
    B. Vertebral fracture
    C. An inherited condition seen in young horses in which the entire spinal cord slowly degenerates
    D. Compression of the cervical spinal cord by malformed or unstable cervical vertebrae
44. Eastern, Western, and Venezuelan viral encephalitis (EVE, WVE, VVE) are transmitted to horses by:
    A. Ticks
    B. Mosquitoes
    C. Inhaling the organism when coughed or sneezed out by an infected horse
    D. Ingestion of moldy feed
45. What set of symptoms indicates brain disease?
    A. Icterus, poor blood clotting, weight loss, anorexia
    B. Profound depression, head pressing, incoordination, aimless wandering, seizures
    C. Urinating and drinking excessively, pain on urination, limb swelling, swollen abdomen
    D. Diarrhea, colic, pale mucous membranes, depression

For the next three questions, match the dermatologic disease with its description.
    A. Equine sarcoid
    B. Melanoma
    C. *Culicoides* spp. hypersensitivity
    D. Dermatophilosis

46. This black tumor occurs commonly in gray horses.
47. This allergic condition causes mane and tail rubbing due to itchiness.
48. This bacterial skin infection causes crusting lesions over wet body areas.
49. Concerning equine anterior uveitis (moon blindness), which statement is true?
    A. It is the most common cause of equine blindness.
    B. The cause is unknown.

C. It cannot be cured.
D. All of the above.

50. Commercial "foal predictor" kits are generally unreliable, and their use by clients should be discouraged.
    A. True
    B. False

51. A newborn foal should pass meconium (first feces) within a few hours after birth.
    A. True
    B. False

52. Routine care of the healthy newborn foal includes (select all that apply):
    A. A foal-side blood test for adequate transfer of immunity (adequate colostrum ingestion) at 1 day of age
    B. Blood cultures at 3 days of age to rule out septicemia (bacterial toxins in the blood)
    C. A packed cell volume to rule out neonatal isoerythrolysis (incompatible blood type with mare)
    D. Dipping the umbilicus in chlorhexidine or iodine solution

53. The most common life-threatening disease of newborn foals is:
    A. Meconium impaction
    B. Neonatal septicemia
    C. Neonatal isoerythrolysis
    D. Ruptured urinary bladder

54. Mr. F calls to say his 2-day-old foal was suckling every 30 minutes for the first day of life and now hasn't suckled for 3 hours. What do you tell him?
    A. Failure to suckle is the first sign of a problem, and the foal should be examined by a veterinarian as soon as possible.
    B. This is normal foal behavior. Expect her to suckle every 6 hours or so from now on. Call us back if she has not suckled after 3 more hours.

55. Concerning the care of recumbent (unable to walk), sick neonatal foals, which statement is most accurate?
    A. These foals require intensive, 24-hour care in a specially equipped facility.
    B. Strict aseptic technique is vital when dealing with intravenous ports.
    C. The technician must be diligent and thorough because a decline in the patient's condition occurs rapidly and without warning.
    D. All of the above.

56. Unless otherwise instructed, a _____ surgery pack should be set up for a cesarean section.
    A. Castration
    B. Colic
    C. Fracture (orthopedic)
    D. Laryngeal

57. The veterinary technician must use caution when handling mares immediately after caudal epidural anesthesia because:
    A. A common side effect is seizures.
    B. The mare's rear legs are uncoordinated.
    C. A common side effect is aggression.
    D. A and C

58. The operation performed on some mares' vulvas to prevent air and feces from entering the vagina is known as:
    A. The modified Whitehouse technique
    B. The perineal-vulvar (PV) operation
    C. Caslick's operation
    D. The postbreeding procedure

59. *Navel ill* refers to:
    A. A patent urachus
    B. An umbilical infection
    C. The absence of an umbilicus
    D. An umbilical hernia

60. What surgical item is designed specifically for castration?
    A. Stainless steel suture material
    B. Silk suture material
    C. Umbilical tape
    D. Emasculators

61. Postoperative care of the equine castration patient involves:
    A. Strict stall confinement for 24 hours and then hand walking 1 or 2 times daily for 1 to 2 weeks to promote drainage
    B. Strict stall confinement for 1 to 2 weeks until drainage ceases
    C. Regular exercise and daily sponging of the incision with dilute chlorhexidine for 1 to 2 weeks
    D. Strict stall confinement for 1 week, then a return to regular exercise

62. What hernia type requires immediate examination by a veterinarian?
    A. Umbilical hernia in a foal in which the contents cannot be pushed back into the abdomen by the owner
    B. Scrotal hernia in an adult stallion
    C. Inguinal hernia in a foal in which the contents can be pushed back into the abdomen by the owner
    D. A and B

63. Which statement concerning laminitis is true? (Select all that apply.)
    A. The disease is caused by inflammation of the sensitive hoof laminae and can lead to coffin-bone rotation.
    B. Even severely affected horses usually return to full athletic function.
    C. Horses with chronic laminitis develop characteristic concentric rings on the hooves as well as an abnormal hoof shape.

D. The disease is extremely painful and often life threatening.
E. Affected horses stand with a characteristic stance with their rear legs camped underneath the torso and their front feet camped out in front.

64. *Bone spavin, high and low ringbone,* and *osselets* are terms that all apply to different forms of:
   A. Tendonitis
   B. Arthritis
   C. Ligament tears
   D. Fractures

65. What disease is frequently treated with arthroscopy?
   A. Subsolar (foot) abscesses
   B. Rhabdomyolysis (tying up)
   C. Osteochondrosis (cartilage abnormalities in young, growing horses)
   D. Laminitis

For the next three questions, match the orthopedic disease with the bandage associated with its treatment or with its stabilization prior to treatment.
   A. Hoof bandage
   B. Kimzey splint
   C. Robert-Jones bandage with splints

66. Foot abscess
67. Lower-limb-only fracture or joint dislocation
68. Upper- or lower-limb fracture or joint dislocation
69. How are feeding and watering usually handled in an adult horse prior to surgery?
   A. Twelve hours prior to surgery, withhold food and water.
   B. Twelve hours prior to surgery, withhold food only.
   C. Twenty-four hours prior to surgery, withhold food only.
   D. Do not withhold food or water prior to surgery.

70. What procedure is performed after anesthetic induction of the equine patient?
   A. Removal of his shoes
   B. Washing out his mouth
   C. Placement of an intravenous catheter
   D. None of the above

71. For most orthopedic surgeries, _____ should be placed in the operating room in addition to the standard surgery supplies.
   A. A 30-ft nylon rope
   B. Radiographs of the affected limb
   C. An emasculator
   D. B and C

72. Horses undergoing surgery lying down are particularly prone to _____ during the procedure.
   A. Kidney damage
   B. Liver damage
   C. Central nervous system damage
   D. Muscle damage

73. Limb bandages placed during orthopedic surgery should be left in place undisturbed (not changed) until the skin sutures are removed.
   A. True
   B. False

74. Only a small percentage of horses with colic require surgery, as most cases respond to medical management.
   A. True
   B. False

75. The majority of colic surgeries are performed with the horse:
   A. In sternal recumbency
   B. In dorsal recumbency
   C. In lateral recumbency
   D. Standing (flank incision)

76. Arthroscopic instruments to be used more than once per day are most often:
   A. Soaked in alcohol
   B. Cold sterilized
   C. Sterilized with ethylene oxide
   D. Not cleaned between procedures

77. Many long-bone fractures in adult horses are correctable due to advances in surgical techniques.
   A. True
   B. False

78. What condition in the postoperative orthopedic patient wearing a limb bandage or cast should be brought to the attention of the veterinarian immediately?
   A. A loose bandage
   B. A wet bandage
   C. A dramatic change in the horse's use of the limb
   D. All of the above

79. To ensure success, _____ is generally more closely regarded in orthopedic surgery than in soft tissue surgery.
   A. Asepsis
   B. Patient positioning
   C. Choice of anesthetic drugs
   D. Choice of suture material

For the next two questions, match the upper respiratory ailment with its description.
   A. Dorsal displacement of the soft palate
   B. Left laryngeal hemiplegia
   C. Epiglottic entrapment
   D. Arytenoid chondritis

80. This condition occurs during exercise, interferes with the horse's breathing, and is first treated by tying the tongue to the lower jaw.
81. Horses with this condition develop exercise intolerance and are called "roarers."
82. Why do animals that have undergone a tracheotomy or tracheostomy need hourly monitoring for the first 24 hours?
   A. There is a risk of airway or tracheostomy obstruction leading to suffocation.

B. There is a risk of bacterial tracheal infection.
C. There is a risk of viral upper respiratory infection.
D. There is a risk of pneumonia.

83. Treatment of flexural and angular limb deformities in foals and young horses may involve (select all that apply):
    A. Corrective shoeing
    B. Surgery
    C. Stall rest
    D. Dietary changes
    E. Bandages, splints, or casts
    F. Antibiotics

84. Life-threatening upper respiratory tract obstruction can be alleviated on an emergency basis by:
    A. Tracheotomy
    B. Pulling the tongue forward and out of the mouth
    C. Administering epinephrine intravenously
    D. Placing finger pressure on the eyeball through the eyelid

85. The minimum acceptable mean arterial blood pressure of a horse during surgery is:
    A. 90 mm Hg
    B. 80 mm Hg
    C. 70 mm Hg
    D. 60 mm Hg

86. How is low blood pressure treated during surgery?
    A. Reduce anesthetic depth.
    B. Increase rate of intravenous fluid administration.
    C. Administer drugs that increase blood pressure.
    D. All of the above

87. Palpation of the hooves for heat and the fetlocks for digital-pulse quality in critically ill horses is performed to detect early:
    A. Founder
    B. Laminitis
    C. Bog spavin
    D. A and B

88. What are the two best sites for intramuscular injections in the horse?

89. In addition to color and turbidity, list three tests frequently performed on bodily fluids such as joint or abdominal fluid.

90. List three ways to help a foal born by cesarean section start breathing.

91. List three possible causes of gastrointestinal-related colic.

92. How is intracarotid injection of medication prevented when administering agents into the jugular vein?

EXTRA CREDIT

93. A client calls and, in an urgent-sounding voice, says his horse is "cast." This means the animal:
    A. Is violently thrashing about due to colic.
    B. Has his hoof trapped and is unable to free it.
    C. Is unable to stand because he has lied down too close to the wall.
    D. Will be acting in a forthcoming feature film.

94. *Ataxia* is:
    A. Circling
    B. Incoordination
    C. A head tilt
    D. An Italian taxi

CHAPTER 30

FOOD ANIMAL MEDICINE AND SURGERY

1. The role of the veterinary technician who works with food animals includes:
   A. Instructing producers about proper technique for placement of growth implants in feedlot cattle
   B. Body condition scoring in cattle and small ruminants
   C. Artificial insemination and corrective footwork
   D. All of the above

2. In situations in which the veterinary staff is having difficulty stimulating a calf to breathe, ____ can be placed under the animal's ____.
   A. Epinephrine; tongue
   B. Doxapram hydrochloride; tongue
   C. Doxapram hydrochloride; upper eyelid
   D. Epinephrine; upper eyelid

3. It is imperative to a calf's survival to receive colostrum within the first ____ of life.
   A. 6 to 8 hours
   B. 1 to 2 hours
   C. Week
   D. Day

4. Anterior uveitis and hypopion in the calf often respond to treatment with:
   A. Antibiotics and prednisone
   B. Antibiotics and cyclosporine
   C. Atropine and antibiotics
   D. Atropine and polymethylmethacrylate

5. Which of the following statements is/are true regarding calves with diarrhea?
   A. Milk and milk products should be warmed before being offered
   B. Stress, poor sanitation, and poor nutrition can contribute to the development of diarrhea:
   C. Warm intravenous fluids should be administered and supplemented with dextrose and bicarbonate as needed.
   D. B and C

6. Actinobacillosis is usually treated with intravenous administration of ____.
   A. Sodium iodide
   B. Penicillin
   C. Oxytetracycline
   D. Dexamethasone
7. Why is it extremely important to exercise caution when using balling guns, dose syringes, and stomach tube in cattle?
   A. To prevent the development of traumatic reticuloperitonitis
   B. To prevent the development of infectious bovine rhinotracheitis
   C. To prevent the development of pharyngeal cellulitis, abscessation, or hematoma
   D. To prevent the development of bovine respiratory syncytial virus
8. Which of the following statements is *false* regarding grain overload in ruminants?
   A. The treatment involves administering thiamine to help prevent liver abscesses, polioencephalomalacia, and laminitis.
   B. Rumen transfaunation may be helpful to reestablish normal rumen microflora and improve appetite during the convalescent period.
   C. The normal color of rumen fluid is olive or brownish-green.
   D. A pH less than 7.5 is suggestive of grain overload.
9. Rumen tympany may be caused by:
   A. Hypocalcemia
   B. Eating large amounts of legumes or grain
   C. Body position (dorsal recumbency)
   D. Proliferation of *Lactobacillus* spp.
10. Which of the following are possible treatment options for ruminants with traumatic reticuloperitonitis?
    A. Exploratory laparotomy and rumenotomy
    B. Administration of broad-spectrum antibiotics
    C. Oral administration of a magnet
    D. All of the above
11. What is the required treatment for abomasal volvulus?
    A. Immediate surgical intervention
    B. Broad-spectrum antibiotics
    C. Administration of mineral oil
    D. Administration of calcium
12. What is the preferred treatment for winter dysentery in ruminants?
    A. Intravenous fluid administration
    B. No treatment is available and most animals recover spontaneously.
    C. Administration of mineral oil
    D. Broad-spectrum antibiotics
13. What is the most frequent cause of chronic diarrhea in adult cattle?
    A. Dietary indiscretion
    B. Bacterial infection
    C. Parasitic infection
    D. Viral infection
14. Which of the following are control programs currently used by producers who want to eliminate Johne disease from their herd?
    A. Cull positive animals and clinically ill animals.
    B. Repeat serologic testing.
    C. Change drinking water frequently.
    D. A and B
15. Vaccination of calves experiencing chronic BVD using the modified live vaccine may result in death of the animal.
    A. True
    B. False
16. Bovine respiratory disease syndrome, commonly called ____, is caused by a combination of respiratory bacteria, viruses, and ____.
    A. Lumpy jaw; enterotoxins
    B. Hardware disease; stress
    C. Founder; poor nutrition
    D. Shipping fever; stress
17. Septic arthritis in calves may be treated with:
    A. Decreasing the amount of grain in the diet
    B. Surgical debridement
    C. Polymethylmethacrylate (PMMA) beads implanted subcutaneously near the infected joints
    D. All of the above
18. In cattle, an infection of the interdigital skin and underlying tissues with an ulcerated, foul-smelling area between the claws and lameness is called:
    A. Interdigital necrobacillosis
    B. Gravel
    C. Foot rot
    D. A and C
19. Acute laminitis may be due to excess, sudden ingestion of ____ or secondary to other diseases, which occur during the ____ period.
    A. Salt; postparturient
    B. Grain; postparturient
    C. Calcium; neonatal
    D. Mycotoxins; neonatal
20. Sole ulcers occur more commonly in the:
    A. Lateral hind claws
    B. Lateral front claws
    C. Medial hind claws
    D. Medial front claws
21. On the hoof, the area of fibrous connective tissue that joins the rigid hoof wall to the more resilient sole is the:
    A. Coronary band
    B. White line
    C. Frog
    D. Sulcus
22. In large ruminants, what are the main weight-bearing claws?
    A. Front lateral and hind lateral
    B. Front lateral and hind medial

C. Front medial and hind medial
D. Front medial and hind lateral
23. What is the single most common disease syndrome in adult dairy cows?
    A. Mastitis
    B. Lymphosarcoma
    C. Bovine respiratory disease syndrome
    D. Periparturient hypocalcemia (milk fever)
24. Infections with *Clostridium chauvoei* and *Clostridium septicum* can be prevented with:
    A. Vaccination with a multivalent bacterium at 2 months of age followed by a booster 4 to 6 weeks later
    B. Aggressive intravenous fluids with broad-spectrum antibiotics
    C. Vaccination with a multivalent bacterium at 6 months of age followed by a booster 4 to 6 weeks later
    D. Reduced grain intake
25. Lymphosarcoma associated with bovine leukemia virus can be managed in most herds with a test and cull program.
    A. True
    B. False
26. Anaplasmosis generally causes _____ and can be treated with ____.
    A. Lameness; NSAIDs
    B. Anemia; tetracycline
    C. Vomiting and diarrhea; penicillin
    D. Seizures; Valium
27. Which of the following statements is/are true regarding anthrax?
    A. If an animal is suspected of having anthrax, a necropsy should be performed and the brain sent to the state veterinarian.
    B. Anthrax-contaminated carcasses should be buried in lime or incinerated.
    C. Contact the area's federal veterinarian immediately if an animal is suspected of having anthrax.
    D. B and C
28. ____ mastitis results when bacteria within reservoirs in the environment gain access to the mammary gland and cause infection.
    A. Environment
    B. Toxic
    C. Contagious
    D. Gangrenous
29. Alternatives to forced or manual fetal extraction of calves include:
    A. Caesarian section
    B. Use of a mechanical calf extractor
    C. Fetotomy
    D. A and B
30. Uterine prolapses are considered emergencies and should be repaired immediately after being noticed.
    A. True
    B. False
31. To initiate uterine involution, is given.
    A. Estrogen
    B. Oxytocin
    C. Progesterone
    D. Carboxymethylcellulose
32. An injection of ___ and ___ 1 month before calving may decrease the incidence of retained placenta in problem herds.
    A. Oxytocin; vitamin E
    B. Antibiotics; selenium
    C. Vitamin E; selenium
    D. Estrogen; oxytocin
33. How should a traumatized prepuce that is swollen be treated?
    A. Soak it in warm water with betadine and epsom salts.
    B. Return the prepuce to the preputial cavity and wrap it with a tube in place to prevent further trauma.
    C. Perform surgery (reefing) once the inflammation and infection are under control.
    D. All of the above
34. Which of the following statements is *false* regarding periparturient hypocalcemia?
    A. It is caused by a severe increase in serum calcium levels.
    B. It usually occurs within 48 hours of calving.
    C. Affected cows often lie in sternal recumbency with their head turned into their flank or may be found in lateral recumbency.
    D. Cows in very early stages of milk fever (before recumbency) often respond to administration of oral calcium gel.
35. Ketosis in dairy cows may result from a primary deficiency of _____ intake or may be secondary to other diseases that cause _____.
    A. Water; dehydration
    B. Calcium; hypocalcemia
    C. Energy; anorexia
    D. Selenium; neurologic signs
36. In cattle, clinical signs of a murmur or thrill, exercise intolerance, congestive heart failure with jugular distension, dependent edema, and fluctuating fever may be indicative of:
    A. Pericarditis
    B. The result of septic emboli from other sites such as omphalophlebitis
    C. Vegetative or valvular endocarditis
    D. B and C
37. Pericarditis should be performed at the ____ rib space, on the ____ side.
    A. Fourth or fifth; right

B. Fourth or fifth; left
C. Fifth or sixth; right
D. Fifth or sixth; left

For questions 38 through 47, choose the disease to which each statement refers. There is only one answer for each statement.

A. Contagious bovine pyelonephritis
B. Cutaneous papillomas
C. Dermatophilus
D. Dermatophytosis
E. Infectious bovine keratoconjunctivitis
F. Listeriosis
G. Obturator and sciatic nerve paresis and paralysis
H. Ocular squamous cell carcinoma
I. Polioencephalomalacia
J. Rabies
K. Thromboembolic meningoencephalitis
L. Urolithiasis

38. Clinical syndromes of this disease are neurological disease, abortion, and septicemia.
39. The cause is *Corynebacterium renale*.
40. The organism is found primarily in the respiratory tract and usually causes pneumonia.
41. This may be caused by dystocia or forced fetal extraction.
42. Pharyngeal and laryngeal paralysis cause an inability to drink.
43. Flies act as vectors for the bacteria.
44. The disease causes a paint brush appearance of the hair.
45. Exposure to ultraviolet light and lack of protective pigmentation around the eye play important roles.
46. Opisthotonos and dorsomedial strabismus are clinical signs.
47. No treatment is necessary because they persist for 3 to 12 months and often spontaneously regress.
48. Most lesions heal on their own, especially calves are turned out to pasture and exposed to light.
49. Dietary management is the key to control and prevention; the calcium to phosphorus ratio of the overall diet should be 21 to 2.51, and a continuous supply of fresh, clean water should be available at all times.
50. Which of the following are true regarding behavior of large ruminants?
    A. Cattle tend to move in open areas or pastures as opposed to along fences.
    B. Cattle tend to move away from bright light.
    C. It is important to invade an animal's flight zone as deeply as possible when moving it to maintain control.
    D. All of the above
    E. None of the above

51. Calves dehorned after 6 months of age are at greater risk of developing ___.
    A. Hemorrhage
    B. Seromas
    C. Sinusitis
    D. Behavior disorders
52. The use of elastrator bands to perform castration of calves has been associated with the development of ___.
    A. Tetanus
    B. Seromas
    C. Hematomas
    D. Sepsis
53. When hand-raising lambs and kids during the first few days after birth, commercial lamb and kid milk replacers should be given in the following amount:
    A. 5% to 10% of their body weight divided into two feedings per day
    B. 5% to 10% of their body weight divided into four feedings per day
    C. 15% to 20% of their body weight divided into three feedings per day
    D. 10% to 15% of their body weight divided into three to four feedings per day
54. Which of the following may predispose small ruminants to enterotoxemia?
    A. Feeding bread or other bakery goods to goats
    B. Sudden, accidental exposure to grain
    C. Turnout to lush pasture
    D. Feeding bran/molasses mash to recently fresh does
    E. All of the above
55. *Pasteurella* pneumonia often causes the formation of fibrous connective tissue in the udder of small ruminants.
    A. True
    B. False
56. Footbaths containing ___ may be the best treatment for *Dichelobacter nodosus* and *Fusobacterium necrophorum* infections in small ruminants because it is least irritating.
    A. Betadine
    B. Copper sulfate
    C. Formalin
    D. Zinc sulfate
57. What is a possible treatment for tetanus in small ruminants?
    A. High doses of tetracycline and NSAIDs
    B. High doses of penicillin and tetanus antitoxin
    C. High doses of ceftiofur and tetanus antitoxin
    D. An anticonvulsant and high doses of penicillin
58. This nutritional myodegeneration disease may be caused by a deficiency of vitamin E and/or selenium.
    A. Caprine arthritis-encephalitis
    B. Johne disease

C. White muscle disease
D. Caseous lymphadenitis
59. Which statement is *false* regarding caseous lymphadenitis (CL) in small ruminants?
    A. Vaccinations are beneficial in goat herds.
    B. Aggressive culling is recommended in herds/flocks with CL.
    C. Practicing good hygiene during tail docking, castration, and shearing can help to prevent the disease.
    D. Differentials include chronic parasitism, caprine arthritis-encephalitis, and Johne disease.
60. Even if lambs survive an acute hemolytic crisis of copper toxicity, there is often irreversible, significant damage to the ____ due to ____.
    A. Liver; hemolysis
    B. Heart; hemoglobinemia
    C. Kidneys; hemoglobinuria
    D. Brain; myoglobinemia
61. When should a pregnancy examination be performed in does to detect pseudopregnancy?
    A. Forty to 70 days after breeding using transrectal ultrasonography
    B. Twenty-five to 40 days after breeding using the transabdominal method
    C. Forty to 70 days after breeding using the transabdominal method
    D. Sixty to 65 days after breeding using the transabdominal method
62. If the urethral process is not present in a small ruminant suspected of having urolithiasis:
    A. It may have necrosed and sloughed.
    B. It may be absent congenitally; this is very common.
    C. It may have already been amputated.
    D. A and C
63. What is the primary route of infection of caprine arthritis-encephalitis?
    A. Through wounds or breaks in the skin
    B. Fecal-oral
    C. Through infected colostrum or milk of the infected dam
    D. Aerosolization
64. ___ is a reportable disease with no known treatment that is only diagnosed through histopathological examination of the brain.
    A. Scrapie
    B. Johne disease
    C. White muscle disease
    D. Tetanus
65. Pinkeye in small ruminants is usually self-limiting and recovery can be expected in a few weeks.
    A. True
    B. False
66. What condition is described? "One technique involves placement of two or three vertical mattress sutures in the lower lid to roll the lid margin out."
    A. Ectropion
    B. Prolapsed third eyelid
    C. Hordeolum
    D. Entropion
67. When removing horn buds with a dehorning iron, what is one serious side effect of leaving the iron on too long?
    A. Abscess formation
    B. Thermal meningitis
    C. Optic neuritis
    D. Facial paralysis
68. When should small ruminants be immunized against erysipelas?
    A. At weaning, then every 6 months
    B. At weaning, then annually
    C. At 2 months of age, then annually
    D. At 1 month of age, then every 6 months
69. Enterotoxigenic *Escherichia coli* is the most important cause of diarrhea in:
    A. Ewes under 4 months of age
    B. Kids under 1 month of age
    C. Lambs under 5 days of age
    D. Piglets under 5 days of age
70. Oral trimethoprim/sulfa and amprolium are the only approved treatments for piglets with *Isospora suis* infections.
    A. True
    B. False
71. What may precipitate malignant hyperthermia (MH) or pale soft exudative pork (PSE)?
    A. Stress
    B. *Escherichia coli*
    C. Halothane
    D. A and C
72. In sows more milk is produced by the ___ mammary glands.
    A. Caudal
    B. Middle
    C. Cranial
    D. None of the above (An equal amount is produced by all mammary glands.)

EXTRA CREDIT

73. Define *extirpation*.
    A. Removal of the lacrimal gland
    B. Removal of the globe
    C. Removal of all the contents of the bony orbit
    D. Removal of ocular masses with cautery
74. When do pot-bellied pigs usually reach their full size?
    A. One year of age
    B. Eight months of age
    C. Twelve to 15 months of age
    D. Two to 3 years of age

CHAPTER 31

NURSING CONCEPTS IN ALTERNATIVE MEDICINE

1. If a muscle spasm is felt while performing the trigger-point massage technique, what should the therapist do?
   A. Immediately move to another area of the body and continue massage.
   B. Increase pressure.
   C. Maintain pressure in that spot until the muscle stops firing.
   D. All of the above

2. Which of the following are benefits of Swedish massage?
   A. Enhanced relaxation and reduced stress
   B. Increased oxygen capacity of the blood
   C. Enhanced blood and lymph circulation
   D. All of the above

3. What massage technique consists of rhythmic lifting, squeezing, and releasing of the tissue?
   A. Effleurage
   B. Friction
   C. Tapotement
   D. Vibration

4. _____ is a form of tapotement used to loosen phlegm congestion in the lungs.
   A. Petrissage
   B. Vibration
   C. Coupage
   D. Friction

5. Contraindications to massage in animals include:
   A. Massage over open wounds or an area of hemorrhage
   B. Massage after a recent high fever
   C. Massaging an apparently healthy animal simply to achieve relaxation
   D. A and B

6. What massage technique is used to lengthen muscles and aid in stretching?
   A. Effleurage
   B. Friction
   C. Tapotement
   D. Vibration

7. Increasing muscle mass without strengthening bone may increase the likelihood of bone fractures.
   A. True
   B. False

8. Swimming is an excellent therapy for dogs if the goal is to strengthen the rear limb(s).
   A. True
   B. False

9. Walking on an underwater treadmill in warm water provides the benefits of improved muscle mobility and ___, enhanced circulation, and facilitation of front-to-rear and side-to-side ___.
   A. Strength; movement
   B. Range of motion; balance
   C. Flexibility; strength
   D. Flexibility; balance

10. The benefits of land treadmills can be maximized by:
    A. Tilting them on an angle as if going up- or downhill
    B. Increasing the speed
    C. Increasing the length of time spent on them
    D. Converting them to underwater treadmills

11. When using ultrasound therapy, the proximity of the bone and the thickness of the tissue determine the ___ to use.
    A. Intensity
    B. Length of time
    C. Frequency
    D. Duty cycle

12. The use of ultrasound therapy is contraindicated:
    A. Over the testes
    B. Over tendons
    C. Over areas of chronic pain
    D. B and C

13. The use of neuromuscular electrical stimulation is contraindicated:
    A. Over neoplasms
    B. Over infection
    C. On animals with seizure disorders
    D. All of the above

14. These joints have rotation as well as flexion and extension.
    A. Carpal and tarsal
    B. Shoulder and hip
    C. Stifle
    C. Elbow

15. For the first ___ after an injury, only cold therapy should be applied to the injured site.
    A. 72 hours
    B. 12 hours
    C. 24 hours
    D. 1 week

16. What homemade device can be used for cold therapy?
    A. A bag of frozen peas
    B. A mixture of alcohol and water in a ziploc freezer bag at a ratio of 21
    C. Frozen water in a paper cup
    D. All of the above

17. What is the recommended maximum time for cryotherapy or heat therapy on horses' limbs?
    A. 1 hour
    B. 15 minutes
    C. 30 minutes
    D. 45 minutes

Copyright © 2006 by Elsevier, Inc. All rights reserved.

18. What is the most common use of acupuncture today?
    A. Gastrointestinal disorders
    B. Pain management
    C. Musculoskeletal disorders
    D. Neurological disorders
19. Which rehabilitation modality is based upon the belief that blockage of energy circulation in the body results in dysfunction or disease and that stagnant energy manifests as spasms or swelling?
    A. Veterinary chiropractic
    B. Hydrotherapy
    C. Physical therapy
    D. Acupuncture
20. The phenomenon of referred pain is part of this theory of acupuncture.
    A. Endogenous opioid theory
    B. Autonomic nervous system theory
    C. Bioelectric theory
    D. Humoral theory
21. Depending on which points are stimulated, acupuncture has been shown to induce systemic increases in:
    A. White blood cells
    B. Red blood cells
    C. Antigens
    D. Cortisol
22. Ultrasound can be performed to stimulate acupuncture points.
    A. True
    B. False
23. Clinical signs of vertebral subluxations include:
    A. Serious organ dysfunction
    B. Mild discomfort
    C. Reduced reflexes
    D. All of the above
24. Situations that warrant other diagnostics/treatment before chiropractic adjustments include:
    A. Active disk disease
    B. The presence of a cranial drawer sign in a dog with rear limb lameness
    C. A horse with neurologic deficits consistent with EPM
    D. B and C
25. Chemical restraint is commonly used on veterinary patients before chiropractic adjustments.
    A. True
    B. False
26. An owner is not able to prepare a balanced home-prepared diet for a pet cat. What can the technician recommend in this case?
    A. Rotate several nutritious and wholesome commercially prepared pet foods, approved by the veterinarian.
    B. Hospitalize the pet so that the staff can prepare and offer the holistic diet.
    C. Prepare a raw diet instead.
    D. Give the pet a multivitamin daily.
27. What are advantages of raw meat as part of a dog's or cat's diet?
    A. It contains fewer enzymes.
    B. It is more easily digested.
    C. These animals are well-equipped to handle potential bacterial contamination.
    D. Raw bones have no potential dangers.
28. What measures can be taken to ensure a balanced, healthy diet for large animals?
    A. Provide proper pasture management.
    B. Provide optimal quality hay and grain.
    C. Supplement the diet with minerals and vitamins to achieve balance.
    D. Perform soil tests and hay analysis for nutrient content regularly.
    E. All of the above.
29. One nutraceutical that is thought to have anticancer properties is:
    A. Shark cartilage
    B. Chondroitin
    C. Sam-E
    D. Taurine
30. Which of the following statements is *false*?
    A. Most herbal therapies are not safe for pregnant animals.
    B. Most herbal therapies are not safe for cats.
    C. Most herbal therapies have a very high margin of safety.
    D. Currently, the United States relies on testing based in Europe and Asia to substantiate the effects of herbal therapy.
31. After steroid therapy, ___ may be given to detoxify the liver.
    A. Gingko
    B. St. John's wort
    C. Milk thistle
    D. Echinacea
32. It is best to administer Western herbs to veterinary patients along with a meal.
    A. True
    B. False
33. Which statement(s) best describe(s) TCM practice?
    A. For more chronic conditions or to help patients maintain health, herbs alone are used.
    B. Acupuncture is considered "stronger" than herbal medicine.
    C. Most TCM practitioners in china use acupuncture only in acute cases.
    D. All of the above
    E. A and C
34. What therapy is based on the belief that things that suppress symptoms actually drive disease deeper into the body or create more imbalance?

    A. Ayurvedic medicine
    B. Traditional Chinese medicine
    C. Humoral therapy
    D. Homeopathy
35. Rescue remedy is a combination of five flower essences that is used to treat animals:
    A. That become nervous when boarding
    B. In times of stress, anxiety, or trauma
    C. Postsurgically
    D. All of the above
36. Pulsed signal therapy is a type of pulsed electromagnetic field therapy that is used to reactivate ____ and increase production of ____ in joints.
    A. Enzymes; synovial fluid
    B. Chondrocytes; proteoglycan and collagen
    C. Collagenase; white blood cells
    D. Electrical fields; protein
37. In aromatherapy, ____ is used to achieve sedation or relaxation.
    A. Lavender oil
    B. Tea tree oil
    C. Thyme oil
    D. Citronella

EXTRA CREDIT

38. Define *phonophoresis*.
    A. Transdermal delivery of medication
    B. The use of sound waves to increase blood flow
    C. Propagation of electric signals in muscles using heat
    D. The use of sound waves to increase a neurologic threshold
39. Define *meridian*.
    A. A spinal tract that transmits pain
    B. An organ system that is stimulated by acupuncture needles
    C. Pathways or channels through which bioelectricity passes in the body
    D. A homeopathic remedy

CHAPTER 32

VETERINARY PRACTICE MANAGEMENT

1. A veterinary technician must be able to work in all areas of the hospital.
    A. True
    B. False
2. The majority of practicing veterinarians:
    A. Are general practitioners.
    B. Offer primary-care level services.
    C. Are specialists at referral practices.
    D. Are tertiary-care providers at veterinary schools.
    E. A and B.
3. What is the purpose of having veterinarians who provide different levels of care at a network of different types of institutions?
    A. To increase the income of each practitioner
    B. To increase the quality of patient care
    C. To provide a foundation of financial support for clinical research at veterinary schools
    D. B and C
    E. All of the above
4. In addition to the AVMA regulations that must be followed in order for a veterinary facility to legally operate, what organization has set standards of excellence that veterinary hospitals must meet in order to be accredited by the organization?
    A. The American Red Cross
    B. The American Medical Association
    C. The American Animal Hospital Association
    D. The Rockefeller Foundation
    E. The United Nations Children's Fund
5. The top two factors in attracting new small animal clients are _____ and _____.
    A. Professional knowledge; facility appearance
    B. Clarity of communication; professional knowledge
    C. Location; recommendations from friends
    D. Animal-handling skills; location
    E. Offering the latest medical technology; recommendations from friends
6. _____ is/are usually acceptable in the reception area and other client-visited areas.
    A. Employee eating and drinking
    B. Employee smoking
    C. Employees out of uniform
    D. Healthy plants
    E. A lot of noise
7. The veterinarian or animal facility cannot be held liable for a pet that escapes.
    A. True
    B. False
8. The ideal small-animal isolation ward has which characteristics? (Select all that apply.)
    A. A separate entrance and exit
    B. An air-handling system separate from the one servicing the rest of the building
    C. Patient care provided by only one or two persons
    D. Patients treated in the main treatment area of the hospital
    E. Strict disinfection and personal-hygiene protocols
9. Why does the practice manager at the hospital where you work insist that employees *not* place any of their food or drinks in the refrigerator where animal food, vaccination, and medications are kept?
    A. This is an Occupational Safety and Health Administration (OSHA) regulation.

B. She is very strict.
C. Molds from human-food spoilage can contaminate vaccines.
D. She doesn't want to deal with spilled drinks and crumbs.
E. Preservatives in some human foods can volatilize and deactivate insulin stored in the refrigerator.

10. Which activity is acceptable in the operating room?
    A. Treatment of isolation-ward patients
    B. Pack preparation and sterilization
    C. Dentistry
    D. Surgery
    E. C and D

11. It is acceptable to place a small animal recovering from anesthesia on the treatment room floor if that is the only place where he can be continuously monitored by the technical staff.
    A. True
    B. False

12. Which statement is true concerning the storage area of the veterinary hospital?
    A. From the management viewpoint, hospital storage space is the most expensive floor space in the building because this space produces the least income.
    B. Supplies and equipment that are no longer used or usable should be removed to make room for the essential items.
    C. Items that can be hung on the wall or from the ceiling should be removed from the floor.
    D. Flammable or toxic material should be safely marked and stored away from foods or drugs.
    E. All of the above.

13. A well-equipped large-animal hospital examination area where a variety of species are treated must be equipped with at least:
    A. Stocks
    B. An alleyway with a squeeze chute and head catch
    C. A variety of sizes of small, indoor pens or stalls
    D. Stocks and large, rotating examination tables designed specifically for restraining cattle on their side
    E. All of the above

14. In a large-animal practice with inpatient services, what functions may all be provided in the same area?
    A. Outpatient examinations and reception/check-in
    B. Inpatient treatments and major surgeries
    C. Outpatient examinations, inpatient treatments, and minor surgeries
    D. A and B
    E. All of the above

15. The most efficient way to manage general cleanliness within the building is to:
    A. Have every duty specifically assigned to a certain person who always performs it.
    B. Hire an after-hours cleaning service for all routine maintenance chores.
    C. Have everyone in the practice assume some of the cleaning responsibility and perform many duties on an as-needed basis.
    D. Have a built-in, central vacuum system for hair removal from the floors.
    E. Keep "extras"—magazine racks, pictures, artwork, shelving—to a minimum, so less cleanup is needed.

16. It is 3 PM at the busy small-animal hospital where you work. The reception area is full of clients. As usual, you have several things that you should be attending to at this moment. Of the five things listed below, which is best attended to immediately?
    A. "Sparky's" cleanup bath for an early-evening discharge
    B. "Little's" 3 PM treatment of 5 mg oral prednisone
    C. The new patient waiting for an initial evaluation and "TPR" in room 1
    D. Dr. B in the treatment room waiting for help to draw blood from a cat
    E. The large pile of feces that "Buddy" just excreted onto the reception-area floor

17. Critical to the successful maintenance of major equipment is:
    A. Assigning one person to its maintenance
    B. Familiarity with electrical-equipment safety rules
    C. A written service file for each piece of equipment containing warranties, maintenance requirements, instructions for use, and a repair representative's telephone number
    D. Task sheets requiring employee initials when regular maintenance and duties are performed
    E. All of the above

18. Which medium-sized-practice situation should be the most cost-effective from a practice-management standpoint?
    A. The veterinarians (DVMs) perform the majority of medical, technical, animal-care, and management duties, with lay staff to help with reception and ward duties.
    B. The same as above but with the addition of a dedicated practice manager (VPM) to attend to the practice-management duties.
    C. The DVMs only diagnose, prescribe treatment, and perform surgery. Certified veterinary technicians perform all technical and nursing duties with the help of veterinary assistants and/or ward attendants. A VPM attends to management duties.

19. In general, it makes the best economic sense to use the lowest-paid employee to do any job that he can competently and legally perform.
    A. True
    B. False
20. If the client is the "lifeblood" of the practice, then the _____ is the staff member perhaps most responsible for keeping the practice "alive" (i.e., clients happy and practice growing)!
    A. Veterinary technician
    B. Veterinary assistant
    C. Ward assistant
    D. Veterinary practice manager
    E. Receptionist
21. The best way to ensure efficient and maximal hospital function when an employee must be absent is to:
    A. Have a list of substitutes who may be able to take that person's place on short notice.
    B. Cross train staff members so they can function in areas to which they are not usually assigned.
    C. Have the veterinarian take over that person's duties for the day.
    D. Reduce the patient load significantly on the days of employee absences.
    E. Terminate employees for unexpected absences to discourage irresponsible behavior.
22. A veterinary technician desiring to become very skilled in one area should seek employment at:
    A. An institutional (veterinary school) teaching-hospital practice
    B. A large (five or more doctors) private hospital, referral facility, or animal medical center
    C. A medium-sized (three to five doctors) private practice
    D. A small (one to two doctors) private practice
    E. A or B
23. Which practice-management technique provides rewards for good employees performing well, guided encouragement for improvement of poor employees, and timely discharge of poor workers?
    A. Proper duty delegation
    B. Having a veterinary practice manager at the hospital
    C. Asking open-ended questions at job interviews
    D. Written job descriptions and periodic performance evaluations
    E. Allowing employees to participate in the hiring process
24. Practice staff meetings:
    A. Should be held at least once monthly.
    B. Should be held at least quarterly.
    C. Should be held at least every 6 months.
    D. Should be held at least annually.
    E. Are only necessary in large practices.
25. If possible, the veterinary technician should delegate _____ tasks to assistants or aides.
    A. Feeding and watering
    B. Restraining
    C. Bathing
    D. Animal exercising
    E. Most non–income-producing (nonbillable or those for which clients do not directly pay)
26. Any case that an owner feels is an emergency is always an emergency case.
    A. True
    B. False
27. Which aspect of patient discharge is most critical to the client's impression of the level of care her pet has received?
    A. The amount she pays for services (*more* equals *better care*)
    B. The efficiency of fee collection by the receptionist
    C. How dry, clean, and odor-free her pet is, along with the neatness of hair removal and appearance of surgery incisions
    D. The appearance of the written home-care instructions
    E. The availability of the veterinarian for questions
28. Which essential aspect of maintaining inventory allows the technician to ensure that items are not staying on the shelf too long before being sold?
    A. Inventory master list of all items in stock
    B. Calculation of turnover rate using a standard mathematical formula
    C. Pharmacy library of all product and ordering information
    D. Making sure that what is received is what was ordered and/or billed
    E. Authorizing payment for shipments
29. Inventory control is generally a large, time-consuming job that should be assigned to one person to manage.
    A. True
    B. False
30. The only unique product that a veterinary practice has to offer is its service.
    A. True
    B. False
31. Critical to client retention is the veterinarian's and the staff's:
    A. Ability to project a concerned, caring personality
    B. Expertise in carefully handling the animals
    C. Clarity of communication
    D. Professional knowledge
    E. A, B, and C
32. A client's appearance should be used to provide a clue about his ability to pay.
    A. True
    B. False

33. Handle negative clients in a(n) _____ manner.
    A. Cautious
    B. Positive and friendly
    C. Similar (negative)
    D. Aggressive
    E. Indifferent
34. During the discharge of most hospitalized cases, it is least confusing to present the pet to the client:
    A. When the client first enters the reception area and states he is there to pick up his pet
    B. During the initial consultation with the technician in the examination room
    C. After the client talks to the veterinarian, when the technician is giving home-care instructions in the examination room
    D. While the client is settling the account with the receptionist
    E. After all consults and instructions have been provided and the account is paid
35. Why are client visits with inpatients best conducted in an examination or treatment room rather than in the ward?
    A. To avoid disturbing other inpatients
    B. To avoid upsetting the client who is sensitive to seeing very sick animals
    C. To prevent hospital liability if the client should trip over a cord or intravenous line
    D. Because the wards usually have a strong odor of urine and feces
    E. To prevent client exposure to radiation in the case of radiographic exposure
36. Concerning how to handle "walk-in" clients in an appointment-based practice, which statement is most accurate?
    A. If an appointment and walk-in client enter the practice at the same time, the appointment is always seen first.
    B. If it is a very busy day, walk-in clients should be gently told they cannot be seen and should schedule an appointment for another time.
    C. Emergency cases are accepted at any time and are given priority over all appointments.
    D. One advantage to the no-appointment system is that it gives greater control over client/patient flow, thus improving work-schedule efficiency.
    E. A and C.
37. In the veterinary-practice field, the most acceptable way to set fee levels is:
    A. To make a competitive guess of how to match or undercut the prices that others charge
    B. To try to estimate what each client can afford
    C. To use accounting methods to establish fees based on the cost of offering the service
38. Which of the following is a direct cost (i.e., not "overhead") of running a business?
    A. Utilities costs
    B. Purchase or rental of the land
    C. Pharmaceutical costs
    D. Facility upkeep
    E. Taxes and interest on any debt
39. The first- and second-largest expense areas of operating a veterinary clinic are ___ and ___, respectively.
    A. Inventory; utilities
    B. Personnel; inventory
    C. Utilities; medical equipment
    D. Accounting/computers; medical equipment
    E. Utilities; personnel
40. Fees for which of the following services should be competitive with neighboring practices? (Select all that apply.)
    A. Fracture repair
    B. Complete blood count
    C. Spay or neuter surgery
    D. Physical examination
    E. Rabies vaccination
41. In most small-animal practices, the practice manager or veterinarian should be involved before services are provided if:
    A. The client pays by credit card.
    B. The client pays by cash.
    C. The client cannot pay the full balance of the bill when services are rendered.
    D. The client pays with a medical credit card.
    E. A and D
42. Which of the following will contribute to a successfully managed practice?
    A. A firm and written credit policy
    B. An appointment (rather than walk-in) system
    C. Review and update of the fee schedule at least every 6 months
    D. Strategic use of an office computer
    E. All of the above
43. All telephone calls should be answered by the ___ ring.
    A. Third
    B. Fourth
    C. Fifth
    D. Sixth
    E. Seventh
44. Adhering to which guideline will improve communication between the staff and clients?
    A. Use scientific terminology so the client knows you are knowledgeable and competent.
    B. Do not discuss information that appears to be "common knowledge" or the client will feel patronized.
    C. Assume a slightly superior manner and tone to build a client's confidence in you.
    D. Let the client talk about her pet's problem, and pay careful attention to both her words and her body language.
    E. All of the above

45. A client should be acknowledged with eye contact, a smile, and a comment:
    A. When he or she first enters the practice
    B. Within 1 minute of entering the practice
    C. Within 5 minutes of entering the practice
    D. When he or she approaches the receptionist's desk
46. The best way to eliminate client complaints about fees is:
    A. To not accept checks
    B. To not accept credit cards
    C. With up-front, open communication
    D. With the use of a written fee-estimate sheet
    E. C and D
47. Which statement is true concerning handling a difficult client? (Select all that apply.)
    A. Try to reduce the level of confrontation.
    B. Try to establish exactly what the complaint is about.
    C. If the client is unreasonable, escort him to an examination room and allow the practice manager or veterinarian to handle him.
    D. If the client seems dangerous or is intoxicated, call the police.
    E. Follow the old adage, "The client is always right, even when he's wrong."
48. Professional marketing can involve:
    A. Advertising in the yellow pages of the telephone book
    B. Sending thank you and sympathy cards to appropriate clients
    C. Providing pet nutritional counseling and dietary management
    D. Writing a newspaper animal column
    E. All of the above
49. A veterinary practice cannot exist without:
    A. Sick animals
    B. A staff who wants to help animals
    C. Satisfied clients
    D. Full-service care
    E. An effective marketing plan

For the next eight questions, classify the marketing technique as internal or external.
    A. Internal
    B. External
50. Practice newsletter
51. Internet Web page
52. Newspapers
53. Client reminders
54. Radio and television
55. Giving a talk at an elementary school
56. Practice appearance
57. Staff appearance
58. "Active" listening involves listening to clients and then verbally rephrasing their messages back to them for verification.
    A. True
    B. False
59. How many reminders are best sent for a specific service?
    A. One
    B. Two
    C. Three
    D. Four
    E. Five
60. It is essential that all staff members handling animals wash their hands:
    A. After every patient
    B. Every 15 minutes
    C. Every 30 minutes
    D. Every 60 minutes
    E. Only before eating
61. Business cards should be made available to clients from both veterinarians and key support staff, especially certified veterinary technicians.
    A. True
    B. False
62. The most effective use of written client information, such as handouts covering specific diseases, is to:
    A. Place them on a rack in the reception area.
    B. Place them on a rack in the examination rooms.
    C. Staple them to the clients' invoices.
    D. Explain the information to clients while pointing it out in the handout and then give the handout to them.
63. Concerning veterinary advertisements in the yellow pages, _____ should be avoided because clients perceive this as less professional.
    A. The use of multiple colors (red and green)
    B. Ads larger than one-fourth page
    C. A photo of the staff members
    D. Listing services offered
    E. A and B
64. Veterinary ethics dictate that a practice's Internet Web site should be used only for:
    A. Information related to that practice, its staff, and services provided
    B. Scheduling appointments
    C. Animal-medical topics only, not general pet care
    D. None of the above (A Web site can be used for all of the above topics and more.)
65. Name the four basic sanitary measures taken by the large-animal veterinarian and veterinary technician at the end of a call to prevent disease transmission between farms.
66. Which of the following clients is best scheduled early in the day, and why? (1) a routine annual checkup, (2) a limping dog, (3) a cat with a "watery eye," (4) a new patient for an annual checkup, (5) a sneezing ferret.
67. Mrs. L's very-well-fed potbellied pig, "Fifi," has fractured her elbow. Prior to hospitalizing her for surgical repair, you provide this client with a

written fee estimate of $1000. Based on the fee-collecting rules used by most animal hospitals, tell Mrs. L what is expected of her financially, regarding payment.
68. You are asked to participate in a practice-wide effort to provide full-service care. List three services in which you would like to participate that could be added to reach this goal. The hospital currently provides basic dental, medical, and surgical services.
69. As a client stands in front of a food-marketing display in the reception area, he slyly asks you why he should purchase his pet food at your practice when it is cheaper elsewhere. How might you answer him?

EXTRA CREDIT

70. *Amortization* is:
    A. Charging bills to clients for future payments
    B. Reduction in value or price
    C. Writing off expenditures by prorating over a fixed period
    D. Naming a newborn animal "Mortimer"

CHAPTER 33

MEDICAL RECORDS

1. Which of the following is not a primary purpose of a medical record?
   A. Supports continuity of patient care across shift changes.
   B. Documents instructions given to the owner(s) when the patient is discharged.
   C. Provides data to conduct retrospective studies.
   D. Helps to develop an effective diagnostic and treatment plan after physical exam findings and patient history have been recorded.
2. Medical records are considered legal documents that insurance companies may require to assess whether a claim is to be paid.
   A. True
   B. False
3. Which form of medical record must be used by hospitals seeking accreditation by the American Animal Hospital Association (AAHA)?
   A. Letter-size folders
   B. 10 × 16 inch cards
   C. Legal-size folders
   D. 5 × 8 inch cards
4. Which type of practice generally uses the carbonized invoice sheets as medical records?
   A. Exotic animal practices
   B. Small animal practices
   C. Feline practices
   D. Ambulatory food and equine practitioners
5. Although impractical, it is required that food animal veterinarians maintain individual medical records for each animal in a herd.
   A. True
   B. False
6. The ___-oriented medical record promotes team-oriented medical care, rapid retrieval of information, and fosters excellent communication.
   A. Source
   B. Patient
   C. Treatment
   D. Problem
7. Medical records that have limited space typically use the ___-oriented patient record format.
   A. Source
   B. Patient
   C. Treatment
   D. Problem
8. If the veterinarian asks you to record the signalment of a new patient, what information about the pet will you obtain?
   A. Primary complaint
   B. Sex and breed
   C. Species
   D. Weight and current medical conditions
   E. Age
   F. A and B
   G. B, C and E
9. In the problem-oriented veterinary medical record, the database consists of the signalment, physical exam, diagnostic tests, and ___.
   A. Primary complaint
   B. Working problem list
   C. History
   D. Logs
10. Which of the following would not be found on a master problem list in a problem-oriented veterinary medical record?
    A. Nystagmus
    B. Congestive heart failure
    C. Osteosarcoma
    D. Pyometra
11. The written process of evaluating and adjusting therapeutic treatment plans is called a ___.
    A. Database
    B. Working problem list
    C. SOAP
    D. Problem-oriented veterinary medical record
12. Which part(s) of the SOAP might the veterinary technician complete?
    A. Plan
    B. Subjective
    C. Assessment
    D. Objective

E. A and C
F. B and D

For questions 13 through 18, choose S, O, A, or P to indicate where each statement belongs in the patient's progress notes.

13. Vomiting and depression following chemotherapy, patient deteriorating
14. Slight bleeding at surgical site 24 hours after onychectomy
15. Bright, alert, barking
16. Abdominal ultrasound to be performed this afternoon
17. Remove urinary catheter and culture the tip. Use shredded newspaper instead of litter; monitor and record volume of urine produced for 24 hours.
18. Temperature = 101.5° F, pulse = 90 beats per minute, respiratory rate = 12 breaths per minute
19. For which of the following procedures is it critical that the owner completes and signs an informed consent form?
    A. Radiographs
    B. Euthanasia
    C. Ear flush
    D. All of the above
20. Which controlled substances must be securely stored in a locked cabinet and inventoried separately from noncontrolled drugs?
    A. Schedule I
    B. Schedule II, III, IV, and V
    C. Schedule II
    D. Schedule IV and V
21. The author recommends that records that have been inactive for ___ or more are moved to storage; records that are ___ or older may be removed from storage and shredded.
    A. 4 years; 7 years
    B. 3 years; 8 years
    C. 4 years; 8 years
    D. 3 years; 7 years
22. The client is, by law, the owner of the medical record.
    A. True
    B. False
23. How should errors be documented in medical records?
    A. Draw a line through the mistake and initial it.
    B. Use erasable ink so that errors can be completely erased.
    C. Obscure the error with white-out, then initial and date it.
    D. Write correct information in the margin, then initial and date it.
    E. None of the above
    F. A and B
    G. A and D

EXTRA CREDIT

24. Which controlled substances must be maintained of a separate inventory?
    A. I
    B. II
    C. III
    D. IV
    E. V
25. By law, how often must controlled drugs must be inventoried?
    A. Annually
    B. Every 6 months
    C. Every 3 years
    D. Every 2 years

CHAPTER 34

COMPUTER APPLICATIONS IN VETERINARY PRACTICE

1. Programs that help the user perform word processing and bookkeeping are considered:
    A. Computer hardware
    B. Operating software
    C. Applications software
    D. Bits
2. Common operating systems include:
    A. UNIX
    B. DOS
    C. Excel
    D. Microsoft Word
    E. Macintosh
    F. A, B, and E
    G. C and D
    H. All of the above
3. Which of the following statements describe features of 32-bit programs?
    A. Thirty-two-bit refers to Windows 3.1, 95, 98, NT, and 2000.
    B. Thirty-two-bit programs allow only one person at a time to manipulate data to avoid confusion in the face of potential litigation.
    C. A revision history is not provided so that changes cannot be tracked.
    D. None of the above
    E. B and C
    F. All of the above
4. Multiple computer terminals in a veterinary clinic are connected through a _____, which manages a _____.
    A. System; network
    B. Server; network
    C. Network; server
    D. Modem; server

5. Computerizing a veterinary clinic can enable better time management so that quality time can be spent with each client and better care can be afforded to each patient.
   A. True
   B. False
6. Basic care of a computer consists of:
   A. Using compressed air to clean inside the computer case every 2 to 3 months
   B. Dusting the computer case at least once a month
   C. Keeping it in an area with good ventilation and plenty of cool air
   D. All of the above
   E. None of the above
7. Practical ways to begin to research various veterinary software companies include:
   A. Meeting with software vendors at national meetings
   B. Reading the trends survey published by the american animal hospital association
   C. Using demo CDs to investigate programs in depth
   D. A and C
   E. All of the above
   F. None of the above
8. Which of the following statements is/are true?
   A. Ideally, only one person in the clinic should be responsible for scheduling appointments.
   B. To date, computer programs are not yet capable of customizing appointment times based upon specific tasks.
   C. In general, 40% of all scheduled appointments are generated from reminders.
   D. To date, veterinary software does not come with predetermined prices of products and services.
   E. A, B, and C
   F. None of the above
9. Usable items such as tape, catheters, and syringes make computerized inventory tracking almost problem free because they are billed separately.
   A. True
   B. False
10. According to the author, how can a veterinary practice prevent computerized medical records from being altered.
    A. Assign one veterinarian to review all tracking changes on a regular basis.
    B. Back up all records on a monthly basis and store them with a data storage facility.
    C. Keep paper files of all computer files.
    D. Allow only one person to enter all data into the computer so that if alterations are suspected later, there is no question as to the responsible person.

EXTRA CREDIT

11. The technician subsidiary of vin.com is:
    A. VSPN.org
    B. AVMA.org
    C. vetmedteam.com
    D. Noah
12. Name three benefits of vetmedteam.com and vspn.org for the veterinary technician, other than the fact that there is no fee to use their services.

CHAPTER 35

ZOONOSES AND PUBLIC HEALTH

1. Cryptococcosis is a _____ organism diagnosed by _____.
   A. Viral; serologic titers of antibody to the organism
   B. Bacterial; culture
   C. Fungal (yeast); direct microscopic examination using India ink as a stain
   D. Fungal (hyphae); direct microscopic examination using potassium hydroxide (KOH) to remove debris from hair samples
2. Which group of individuals is at high risk for developing severe complications from a minor wound or zoonotic disease?
   A. Pregnant women
   B. Persons positive for the human immunodeficiency virus (HIV) or who have acquired immunodeficiency syndrome (AIDS)
   C. People receiving long-term corticosteroid therapy
   D. All of the above

For the next five questions, match the zoonotic disease with the species most likely to transmit the disease to veterinary personnel in the course of their workday
   A. Reptiles
   B. Cats
   C. Cattle
   D. Dogs
   E. Sheep
3. Pasteurellosis
4. Q fever (*Coxiella burnetii*)
5. Campylobacteriosis
6. Brucellosis
7. Salmonellosis

Use the following scenario to answer the next three questions. You and the veterinarian for whom you work are walking through a field investigating a case of "sudden death" in several beef cattle. You come across a couple of carcasses with a bloody discharge from their nostrils and ears. (*Note:* There is no possibility of a lightning strike.)

8. What zoonotic disease will most likely cause these signs?
   A. Q fever
   B. Anthrax
   C. Brucellosis
   D. Rabies
9. After diagnostic samples not requiring a necropsy are obtained, what precautions will help protect you and others from infection with the suspected zoonotic disease?
   A. Do not perform a necropsy and burn the carcass at the site.
   B. Wear heavy gloves to avoid contamination of any skin cuts during the necropsy.
   C. Wear a mask to prevent inhalation of microorganisms during the necropsy.
   D. Remove the carcass to a veterinary facility for a necropsy and soak the hair in chlorhexidine prior to the necropsy.
10. In addition to veterinary personnel, workers in what other occupation are at high risk for acquiring a fatal form of this disease?
    A. Laboratory-rodent care
    B. Chicken processing
    C. Wool processing
    D. Primate care

For the next five questions, match the zoonotic disease with the route by which a veterinary technician at work would most likely contract the disease.
   A. Ornithosis (psittacosis)
   B. Rabies
   C. Contagious ecthyma (orf)
   D. Dermatophytosis (tinea or ringworm)
   E. Cryptosporidiosis
11. Bite wound or contact with saliva
12. Direct contact with infective material
13. Fecal-oral
14. Inhalation of agent excreted in bird feces
15. Direct contact with infected animal or spores on hair or dander
16. Another term for Newcastle disease in birds is *chlamydiosis*.
    A. True
    B. False
17. Avoiding contact with the placentas and birth fluids of aborted ruminant fetuses prevents the possibility of contracting:
    A. Q fever
    B. Brucellosis
    C. *Capnocytophaga* infection
    D. A and B
18. _____ occurs worldwide in all age-groups, is probably the most common cause of food- or waterborne diarrhea in the world and accounts for more than 2 million cases in the United States alone.
    A. Campylobacteriosis
    B. *Capnocytophaga* infection
    C. Cat-scratch disease
    D. Cutaneous anthrax

Use the following scenario to answer the next two questions. An otherwise healthy veterinary technician, Anna, is bitten by a 2-year-old mixed-breed dog, "Tow Tow," while restraining him for a pedicure. The bite does not cause severe tissue damage, but the canine teeth penetrate her skin and she does bleed. Tow Tow is current on all of his vaccinations including rabies. He lives primarily in the backyard of his owner's suburban home.

19. What is the best, first action Anna should take following the bite?
    A. Wash the wound with soap and water, then with povidone-iodine, and follow with a thorough irrigation with water.
    B. Place Tow Tow in the run reserved for dogs needing quarantine due to suspected rabies.
    C. Call the local county or city rabies-control department to find out how to deal with Tow Tow.
    D. Administer the antidote to rabies, which should be in the clinic refrigerator, intramuscularly in her triceps muscle.
20. What disease should Anna be most concerned about contracting?
    A. Pasteurellosis
    B. Rabies
    C. *Capnocytophaga* infection
    D. A or C
21. Frequent hand washing with disinfectant soaps or detergents by those working with _____ can lessen the chance of contracting erysipeloid at work.
    A. Dogs and cats
    B. Swine, domestic fowl, fish, or shellfish
    C. Ruminants
    D. Primates
22. _____ causes both "fowl cholera" and rabbit "snuffles."
    A. *Toxoplasma gondii*
    B. *Chlamydia psittaci*
    C. *Coxiella burnetii*
    D. *Pasteurella multocida*
23. What is a "reportable" disease?
    A. *Reportable* is another term for zoonotic.
    B. A confirmed diagnosis of a reportable disease must be reported to local health authorities.
    C. A reportable disease is any disease potentially fatal to humans.
    D. A reportable disease is any foreign disease not usually seen in the United States.
24. If you develop a sudden headache, vomiting, malaise, fever, and chills followed by a rash on your extremities, and you work with rats or rodents,

you should report this to your physician so that she can initiate the proper diagnostic methods for potential:
   A. Streptobacillosis or spirillosis
   B. Newcastle disease
   C. Dermatophytosis
   D. Cryptococcosis

25. Which agent causes dermatophytosis (tinea or ringworm)?
   A. *Trichophyton mentagrophytes*
   B. *Trichophyton verrucosum*
   C. *Microsporum canis*
   D. All of the above

26. Which agent can cause diarrhea in humans who accidentally ingest the diarrheic fecal material of an infected animal?
   A. *Cryptococcus neoformans*
   B. *Cryptosporidium parvum*
   C. *Trichophyton mentagrophytes*
   D. *Erysipelothrix rhusiopathiae*

27. Pregnant women should be counseled to _____ in order to avoid toxoplasmosis.
   A. Avoid contact with or wash hands thoroughly after contact with cat feces or dirty litter
   B. Wash hands thoroughly after gardening or any contact with soil
   C. Avoid consumption or handling of undercooked or raw meat
   D. All of the above

28. Contagious ecthyma (orf) is most commonly seen in people coming into contact with:
   A. Rodents
   B. Swine
   C. Sheep or goats
   D. Horses

29. In humans, herpesvirus simiae (B-virus) infection causes:
   A. A mild upper respiratory infection that usually resolves on its own in 1 to 2 weeks
   B. Genital ulcers
   C. Ulcers, sores, and blisters around the mouth
   D. A severe and usually fatal neurologic disorder

30. How is herpesvirus simiae (B-virus) infection acquired?
   A. By accidental ingestion of infected feces (fecal-oral)
   B. By infected aerosols (microsize droplets) contacting human eyes or nasal or oral mucosa
   C. By a bite wound or any salivary contact with broken skin
   D. B and C

31. "Haverhill fever" is one form of:
   A. Streptobacillosis
   B. Anthrax
   C. Cat-scratch disease
   D. Herpesvirus simiae (B-type) virus

32. Which statement concerning rabies is most accurate?
   A. In the live animal, rabies is diagnosed by an in-house ELISA performed on feces.
   B. Behavioral changes with profuse salivation, aggression, a change in voice, and/ or paralysis may suggest a presumptive diagnosis of rabies.
   C. In the case of a dead animal, the liver is submitted to a laboratory for diagnosis.
   D. Cattle and horses are not susceptible to rabies.

33. Most cases of human rabies are attributable to _____ because the virus is most abundant in _____.
   A. A bite by an infected animal; saliva
   B. A scratch by the claws of an infected animal; epithelial tissue
   C. Casual contact with an infected animal; saliva
   D. Accidental ingestion of feces; feces

34. Rabies is always fatal once clinical disease has developed.
   A. True
   B. False

35. Which statement concerning dealing with potential human exposure to rabies is true?
   A. Local laws may vary but, in general, a dog or cat that has bitten a person should be quarantined and observed for at least 10 days.
   B. One of the most effective means of preventing rabies in humans is to cleanse any animal bite or scratch wound immediately and thoroughly.
   C. Preexposure immunization (a rabies vaccine) is recommended for all persons coming into contact with wild or unvaccinated domestic animals.
   D. All of the above

36. All cases of animal and human rabies should be reported to health authorities.
   A. True
   B. False

37. The primary reason for the 30-day quarantine period for birds entering the United States from foreign countries is Newcastle disease–outbreak prevention.
   A. True
   B. False

38. Which of the following statements is/are true regarding *Coxiella burnetti* (Q fever)?
   A. Farm animals are the most common sources of Q fever, but cats, dogs, and rabbits may also transmit the disease.
   B. Exposure to newborn or stillborn pet animals has been linked to Q fever in urban areas.
   C. The agent can be present in infected birth fluids and ruminant placentae, or in wool or hides, and soil in areas where livestock are kept.
   D. None of the above
   E. All of the above

39. The most serious forms of tularemia, ___ and ___, can be treated with antibiotics; ___ is the drug of choice.
    A. Typhoidal, pneumonic; streptomycin
    B. Pneumonic, ulceroglandular; clavamox
    C. Pneumonic, typhoidal; penicillin
    D. Ulceroglandular, pneumonic; streptomycin
40. In 2003, the first reported case of monkeypox in the United States was reported. The virus was transmitted from rats to ___ to humans by direct contact.
    A. Rabbits
    B. Deer
    C. Prairie dogs
    D. Bats
41. In humans, this disease presents as a raised, purplish lesion accompanied by severe pain and swelling.
    A. Cat-scratch disease
    B. Toxoplasmosis
    C. *Campylobacter*
    D. Erysipelothrix
42. This disease can be isolated from fecal specimens; clinical signs in humans include acute enterocolitis 12 to 36 hours after ingestion, headache, abdominal pain, diarrhea, nausea, and fever.
    A. Tularemia
    B. Salmonellosis
    C. Newcastle disease
    D. West Nile virus
43. How do humans contract avian chlamydiosis?
    A. By eating undercooked bird (chicken, turkey)
    B. Through bites of infected birds that break the skin
    C. Inhalation of the organism in dried bird feces, ocular or nasal secretions of birds, dust from feathers
    D. All of the above

Use the following scenario to answer the next three short-answer questions. A client who has just purchased a box turtle for her 7-year-old son calls to ask what she should know about "that disease" she's "heard that reptiles carry."

44. To what disease is she most likely referring?
45. What are the signs of this disease in most reptiles?
46. How can she best prevent her child from contracting the disease (apart from getting rid of the turtle)?
47. How does a person become infected with cat-scratch disease?
48. Other than dogs and cats, name four species that are usually responsible for the transmission of rabies.

EXTRA CREDIT

49. A *snood* is a:
    A. Group of hens
    B. Cone-shaped mass of red vascular tissue that lies across the base of a turkey's beak
    C. Place where pigs wallow to stay cool.
    D. Short nap taken by a student during lecture
50. *Velogenic* is:
    A. A term meaning "highly virulent."
    B. A disease in which direct contact is not required for infection transmission.
    C. A term meaning "predisposed to infecting the viscera."
    D. A term describing a raceway for bicycles without brakes.

CHAPTER 36

OCCUPATIONAL HEALTH AND SAFETY

1. Who is the most important person in ensuring your safety on the job?
    A. Management
    B. The veterinarian
    C. *You*
    D. The technical staff
2. OSHA laws require employers to:
    A. Provide employees with appropriate safety equipment.
    B. Train employees in safety procedures and the proper use of safety equipment.
    C. Have a safety program, which includes educating employees about the inherent risks of their jobs.
    D. All of the above
3. What should an employee do if a complaint is not taken seriously by an employer or if there is a dangerous situation that is not adequately addressed?
    A. Seek employment elsewhere.
    B. Notify the regional OSHA office.
    C. Try to correct the situation yourself.
    D. Avoid the problem area and just try to work around it.
4. In most states, an employee who is terminated for willful violation of safety rules will likely be denied _____.
    A. Unemployment benefits
    B. Social security benefits
    C. Health insurance
    D. All of the above
5. An employee must always admit an OSHA representative into the building for an inspection.
    A. True
    B. False
6. The proper way to lift heavy objects is to:
    A. Keep your legs straight and bend at the waist.
    B. Keep your back straight and bend at the waist and lift with your back.

C. Keep your back straight and lift with your legs.
D. Recruit help is the object is too heavy, especially if it weight over 40 lb.
E. C and D.

7. What is the best way to prevent ergonomic injuries?
   A. Take antiinflammatory medication at the first sign of pain.
   B. Apply ice to painful areas.
   C. Change your posture and routine frequently.
   D. Try to consistently perform the same duties as often as possible.

8. How should chemicals be stored?
   A. With tight-fitting lids, on shelves at or below eye level
   B. With tight-fitting lids, on shelves at or above eye level
   C. On the top shelf to avoid spills
   D. With tight-fitting lids, in the basement

9. Which of the following precautions must be followed when opening an autoclave?
   A. Before opening an autoclave, activate the "vent" device.
   B. Always keep hands and face away from the steam.
   C. Always let steam dissipate completely before opening the door fully.
   D. Be careful when removing packs because they may still be hot.
   E. All of the above

10. With which of the following should surge suppressors *not* be used?
    A. Autoclaves or coffee pots
    B. Computers
    C. Portable heaters
    D. A and C

11. Overloaded or faulty electrical cords can overheat or short out and start a fire, even when the equipment is turned off.
    A. True
    B. False

12. Flammable material such as newspapers, boxes, and cleaning chemicals must be stored at least ____ away from an ignition source such as a water heater, furnace, or stove.
    A. 10 feet
    B. 5 feet
    C. 3 feet
    D. 20 feet

13. How many clear exits from the building must be available at all times?
    A. Two
    B. Three
    C. One on each floor

14. When using a fire extinguisher:
    A. Be sure to call the fire department immediately afterward.
    B. Be sure that several co-workers remain in the building with you in case of an accident.
    C. Make sure that the alarm has been sounded.
    D. None of the above.

15. If someone demands money, drugs, or other material items while threatening your personal safety in the clinic, what is recommended?
    A. Do not withhold the things that they demand.
    B. Attempt to withhold the things they demand while you try to notify a co-worker or passerby.
    C. Attempt to contact the police if it can be safely done without the person's knowledge.
    D. All of the above.
    E. A and C.

16. What must be included in the hazardous material plan?
    A. An up-to-date list of products containing hazardous chemicals known to be in the hospital
    B. Instructions for organizing and filing material safety data sheets
    C. Specifications for a secondary container labeling system
    D. List of the people responsible for ensuring that all employees have received the necessary safety training
    E. B and C
    F. All of the above

17. Historically used as a tissue preservative, this potentially human carcinogen should be obtained in small, premeasured containers whenever possible.
    A. Formalin
    B. Glutaraldehyde
    C. Ethylene oxide
    D. Alcohol

18. When using this chemical to cold sterilize instruments, be sure to wash your hands after handling instruments exposed to the solution and keep the trays covered to minimize evaporation.
    A. Formalin
    B. Glutaraldehyde
    C. Ethylene oxide
    D. Alcohol

19. You have been asked to purchase hearing protectors for the veterinary staff. When reading the packaging, you know that the product must be rated to filter the noise by at least ____.
    A. 40 dB
    B. 10 dB
    C. 20 dB
    D. 50 dB

20. Sometimes ____ restraint if safer than physical restraint for both the personnel and the animal.
    A. Aggressive
    B. Chemical

C. No
D. None of the above
21. What personal protective equipment must always be worn when bathing or dipping pets?
   A. Goggles
   B. Gloves
   C. Protective apron
   D. Hearing protectors
   E. All of the above
22. Rabies may be spread through contact with the animal's _____.
   A. Blood
   B. Urine
   C. Saliva
   D. Feces
23. Lyme disease is spread through bites from ____.
   A. Dogs
   B. Ticks
   C. Fleas
   D. Mites
24. It is believed that fungal spores (such as ringworm) can be carried to other locations (such as your home) on clothing and infect other animals or other people.
   A. True
   B. False
25. A zoonotic disease that appears as small, red lines on the skin in the regions where the parasite has burrowed into the skin from the soil is _____ and is caused by _____.
   A. Cutaneous larval migrans; hookworms
   B. Visceral larval migrans; hookworms
   C. Cutaneous larval migrans; roundworms
   D. Lyme disease; ticks
26. It is important to wash raw vegetables thoroughly and to avoid raw and undercooked meat, especially lamb, in order to avoid this zoonotic disease.
   A. Visceral larval migrans
   B. Rabies
   C. Sarcoptic mange
   D. Toxoplasmosis
27. In the veterinary profession, as in the human medical profession, exposure to animal blood and other animal secretions is considered a serious health risk to the staff.
   A. True
   B. False
28. This organism has been linked to cardiac and pulmonary problems in humans and animals and may be aerosolized during dental procedures.
   A. *Salmonella* spp.
   B. *Escherichia coli*
   C. *Borrelia burgdorferi*
   D. *Pasteurella multocida*
29. On an x-ray machine, the ____ cones down the area to be radiographed so that ____ radiation is minimized.
   A. Grid; exposure to
   B. Collimator; scatter
   C. Tube; scatter
   D. Cathode; exposure to
30. Which of the following procedures can help to minimize exposure to waste anesthetic gases?
   A. When a surgical procedure is finished, turn off the vaporizer and decrease the flow of oxygen to the patient.
   B. Never use funnels to fill a vaporizer because this increases the likelihood of the liquid overflowing and dripping down the machine.
   C. Always perform a leak check before using the anesthetic machine.
   D. Inflate the cuff of the endotracheal tube (already placed in the animal) before connecting the animal to the anesthesia machine.
   E. A and B
   F. C and D
31. Regardless of the size of the compressed gas cylinder, always place them in a cool, dry place, away from potential heat sources.
   A. True
   B. False
32. When disposing of a needle and syringe, ____ remove the needle first, ____ try to destroy the needle, and ____ dispose of the needle and syringe together.
   A. Always; never; never
   B. Never; never; always
   C. Never; always; always
   D. Always; always; never

EXTRA CREDIT

33. Place the following statements in the correct order (number 1 through 4) to describe the proper use of a fire extinguisher:
   ____ Squeeze the handle.
   ____ Aim low.
   ____ Sweep from side to side.
   ____ Pull the pin.

CHAPTER 37

EUTHANASIA

1. *Euthanasia* was defined by the 1986 American Veterinary Medical Association (AVMA) Panel on Euthanasia as "the act of inducing painless death."
   A. True
   B. False
2. Although euthanasia is an emotionally charged issue, most members of the veterinary profession are

unified in their acceptance of the practice and hold the same view of its utility.
A. True
B. False

3. The decision to euthanize a pet is often made more difficult because few pet owners have an adequate support group available that understands the bond that develops between an animal and its caretaker.
A. True
B. False

4. The most important help the veterinary technician can provide an owner is answering their questions about euthanasia.
A. True
B. False

5. If an owner makes a decision to euthanize that the veterinary staff believes is not in the best interest of the pet, the staff should gently but firmly try to convince the owner to change his decision.
A. True
B. False

6. As many as 40% of clients change veterinarians after a pet has died. This figure probably approaches 100% if euthanasia is handled in a manner that causes the client to perceive a lack of care, concern, or respect on the part of the veterinarian or other staff members.
A. True
B. False

7. In general, slang terms such as "put to sleep" or "put down" are preferred over the formal medical term *euthanasia* when discussing the subject with owners.
A. True
B. False

8. Allowing a client to be present for the euthanasia is often too graphic and shocking for them; it interrupts a healthy grief process and should be avoided.
A. True
B. False

9. Euthanasia appointments should be scheduled when interruptions are unlikely and placed in a time slot of at least 30 minutes.
A. True
B. False

10. If the procedure is to be performed in an examination room, the pet should *not* be placed on a blanket because of the risk posthumous urination or defecation.
A. True
B. False

11. Always take payment or make arrangements for payment and make arrangements for care of the pet's remains prior to the euthanasia procedure.
A. True
B. False

12. Perceived lack of caring or insensitivity by the veterinary staff and the thought of having to return to the room where their previous pet was euthanized are two major reasons that clients do not return to the euthanizing veterinarian with their next pet.
A. True
B. False

13. Clients wishing to be present for their pet's euthanasia should also be allowed to observe the placement of the intravenous catheter that will be used for the injection.
A. True
B. False

14. Preeuthanasia sedatives or general anesthetics are often used to calm an agitated patient or shorten the "excitement" phase that occurs as the euthanasia solution takes effect.
A. True
B. False

15. Diazepam is the most commonly used euthanasia solution.
A. True
B. False

16. The euthanasia solution should be administered very slowly to prevent perivascular infiltration and resulting lack of effect.
A. True
B. False

17. One of the most important aspects of creating a smooth client experience of the euthanasia process is informing them, before the procedure, of every detail, what to expect, and every possible complication that can occur.
A. True
B. False

18. When returning a pet's body to a client, you should clean any blood off the fur, remove any catheters or bandages, place the tongue in the mouth, and close the pet's eyes.
A. True
B. False

19. Do *not* call a client who has lost a pet; simply send a condolence card signed by everyone on the hospital's staff.
A. True
B. False

20. If the client wishes to know what will be done with a pet's body left with the veterinarian for disposal, it is best to tell them the body will go into a "mass cremation with other animals" regardless of how the remains will actually be handled.
A. True
B. False

21. Successful strategies for coping with the stress of performing euthanasia include staff discussions

about feelings, rotation of euthanasia responsibilities, and dark humor.
A. True
B. False

22. The best and safest vein to use for large-animal euthanasia is the cephalic vein.
A. True
B. False

23. Technicians performing the frequent euthanasia procedures often required in animal shelters are actually less affected by the stress that normally accompanies the procedure because they become emotionally acclimatized to death.
A. True
B. False

24. Frequent performance of euthanasia is a primary cause of burnout in small animal practices and can be even more stressful to the technical staff than it is to the veterinarian because staff members usually have little control over the situation.
A. True
B. False

CHAPTER 38

CLIENT BEREAVEMENT AND THE HUMAN-ANIMAL BOND

1. Due to changing family structures and an increasing number of people who live alone, companion animals have taken on larger roles in people's support systems and are often considered members of their owner's family.
A. True
B. False

2. In the 1990s, the dog supplanted the cat as the most popular pet in the United States.
A. True
B. False

3. When pet loss occurs, the veterinary staff can expect the same level of intensity of grief from all owners.
A. True
B. False

4. Because people who make up client support systems often do not understand the full extent of attachment between a pet owner and pet, pet owners often turn to veterinary professionals as sources of support, comfort, and understanding at and around the time of their pet's death.
A. True
B. False

5. Crying, taking time away from work, and wanting to memorialize a pet are unhealthy responses to the death of a pet and are a sign of an interrupted, or blocked, grief process.
A. True
B. False

6. The five stages of the grief process are denial, bargaining, anger, depression, and resolution.
A. True
B. False

7. All client-grieving behaviors should be met with acceptance and reassurance that the client's feelings are normal, but severe depression can be addressed by referral to a professional counselor.
A. True
B. False

8. Never attempt to force a client who is in denial about a pet's illness or death to "come to her senses" or move out of denial.
A. True
B. False

9. When helping a client find a new animal to replace a dead pet, encourage them to choose one of the same breed, gender, and color.
A. True
B. False

10. Denial is best met with patient repetition of the facts until the client is ready to accept them.
A. True
B. False

11. Due to the volatile nature of this emotion and the risk of liability, angry clients should be avoided until they have moved through this stage of the grief process.
A. True
B. False

12. Many veterinary schools offer free pet-loss support hotlines for clients needing support after the death of a pet.
A. True
B. False

13. Because young children do not fully understand the permanence of death, they should be protected from the truth about a pet's illness possibly by telling them the family pet "went to live on a farm."
A. True
B. False

14. Children under the age of 12 do not really understand that death is final.
A. True
B. False

15. Straightforward explanations and concrete words like "dead" and "died" should be used when talking to children about death.
A. True
B. False

16. The veterinary technician can play a vital role in helping a bereaved client by being available; listening; assuring the client that his feelings, emotions, and struggles are normal; and offering referral when the client thinks he needs more help than his available support group is able to provide.
    A. True
    B. False
17. Technicians must not forget to apply the principles learned about the grieving process to themselves, as they too will experience grief when their work duties bring them into close association with euthanasia and pet loss.
    A. True
    B. False
18. List three suggestions you might make to an owner needing or wishing to memorialize a pet.
19. A client who responds to a diagnosis of cancer with a request that the pet's toenails be clipped is exhibiting which stage of grief? Can this behavior be considered normal?
20. Name three factors that may complicate, prolong, or intensify the grief process.

CHAPTER 39

STRESS AND SUBSTANCE ABUSE IN PRACTICE

1. According to current research, stress can be responsible for
   A. Physical illness
   B. Mental illness
   C. Death
   D. Pleasure
   E. All of the above
2. In general, veterinary medicine is a field known for its _____ potential for daily stress.
   A. Very low
   B. Low
   C. Moderate
   D. High
3. What factors most determine whether stress has a negative or positive impact?
   A. External stressors, such as workload or time schedule, are most often negative.
   B. Internal stressors, such as emotions and sensitivities, are most often negative.
   C. Environmental stressors, such as a hot room or noise, are most often negative.
   D. Stressors that are perceived as not self-chosen, out of a person's control, or unpredictable are most often negative.
4. Stress, whether good or bad, is a nonspecific response of the:
   A. Autonomic nervous system (fight or flight)
   B. Cerebral cortex (emotions)
   C. Cerebral cortex (thoughts)
   D. Peripheral nervous system (muscles and nerves)
5. Moods are affected by a shortage or excess of one or more _____.
   A. Medications
   B. Stressors
   C. Neurotransmitters
   D. Hormones
6. Which statement concerning the body's response to stress is most accurate?
   A. Negative stress always results in a stress-related illness.
   B. Stress-related illnesses only occur if the body cannot adequately adapt to the stress or the stress occurs without interruption for a long period.
   C. The stress response follows a predictable three-phase pathway alarm reaction, then adaptation or resistance, then exhaustion or illness.
   D. B and C
7. What personality type is more resistant to stress-related illness?
   A. Is competitive, impatient, perfectionistic.
   B. Has realistic expectations, takes and enjoys time off for relaxation, comfortable delegating responsibilities to others.
   C. Believe they are in control of their life and responses; do not withdraw from situations; believe challenges are exciting.
   D. B and C.
8. It is important to take into account the total number of stressors on an individual to determine his or her true risk for stress-related illness.
   A. True
   B. False
9. The life event determined to cause most people the most stress is:
   A. Trouble with a boss
   B. Beginning or ending school
   C. Death of a spouse
   D. Marriage
10. Increased frequency of breaks will most effectively relieve which workplace stressor?
    A. Space limitations
    B. Inadequate equipment
    C. Excessively high noise levels
    D. Unpredictable schedule changes
11. A person _____ will find almost every situation stressful.
    A. With low self-esteem
    B. Who is inflexible
    C. Who prefers animals to people
    D. Who is empathetic

12. Veterinary technicians who are empathetic are able to:
    A. Feel pity (feel sorry) for a suffering animal or person
    B. Relieve animal or human suffering through emotional or physical means
    C. Share in an animal's or human's feelings or emotions (actually feel them as if they were their own)
    D. Figure out what is causing an animal or human pain

For the next three questions, match the type of client with the best way to handle them and reduce the staff member's frustration with them.
    A. Elderly clients
    B. Angry clients
    C. Independent clients (who consult a veterinarian but continue to treat their animals in their own predetermined fashion)
13. Listen to them, do not become defensive, and get support from other staff members after interacting with them.
14. Treat them as if their opinions are important and explain, in terms that they understand, your opinion as to diagnosis, justification of the diagnosis, and treatment.
15. Schedule more time for them, take a deep breath, and be very patient.
16. The ideal amount of sleep to increase a person's stress resistance is:
    A. Whatever amount makes a person feel his or her best, work best, and enjoy rising in the morning
    B. 7 hours
    C. 8 hours
    D. 9 hours
17. How does regular exercise combat stress?
    A. It causes a release from tension.
    B. It restores normal body chemical balance.
    C. It relieves depression.
    D. All of the above
18. Which way of seeking emotional support from others will provide the most long-term benefit to all involved?
    A. Seek support exclusively from one or two people, making one of those a spouse if you are married.
    B. Seek support only from those in your personal life; avoid revealing feelings to and asking for help from those at work.
    C. If you need support, use the services of a well-trained and compatible professional counselor.
    D. Seek support from a wide variety of sources including, but not limited to, friends, family members, and co-workers; do not rely exclusively on one or two people.
19. The terms *substance abuse* and *substance dependence* are equivalent.
    A. True
    B. False
20. Factors that may contribute to the abuse of a substance are:
    A. Environmental factors such as high-stress
    B. Sociocultural factors such as ethnicity, culture, age, occupation, and social class
    C. Genetic vulnerability
    D. Chronic pain and self-medication
    E. All of the above
    F. B and C
    G. None of the above
21. Which of the following statements is/are true regarding substance abuse in the veterinary professional environment?
    A. If a co-worker is suspected of having a substance abuse problem that interferes with his or her ability to work, the proper initial action is to report the impairment to the appropriate governing board.
    B. In general, veterinary staff members with substance abuse issues are very adept at hiding their problem and co-workers are rarely able to intervene and help.
    C. An entire practice may be at risk of malpractice due to a substance abuser.
    D. Currently, 15 states have a board of veterinary medicine that awards, reviews, and can suspend licenses for veterinarians of that state.

WRITTEN EXERCISES

1. Fill out Table 37-3 to determine whether your personality is a strong type A, a strong type B, or somewhere in the middle. Then write three examples in which you exhibited characteristics consistent with your dominant personality type and (if possible) three in which you responded according to your nondominant personality type.
2. What causes you the most stress? Turn an $8 \frac{1}{2} \times 11$ inch sheet of paper sideways and divide it into four columns. Use the discussion of different types of stressors under "identifying stressors" in the chapter. In the first column, list one or two recent things you perceived as "very stressful" in each category life event: environmental, personal, client or classmate, and career or school. In the second column, write down why you believe this caused you stress. In the third column, write down whether you were happy with the way you responded to each stressor. Now, using the "coping with stress" discussion in the chapter, write down in the fourth column some ways you could have modified your response or handled the situation differently so that, in the future, each stressor can become positive rather than negative, or may even be prevented.

3. Using the stress resistor habits section in the chapter, record your own nutritional, sleep, exercise, and mental-recreation habits for 5 days. Are there areas in which you can improve or reduce your stress level? If so, list two changes you can make in each problem area to increase your resistance to stress.

INTERACTIVE EXERCISES LED BY THE INSTRUCTOR

1. **Developing relaxation skills.** As a class, perform one of the relaxation exercises listed in Tables 37-7 and 37-8. Afterwards, have a class discussion of how the exercises made the class feel. Did the exercises increase their feeling of relaxation? Have everybody read the section entitled "relaxation techniques" in the chapter, which lists some other methods of relaxing. Discuss whether they use any of these techniques and what other things they do to relax.

2. **Exploring personality-type recognition.** Break the class into small groups of two or three. Have each person write down secretly what his or her personality type was determined to be in the first written exercise and what he or she believes is the personality type of the other members of the group. Then have everyone reveal his or her response, and discuss why he or she classified each person as they did. If there were discrepancies in answers, have them discuss why people may perceive a person differently than the quiz classifies him or her.

Answer Key

INTRODUCTION

1. C	12. A	23. D	33. A
2. C	13. A	24. B	34. B
3. E	14. B	25. B	35. C
4. A	15. A	26. D	36. B
5. B	16. D	27. A	37. A
6. A	17. E	28. E	38. A
7. D	18. E	29. D	39. E
8. C	19. C	30. A	40. B
9. D	20. C	31. B	41. A
10. A	21. D	32. B	42. E
11. D	22. D		

EXTRA CREDIT
43. A

CHAPTER 1

1. B	13. A	24. B	35. D
2. A	14. C	25. D	36. B
3. D	15. A	26. D	37. C
4. C	16. C	27. C	38. B
5. B	17. B	28. A	39. C
6. B	18. A	29. B	40. B
7. D	19. A	30. A	41. D
8. A	20. B	31. C	42. A
9. B	21. D	32. D	43. C
10. D	22. C	33. C	44. A
11. C	23. A	34. B	45. A
12. D			

46. Avoiding direct eye contact with the head down, lips pulled back horizontally, ears flattened, and tail between the legs
47. Control of the head: kneeling on the neck near the head
48. (1) Try to keep the dog in sight until there is an opportunity to capture it. (2) Corner it. (3) Use a high-pitched voice to reassure the dog. (4) Squat in front of the dog, move slowly and deliberately, and offer the back of your hand for the dog to sniff. (5) Reassure the dog with some general petting and gently grab its collar.
49. Head too far forward or head too far back
50. Jugular, cephalic, medial saphenous
51. Because snakes attack on the basis of smell

EXTRA CREDIT
52. C
53. B

CHAPTER 2

1. A	12. B	23. B	34. C
2. E	13. D	24. D	35. A
3. B	14. E	25. D	36. A
4. C	15. B	26. B	37. B
5. A	16. A	27. B	38. D
6. B	17. C	28. D	39. B
7. D	18. A	29. D	40. D
8. B	19. A	30. A	41. E
9. C	20. A	31. D	42. F
10. A	21. D	32. A	43. F
11. C	22. B	33. D	

44. Popliteal, prescapular, submandibular
45. Axillary, inguinal
46. Divide the lung lobes into quadrants and auscult each quadrant individually and bilaterally.
47. Tricuspid
48. Possible answers: sniff; recoil after a sniff; nose lick; blink; direct and consensual pupillary light responses present; normal eye movement or eye position; can close jaw; normal facial muscle tone; eye blink; facial symmetry; startle response; normal nystagmus; normal head posture; normal righting; swallow; cough; retraction of tongue
49. Mitral, holosystolic, crescendo, grade 3/6 murmur

EXTRA CREDIT
50. A

Copyright © 2006 by Elsevier, Inc. All rights reserved.

CHAPTER 3

1. A	25. B	49. B
2. D	26. A	50. B
3. B	27. D	51. A, B, D
4. C	28. C	52. A
5. B	29. A	53. C
6. A	30. B	54. D
7. D	31. D	55. D
8. B	32. D	56. C
9. D	33. C	57. B
10. C	34. D	58. D
11. A	35. D	59. C
12. B	36. B	60. B
13. D	37. C or D	61. A
14. C	38. A	62. D
15. C	39. D	63. C
16. C	40. B	64. D
17. A	41. C	65. D
18. D	42. D	66. B
19. B	43. C	67. A
20. A	44. A	68. A
21. C	45. C	69. D
22. D	46. B	70. B
23. B, C, D	47. D	71. A
24. B	48. B	72. D

73. Draw blood because fluid administration and recent ingestion of a high-fat or high-protein meal may alter blood laboratory values.
74. (1) Place bitch in standing or laterally recumbent position. (2) Wipe vulvar region with warm water. (3) Use gloved hand to separate labia so a cotton swab can be inserted and rolled against the vaginal wall. (4) Remove swab from vagina and roll across a glass slide.
75. (1) Place animal in tub. (2) Place end of long, lubricated tubing into rectum. (3) Raise tube end, insert funnel, and pour water into funnel so it enters intestines. (4) Gradually move tube back and forth and advance it up intestinal tract as fecal material is expelled.
76. Nuchal ligament, cervical spine, scapular spine
77. The introduction of microorganisms into the udder

EXTRA CREDIT
78. B
79. C

CHAPTER 4

1. A	13. B	24. B	35. A
2. C	14. E	25. A	36. C
3. d	15. D	26. C	37. B
4. C	16. B	27. D	38. A
5. A	17. B	28. B	39. A
6. b	18. A	29. A	40. C
7. B	19. A	30. A	41. C
8. B	20. B	31. D	42. D
9. E	21. E	32. C	43. B
10. B	22. B	33. C	44. A
11. A	23. B	34. B	45. C
12. E			

46. Possible answers: It fills the tissue defect; it protects the wound; it provides a barrier to infection; it provides a surface for new epithelial cells to form across; it provides a source of special fibroblasts called *myofibroblasts*.
47. (1) Application of anchoring tape strips (stirrups) to the distal portion of the limb; (2) application of the padded secondary layer over the stirrups; (3) application of the gauze tertiary layer; (4) application of the splint; (5) reflection and twisting of the stirrups to adhere to the gauze layer; (6) application of the protective tertiary layer of tape
48. Burns from cage dryers and prolonged contact with heating pads
49. A wooden, wedge-shaped block is placed under the heel and incorporated into the last cast layer. The wedge allows the horse to walk more easily when wearing a cast.
50. Place a pad of orthopedic felt, with holes cut out for the dewclaws, over the dewclaws.

EXTRA CREDIT
51. C
52. C

CHAPTER 5

1. B	8. C	15. A	21. A
2. A	9. A	16. D	22. D
3. B	10. B	17. B	23. A
4. C	11. B	18. B	24. D
5. A	12. A	19. D	25. B
6. C	13. B	20. C	26. C
7. C	14. B		

27. Signalment, history, clinical findings
28. The head
29. Individually in separate, labeled containers

30. In left lateral recumbency; this positions the rumen on the down side, which facilitates removal of the abdominal organs.
31. The entire vertebral column with the spinal cord inside should be collected and fixed after the limbs, head, and surrounding muscles are removed. The vertebral column and spinal cord are submitted whole to the laboratory.

EXTRA CREDIT
32. C

CHAPTER 6

1. B	13. A	24. B	35. B
2. E	14. A	25. E	36. D
3. C	15. D	26. A	37. A
4. B	16. A	27. D	38. D
5. E	17. E	28. C	39. C
6. C	18. A	29. A	40. C
7. D	19. B	30. B	41. C
8. B	20. D	31. C	42. A
9. A	21. F	32. A	43. B
10. B	22. C	33. A	44. C
11. D	23. B	34. B	45. B
12. A			

46. (1) Fill a plain microhematocrit tube with anticoagulated blood; (2) seal one end of the tube with a specific clay; (3) centrifuge the sample in a microhematocrit centrifuge; (4) apply the sample to a chart to determine the PCV.
47. Color, turbidity, specific gravity
48. (1) Pour 10 ml of urine into a conical-tip centrifuge tube; (2) centrifuge tube at slow speed; (3) decant supernatant; (4) tap tube to resuspend the sediment in the bottom of the tube; (5) transfer a drop of suspended sediment to a slide with a pipette (6) place coverslip.
49. Possible answers: poor-quality or outdated reagents; failure to calibrate or run controls; improper pipetting techniques; improper maintenance of instrument; lipemic or hemolyzed samples; allowing serum to sit on clot; use of inappropriate cuvettes; power surges or failure
50. The presence in the blood of erythrocytes that vary considerably in size

EXTRA CREDIT
51. C
52. B

CHAPTER 7

1. B	13. A	24. D	35. A
2. A	14. C	25. A	36. B
3. D	15. D	26. D	37. B
4. D	16. C	27. D	38. A
5. D	17. C	28. B	39. C
6. B	18. C	29. C	40. B
7. A	19. B	30. D	41. B
8. C	20. A	31. A	42. C
9. B	21. D	32. C	43. A
10. A	22. A	33. E	44. D
11. B	23. A	34. B	45. C
12. A			

46. Large roundworm; *Ascaris suum*
47. Egg: laid in fur and falls out to land where pet sleeps or plays; larvae: live where eggs have hatched (i.e., where the pet sleeps or plays) and feed on organic debris, especially flea dirt; pupae: larvae molts into a dormant pupae encased in a cocoon; adult: adults emerge from cocoon and feed on blood of host
48. The chemical solutions used have a higher specific gravity (are heavier) than water, which causes the eggs to float to the top.
49. The eggs are too heavy to float.
50. This can occur during the prepatent period.

EXTRA CREDIT
51. A
52. C

CHAPTER 8

1. C	17. D	32. B	47. A
2. A	18. A	33. C	48. B
3. B	19. C	34. G	49. A
4. B	20. C	35. D	50. D
5. B	21. D	36. H	51. D
6. D	22. A	37. A	52. D
7. D	23. C	38. C	53. C
8. A	24. D	39. D	54. C
9. A	25. A	40. A	55. A
10. C	26. A	41. B	56. C
11. A	27. E	42. C	57. C
12. C	28. J	43. A	58. A
13. D	29. I	44. D	59. B
14. C	30. A	45. B	60. D
15. A	31. F	46. C	61. D
16. D			

62. Patient identification (name, species, case number, or owner), name of veterinarian, source of the sample, and additional clinical history

63. Asymptomatic carriers are brushed all over with a sterile or new toothbrush to gather hair and scales. The hair and debris are scraped or plucked directly from the lesion in symptomatic patients.
64. Failure of the neonatal animal to obtain and absorb adequate colostral immunoglobulins

EXTRA CREDIT
65. B
66. B

CHAPTER 9

1. D	15. D	29. B	43. A
2. A	16. A	30. D	44. B
3. B	17. A	31. A	45. B
4. C	18. B	32. B	46. B
5. A	19. D	33. C	47. A
6. D	20. C	34. B	48. C
7. B	21. B	35. B	49. D
8. B	22. A	36. D	50. C
9. D	23. C	37. B	51. D
10. A	24. D	38. A	52. B
11. D	25. B	39. A	53. A
12. D	26. A	40. B	54. D
13. A	27. C	41. C	55. B
14. C	28. A	42. B	

56. The first step starts the anode rotating. The second step activates the high-voltage circuit, resulting in x-ray production.
57. At least every 90 days
58. Possible answers: collimator; smallest possible aperture; aluminum filter; avoid retakes with proper exposure factors and animal position; no human body parts in the primary x-ray beam; wear lead apron and gloves; use cassette holders, restraining devices, and positioning devices; use anesthesia for unmanageable patients; only required personnel in room; use good, fast screens.
59. These practices remove air, through which the ultrasound beam cannot travel.

EXTRA CREDIT
60. D
61. A

CHAPTER 10

1. A	8. C	15. B	22. B
2. C	9. D	16. C	23. D
3. C	10. D	17. A	24. B
4. B	11. A	18. B	25. A
5. D	12. D	19. A	
6. C	13. B	20. A	
7. B	14. B	21. D	

26. Possible answers: abnormal swellings that persist or continue to grow; sores that do not heal; weight loss; loss of appetite; bleeding or discharge from any body opening; offensive odor; difficulty eating or swallowing; hesitation to exercise or loss of stamina; persistent lameness or stiffness; difficulty breathing, urinating, or defecating
27. Paint the outside of the sample with tissue paint, slice it so that no area is thicker than 1 cm (as if cutting a loaf of bread), and leave one edge intact.
28. Find out which drug was last administered and when that treatment was given.

CHAPTER 11

1. B	16. B	31. C	46. C
2. D	17. E	32. A	47. B
3. C	18. A	33. B	48. D
4. A	19. D	34. C	49. A
5. D	20. C	35. D	50. D
6. C	21. D	36. B	51. A
7. D	22. B	37. B	52. A
8. C	23. A	38. A	53. B
9. C	24. A	39. E	54. B
10. B	25. B	40. B	55. C
11. A	26. D	41. C	56. B
12. B	27. D	42. D	57. D
13. C	28. D	43. A	
14. A	29. D	44. A	
15. A	30. B	45. A	

58. D, canine distemper; A_2, canine adenovirus, type 2 (infectious canine hepatitis); P, canine parainfluenza; L, leptospirosis; P, canine parvovirus, type 2 disease; C, canine coronavirus disease
59. FVR, feline viral rhinotracheitis; C, feline calicivirus infection; P, feline panleukopenia
60. (1) Controls flies and internal parasites; (2) Prevents the spread of infectious disease.
61. Clip needle teeth, dock tails, castrate, ear notch, and inject iron dextran
62. Frequent foot trimming, footbaths or soaks, and vaccination

EXTRA CREDIT
63. B
64. A

CHAPTER 12

1. D	9. C	16. A	23. A
2. A	10. B	17. B	24. B
3. A	11. D	18. B	25. B
4. D	12. B	19. B	26. C
5. B	13. A	20. A	27. B
6. B	14. C	21. A	28. D
7. C	15. A	22. B	29. A
8. D			

30. Swab the anogenital area with moistened cotton or dry, soft tissue paper to manually stimulate the elimination reflex. This should be done until the animal is 3 weeks old.
31. External heat source for 1 to 3 weeks; bedding: padded, disposable, or washable flooring such as indoor-outdoor carpeting and disposable diapers or cotton towels to keep them warm and dry; container: a small box raised slightly off the floor with sides high enough to keep them inside and prevent drafts; keep them at 35.5° C to 36.1° C (96° F to 97° F) for the first week and 36.1° C to 37.7° C (97° F to 100° F) for the second through fourth weeks of life.
32. IV catheters are a primary iatrogenic portal of infection and must be placed and maintained under conditions of rigid asepsis. Allow the equine umbilicus to tear on its own; apply a 2% to 3.5% iodine solution four times daily for 1 week or until umbilical disease abates.

EXTRA CREDIT
33. C
34. A

CHAPTER 13

1. C	11. C
2. A	12. B
3. D	13. A
4. A	14. See Box 13-3.
5. D	15. See Box 13-3.
6. B	
7. A	
8. A	
9. D	
10. D	

EXTRA CREDIT
16. B

CHAPTER 14

1. D	11. A	21. B
2. D	12. A	22. C
3. B	13. D	23. D
4. B	14. C	24. C
5. C	15. D	25. A
6. B	16. B	
7. B	17. A	
8. D	18. B	
9. B	19. A	
10. D	20. D	

EXTRA CREDIT
26. A

CHAPTER 15

1. C	18. A	36. D
2. A	19. C	37. B
3. D	20. C	38. A
4. D	21. A	39. C
5. B	22. D	40. D
6. A	23. B	41. B
7. A	24. D	42. A
8. A	25. D	43. Captive tortoises
9. Water-soluble vitamins	26. C	44. Gerbils
10. Vitamin K	27. A	45. Guinea pigs
11. Calcium	28. D	46. Snakes
12. Iron	29. B	47. Rabbits
13. Vitamin E	30. C	48. Horses
14. Phosphorus	31. D	49. Chinchillas
15. C	32. D	50. Horses
16. B	33. D	51. B
17. B	34. A	
	35. A	

EXTRA CREDIT
52. D

CHAPTER 16

1. D	10. C	19. C	28. D
2. B	11. B	20. B	29. B
3. D	12. C	21. D	30. C
4. A	13. B	22. A	31. A
5. D	14. D	23. D	32. C
6. B	15. A	24. A	33. A
7. D	16. B	25. A	34. B
8. A	17. A	26. D	35. B
9. D	18. A	27. A	

36. (1) Total mixed ration: all feedstuffs are weighed and measured into a complete ration. (2) Animals

are provided hay free choice at all times, silage is offered once or twice a day, and feed concentrates are fed twice daily.
37. Calcium and phosphorus
38. The time in the growth phase of growing cattle when they are fed to produce beef that is desirable to the food consumer
39. Copper

EXTRA CREDIT
40. C

CHAPTER 17

1. C	16. D	31. A	46. B
2. B	17. B	32. B	47. C
3. D	18. D	33. D	48. H
4. C	19. C	34. B	49. G
5. A	20. A	35. B	50. A
6. D	21. C	36. D	51. D
7. C	22. A	37. D	52. F
8. B	23. B	38. A	53. I
9. A	24. A	39. C	54. C
10. A	25. D	40. C	55. A
11. D	26. A	41. D	56. D
12. C	27. A	42. D	57. B
13. C	28. C	43. C	
14. B	29. D	44. A	
15. C	30. D	45. E	

58. 100% cornified cells: angular cell borders and nucleus pyknotic or not visible.
59. The queen is in estrus; spay her.
60. Uterine prolapse; immediately (emergency)
61. The harness is fitted with a marking crayon that detects ewes returning to estrus (not pregnant).
62. The final, clear, prostatic portion

EXTRA CREDIT
63. C
64. A

CHAPTER 18

1. D	11. D	21. C	31. B
2. D	12. A	22. D	32. A
3. D	13. D	23. C	33. B
4. A	14. C	24. A	34. C
5. D	15. C	25. A	35. C
6. B	16. A	26. B	36. B
7. A	17. A	27. A	37. A
8. B	18. D	28. D	38. A
9. C	19. A	29. B	39. D
10. A	20. C	30. C	40. D

41. A cotton swab is moistened, inserted into the cloaca, and gently rotated.
42. Cutaneous ulnar vein, right jugular vein, medial metatarsal vein, and toenail clipping
43. Harderian gland secretions

EXTRA CREDIT
44. A
45. C

CHAPTER 19

1. D	12. B	23. D	34. A
2. B	13. A	24. C	35. D
3. D	14. D	25. A	36. B
4. D	15. D	26. B	37. B
5. B	16. B	27. A	38. A
6. A	17. C	28. D	39. B
7. B	18. D	29. B	40. C
8. D	19. D	30. D	41. A
9. D	20. D	31. D	
10. C	21. B	32. D	
11. D	22. A	33. A	

EXTRA CREDIT
42. A
43. B

CHAPTER 20

1. C	11. B	21. A	31. D
2. D	12. A	22. C	32. D
3. B	13. A	23. D	33. C
4. B	14. B	24. C	34. C
5. A	15. D	25. D	35. B
6. A	16. C	26. A	36. B
7. D	17. A	27. A	37. A
8. B	18. D	28. D	
9. C	19. B	29. A	
10. A	20. A	30. B	

38. Clip hair over lateral thorax or dorsal neck and press patch to skin for 30 seconds; place bandage over patch for canine patients.
39. Carprofen causes less gastrointestinal ulceration than aspirin, which means greater doses can be given, making carprofen much more effective.
40. This technique produces analgesia of longer duration and without additional side effects.
41. Labrador retriever; hepatic toxicosis

EXTRA CREDIT
42. C

CHAPTER 21

1. B	13. D	25. A	37. A	49. B
2. A	14. F	26. D	38. C	50. D
3. D	15. H	27. A	39. D	51. A
4. C	16. I	28. A	40. B	52. C
5. B	17. A	29. A	41. E	53. B
6. A	18. J	30. C	42. F	54. C
7. D	19. L	31. D	43. B	55. D
8. A	20. B	32. B	44. B	56. E
9. D	21. J	33. A	45. C	57. A
10. A	22. C	34. C	46. D	58. C
11. B	23. D	35. D	47. C	59. D
12. G	24. A	36. A	48. A	

60. In geriatric patients, decreased biotransformation by the liver and decreased renal function cause slow elimination of most drugs from the body.
61. Preanesthetic, mydriatic, antidote for organophosphate poisoning
62. 1 kg
63. 1/3 or 0.3 ml
64. Labeling requirements vary between states but may include name, address, and telephone number of clinic; name of client; animal identification; species of animal; date; prescribing veterinarian; name of medication; quantity of medication dispensed; adequate directions for proper administration of medication; number of refills authorized; and prescription transaction number (optional).

EXTRA CREDIT
65. C

CHAPTER 22

1. C	11. C	21. A	31. B	41. B
2. D	12. D	22. D	32. A	42. D
3. D	13. A	23. B	33. B	43. C
4. B	14. D	24. B	34. D	44. C
5. C	15. A	25. B	35. C	45. B
6. A	16. C	26. A	36. C	46. A
7. B	17. C	27. B	37. C	
8. D	18. D	28. C	38. A	
9. B	19. D	29. D	39. A	
10. A	20. A	30. C	40. A	

47. Roeder and Backhaus; Roeder might be preferred because the ball stop on jaws prevents deep tissue penetration and prevents the towel from slipping toward box lock.
48. Sterilization is the destruction of all organisms and spores on an object; disinfection is the destruction of the vegetative forms of bacteria but not the spores.
49. Autoclave tape, fusible melting pellet glass type, culture tests, chemical sterilization indicators
50. Open and closed
51. They filter bacteria exhaled out of mouth and nose.

EXTRA CREDIT
52. B
53. C

CHAPTER 23

1. D	9. B	16. A	23. D	30. D
2. A	10. D	17. A	24. A	31. B
3. C	11. C	18. A	25. D	32. A
4. C	12. A	19. C	26. B	33. B
5. A	13. D	20. B	27. D	34. A
6. D	14. A	21. B	28. B	35. A
7. C	15. B	22. C	29. B	36. C
8. A				

37. Blotting motion
38. To provide an open site of discharge in infected tissues, to evacuate dead space, and to remove lavage solutions
39. To prevent retrograde infection and because drainage travels around outside of drain so cleanliness keeps area open for drainage

EXTRA CREDIT
40. A
41. B

CHAPTER 24

1. B	15. H	29. N
2. D	16. C	30. P
3. B	17. M	31. K
4. C	18. B	32. G
5. C	19. K	33. J
6. C	20. M	34. N
7. A	21. N	35. B
8. D	22. D	36. B
9. C	23. L	37. B
10. D	24. E	38. D
11. A	25. Q	39. A
12. A	26. A	40. D
13. C	27. F	
14. I	28. O	

EXTRA CREDIT
41. Direct contact may damage cartilage and cartilage has a relatively poor response to trauma. Instead, it is recommended to retract the joint capsule to decrease trauma and increase exposure.
42. Onychectomy, urethrostomy, castration

CHAPTER 25

1. D	35. A	69. A
2. C	36. A	70. D
3. B	37. D	71. B
4. A	38. B	72. C
5. C	39. B	73. C
6. B	40. C	74. B
7. D	41. A	75. A
8. C	42. A	76. B
9. C	43. C	77. D
10. A	44. D	78. D
11. D	45. B	79. A
12. C	46. A	80. B
13. A	47. D	81. D
14. D	48. B	82. A
15. B	49. B	83. B
16. D	50. A, B, C, D, F	84. D
17. A	51. C	85. C
18. A	52. A	86. A
19. D	53. A	87. D
20. B	54. C	88. D
21. C, D, E, F, H	55. B	89. D
22. A	56. A	90. C
23. B	57. B	91. A
24. C	58. B	92. B
25. C	59. A	93. A
26. B	60. A	94. D
27. C	61. C	95. A
28. A	62. A	96. A
29. D	63. D	97. D
30. B	64. A	98. D
31. D	65. C	99. B
32. D	66. B	100. A
33. A	67. A	101. A
34. C	68. B	

102. Possible answers: clean cage; food and water if indicated; exercise; grooming; treatment with respect; relief of suffering; stress-free environment
103. TPR, mucous-membrane color, CRT
104. Drug, time, dose, route, and possibly the initials of the person giving the drug
105. To overcome gradually declining maternal-antibody interference with vaccination
106. Possible answers: rear-leg weakness; generalized weakness; focal or diffuse muscle twitching; incoordination; blindness; generalized seizures; behavioral changes

EXTRA CREDIT

107. A
108. C
109. A

CHAPTER 26

1. D	15. D	29. C	43. B
2. A	16. B	30. G	44. A
3. E	17. D	31. B	45. D
4. B	18. B	32. B	46. A
5. A	19. C	33. D	47. D
6. F	20. B	34. C	48. C
7. E	21. E	35. F	49. C
8. B	22. D	36. E	50. B
9. C	23. B	37. A	51. B
10. D	24. A	38. B	52. G
11. A	25. E	39. G	53. A
12. C	26. D	40. D	
13. A	27. A	41. F	
14. A	28. B	42. B	

EXTRA CREDIT

54. (1) By blowing air into the patients mouth and/or nose; (2) face mask; (3) nasal oxygen cannula; (4) endotracheal tube
55. D

CHAPTER 27

1. B	11. B	21. G	31. D
2. D	12. L	22. M	32. B
3. C	13. J	23. A	33. H
4. B	14. K	24. N	34. A
5. C	15. B	25. C	35. C
6. A	16. F	26. H	36. F
7. D	17. O	27. D	37. J
8. C	18. I	28. D	38. E
9. D	19. D	29. B	39. L
10. C	20. E	30. I	40. G

EXTRA CREDIT

41. K
42. B
43. A

CHAPTER 28

1. C	18. A	35. D	52. B
2. A	19. B	36. A	53. F
3. B	20. D	37. D	54. D
4. C	21. A	38. A	55. D
5. A	22. B	39. B	56. F
6. D	23. C	40. G	
7. A	24. D	41. C	
8. B	25. B	42. I	
9. D	26. C	43. H	
10. A	27. A	44. A	
11. B	28. C	45. K	
12. B	29. D	46. J	
13. A	30. B	47. E	
14. B	31. C	48. B	
15. C	32. A	49. F	
16. D	33. B	50. D	
17. A, B, C, D, E	34. C	51. D	

57. Proper diet, routine dental scaling and polishing, and daily teeth brushing or mouth rinsing
58. (1) Disconnect the animals from the anesthesia circuit when repositioning them. (2) Minimize movement of the endotracheal tube. (3) Inflate the cuff just enough to stop anesthetic-gas leaks.
59. Possible answers: ulcerated areas; loose teeth; periodontal pockets; receded gingivae; degree of periodontal disease; fractured teeth
60. Fluoride strengthens enamel, decreases tooth sensitivity, has antimicrobial properties, and decreases the rate of plaque reattachment.
61. To save a "dead" or dying tooth

EXTRA CREDIT
62. A

CHAPTER 29

1. B	30. C	59. B	
2. B	31. B	60. D	
3. C	32. A	61. A	
4. D	33. D	62. D	
5. A	34. C	63. A, C, D, E	
6. B	35. B	64. B	
7. A	36. B	65. C	
8. B	37. C	66. A	
9. D	38. A	67. B	
10. B	39. B	68. C	
11. B	40. C	69. B	
12. A	41. B	70. D	
13. B	42. A	71. B	
14. D	43. D	72. D	
15. A	44. B	73. B	
16. D	45. B	74. A	
17. A, C, D, F, H, I	46. B	75. B	
18. D	47. C	76. B	
19. D	48. D	77. A	
20. D	49. D	78. C	
21. A, B, C, D	50. B	79. A	
22. B	51. A	80. A	
23. C	52. A, D	81. B	
24. A	53. B	82. A	
25. D	54. A	83. A, B, C, D, E, F	
26. C	55. D	84. A	
27. B	56. B	85. C	
28. B	57. B	86. D	
29. C	58. C	87. D	

88. Semimembranosus or semitendinosus muscle and lateral neck
89. Possible answers: total protein; total nucleated cell count; differential cell count; bacterial culture
90. Possible answers: respiratory-stimulant drugs; straw in the nose; mouth-to-nose ventilation; Ambu bag and cone-shaped face mask with oxygen; vigorous rubbing and drying, sucking mucus and stomach contents from airway
91. Possible answers: volvulus; intestinal incarceration; feed or foreign-body impactions; enterolith obstruction; parasitic infection; intestinal displacement; tympany; inflammatory bowel disease
92. Insert needle unattached to syringe: slowly oozing blood is venous and blood exiting in a pulsatile manner is arterial.

EXTRA CREDIT
93. C
94. B

CHAPTER 30

1. D	19. B	37. B	55. B
2. B	20. A	38. F	56. D
3. A	21. B	39. A	57. B
4. C	22. D	40. K	58. C
5. D	23. A	41. G	59. A
6. A	24. A	42. J	60. C
7. C	25. B	43. E	61. C
8. D	26. B	44. C	62. D
9. B	27. D	45. H	63. C
10. D	28. A	46. I	64. A
11. A	29. D	47. B	65. A
12. B	30. A	48. D	66. D
13. C	31. B	49. L	67. B
14. D	32. C	50. E	68. A
15. A	33. D	51. C	69. C
16. D	34. A	52. A	70. B
17. C	35. C	53. D	71. D
18. D	36. D	54. E	72. C

EXTRA CREDIT
73. C
74. D

CHAPTER 31

1. C	14. B	27. B
2. D	15. A	28. E
3. A	16. D	29. A
4. C	17. B	30. C
5. D	18. B	31. C
6. A	19. D	32. B
7. A	20. B	33. E
8. B	21. A	34. D
9. D	22. A	35. D
10. A	23. D	36. B
11. C	24. A	37. A
12. A	25. B	
13. D	26. A	

EXTRA CREDIT
38. A
39. C

CHAPTER 32

1. A	17. E	33. B	49. C
2. E	18. C	34. E	50. A or B
3. D	19. A	35. A	51. B
4. C	20. E	36. E	52. B
5. C	21. B	37. C	53. A
6. D	22. E	38. C	54. B
7. B	23. D	39. B	55. B
8. B, C, E	24. A	40. C, D, E	56. A
9. A	25. E	41. C	57. A
10. D	26. A	42. E	58. A
11. A	27. C	43. A	59. C
12. E	28. B	44. D	60. A
13. E	29. A	45. A	61. A
14. C	30. A	46. E	62. D
15. C	31. E	47. A, B, C, D, E	63. E
16. E	32. B	48. E	64. D

65. Washing hands, changing to clean coveralls, chemical disinfection of boots, cleaning of equipment
66. The limping dog because if he needs to be left for x-rays, an early appointment will enable diagnosis by the end of the day
67. "It is hospital policy for us collect a 50% deposit now, which is $500, and the balance of the account is due when you pick up Fifi after her surgery."
68. Possible answers: pet prepurchase counseling; human-animal-bond and behavioral-problem counseling; pediatric care; preventive medicine; nutritional counseling or management; veterinary-supervised boarding; geriatric care; advanced dentistry; bereavement counseling; cremation service
69. Suggested answer: "Because only we can provide you with professional advice concerning how to feed your pet for her best health and according to her changing needs. You have medical advice from a veterinarian anytime you ask, and we are all specially trained in the nutritional content and function of, as well as how to feed, each diet."

EXTRA CREDIT
70. C

CHAPTER 33

1. C
2. A
3. A
4. D
5. B
6. D
7. A
8. G
9. C
10. A
11. C
12. F
13. A
14. A
15. S
16. P
17. P
18. O
19. B
20. B
21. C
22. B
23. G

EXTRA CREDIT
24. B
25. D

CHAPTER 34

1. C
2. F
3. D
4. B
5. A
6. D
7. E
8. D
9. B
10. B

EXTRA CREDIT
11. A
12. (1) Both have libraries with search engines; (2) both offer classes for continuing education; (3) both have message boards on every veterinary discipline.

CHAPTER 35

1. C
2. D
3. B
4. E
5. D
6. C
7. A
8. B
9. A
10. C
11. B
12. C
13. E
14. A
15. D
16. B
17. D
18. A
19. A
20. D
21. B
22. D
23. B
24. A
25. D
26. B
27. D
28. C
29. D
30. D
31. A
32. B
33. A
34. A
35. D
36. A
37. A
38. E
39. A
40. C
41. D
42. B
43. C

44. Salmonellosis
45. There are no symptoms.
46. (1) Wash hands thoroughly after contact with pet or cage items (fecal-oral transmission). (2) Keep turtle out of kitchen, eating, and bathing areas.
47. Infected-flea (from an infected cat) feces makes contact with a break in human skin.
48. Possible answers: foxes; coyotes; skunks; raccoons; bats

EXTRA CREDIT
49. B
50. A

CHAPTER 36

1. C
2. D
3. B
4. A
5. B
6. E
7. C
8. A
9. E
10. D
11. A
12. C
13. A
14. C
15. E
16. F
17. A
18. B
19. C
20. B
21. A
22. C
23. B
24. A
25. A
26. D
27. B
28. D
29. B
30. F
31. A
32. B

EXTRA CREDIT
33. 3, 2, 4, 1

CHAPTER 37

1. A
2. B
3. A
4. A
5. B
6. A
7. B
8. B
9. A
10. B
11. A
12. A
13. B
14. A
15. B
16. B
17. A
18. A
19. B
20. B
21. A
22. B
23. B
24. A

CHAPTER 38

1. A
2. B
3. B
4. A
5. B
6. A
7. A
8. A
9. B
10. A
11. B
12. A
13. B
14. B
15. A
16. A
17. A

18. Possible suggestions include having the owner make a scrapbook, plant a tree, write a letter to the pet, write the pet's life story, or have the pet cremated with the ashes returned.
19. Denial; yes
20. Possible answers can be found in Table 20-5.

CHAPTER 39

1. E
2. D
3. D
4. A
5. B
6. D
7. D
8. A
9. C
10. C
11. A
12. C
13. B
14. C
15. A
16. A
17. D
18. D
19. B
20. E
21. C

22. She is experiencing burnout. Possible answers: offer support, readings, gentle confrontation and observations, and personal experiences; listen; encourage vacations; start an office exercise program or other staff activities away from the office; use judgment in suggesting counseling. (There are many other possible answers)